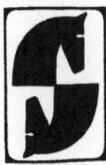

Georg Eisner

Biomicroscopy of the Peripheral Fundus

An Atlas and Textbook

Foreword by Professor Dr. Hans Goldmann

With 121 Partly Colored Figures

Drawings by Willy Hess

Springer-Verlag New York · Heidelberg · Berlin 1973

Privatdozent Dr. G. Eisner
Chefarzt an der Universitäts-Augenklinik Bern

ISBN 978-3-642-85805-5   ISBN 978-3-642-85803-1 (eBook)
DOI 10.1007/978-3-642-85803-1

Foreword

It gives me particular pleasure to write the foreword to this book; this is largely due to the fact that I have devoted a substantial part of my life to the improvement of the methods used in ophthalmic research. Rarely has one of my students taken the opportunity of dealing systematically with the possibilities of these methods. Dr. Eisner is, however, one of these exceptions. First, he has substantially improved the indentation contact glass; secondly, he has, with untiring enthusiasm, made a systematic collection of the normal and pathologic findings, which, with the help of the indentation contact glass and the slit lamp, can be observed in the outermost periphery of the fundus and the ciliary body. He has compared them to findings obtained with slight magnification in autopsy eyes and to histological sections. Owing to a fortunate circumstance, W. Hess, who is both an excellent draughtsman and a master of the special examination technique, was able to reproduce the visual phenomena faithfully. The reader who tries to interpret these illustrations spatially will discover that this was often not easy. It is a process which requires a certain effort of imagination of space, but which is very rewarding. Dr. Eisner's monograph is an introduction to a little-known branch of biomicroscopy which broadens our means of diagnosis and promises further interesting aspects for the future. I wish him well-earned success.

Berne, August 1973   HANS GOLDMANN

Preface

This book is intended as an introduction to a new method of examination. To make it easier to use, we have chosen a smaller size than is usual for an atlas and kept the illustrations separate from the text. It is thus easier to find the pictures referred to more than once, and the illustrations can be used independently.

The drawings showing biomicroscopic findings are accurate reproductions of actual eyes seen with the contact glass. Had we illustrated the atlas with semi-schematic drawings, interpretation would no doubt have been much easier for the reader. We felt, however, that if the illustrations were presented like photographs the reader would become familiar with the difficulties he was likely to see in living eyes.

Indentation biomicroscopy is a relatively new method of examination. No doubt new knowledge confirming or negating the findings described in this atlas will come to light as the technique becomes more widely used. The author would appreciate any reports of observations obtained with this method, and especially any reports of findings that contradict the concepts explained here.

With a view to later editions, we should be grateful for any constructive criticism.

Berne, August 1973   GEORG EISNER

Acknowledgements

This book deals with indentation biomicroscopy, a new examination technique used over the past ten years at Berne University Eye Hospital. It was encouraged to write it by Prof. Hans Goldmann, under whom I had the privilege to study ophthalmology. My deepest gratitude goes to him for teaching me the pleasures of exploring new scientific fields, and for his constant support in this task.

I should like to thank his successor, my friend Prof. Peter Niesel, for his untiring assistance. He reviewed the manuscript with close attention and gave me valuable suggestions and advice.

Especial thanks go to Mr. Willi Hess, the medical illustrator, who contributed a great deal to this book. He took an active part in its creation, not only because of his superb draughtsmanship, but also thanks to his sharp powers of observation in the critical interpretation of biomicroscopic findings. We spent many hours in fierce discussion but eventually had the great satisfaction of seeing our interpretations confirmed by subsequent examinations of autopsy eyes.

I am grateful to Dr. Basil Daicker (Basle), who has covered the same field from the pathologic point of view, for generously allowing me to read his textbook "Anatomie und Pathologie der menschlichen retino-ziliaren Fundusperipherie" before it went to press. He and Dr. R. Y. Foos provided me with a number of valuable pathologic illustrations. Dr. Daicker's illustrations are reproduced by courtesy of S. Karger.

I thank my colleagues at the Berne University Eye Hospital, Dr. Denise Gränicher, Dr. Balder Gloor, and Dr. Walter Plüschke, for all their great help.

The manuscript was originally written in German and its translation into English proved extremely difficult. Besides the linguistic aspects, there were many factual problems, since the subject matter dealt with here is in many respects new. A first attempt was made by Professor Britta M. Charleston and her assistant, Miss Elizabeth L. Wilson, of the Berne University English Department. Their translation was reviewed by Emanuel Rosen, M.D., Allenhurst N.J., who in his own scientific work has contributed to the knowledge of the anterior vitreous and the ciliary body. I am especially indebted to him for, notwithstanding the many calls on his time, he spent a great deal of his spare time on the manuscript, eliminating stylistic and terminological errors. My warmest thanks to him for his endeavours in this ungrateful task.

The final editorial work was done by my wife, Susanne Eisner-Kartagener, who worked long and hard to make the text clear and readable. Most of all I am grateful to her that in all the years spent on this book she did everything possible to keep the author in good spirits.

Further, I thank all those who did the secretarial work, especially Miss Margrit Sauerländer, and Mrs. Rosemarie Doebeli and Miss Eva Bachmann for their technical assistance.

Finally, we are greatly indebted to Springer-Verlag and its employees for their untiring assistance in the preparation of this book.

GEORG EISNER

Contents

Introduction

One of the most fascinating features in ophthalmology is the facility with which the living eye can be examined microscopically. Only the most peripheral portions of the fundus in the normal eye could not, until recently, be visualized. This fact is of distinct disadvantage in clinical practice, since so many pathological conditions originate in the periphery of the fundus. Early detection could lead to early prophylaxis or therapy. However, these peripheral changes situated beyond the limits of the visual field produce no symptoms. If they are to be detected early, it is only by a routine examination of this region. Proper peripheral fundus examination demonstrates where and when therapeutic measures are necessary, as well as when these measures should be discontinued. This is of special importance today, since, while modern treatments are more effective, their side effects are also more dangerous. In order to estimate the therapeutic risks, however, a reliable prognosis of the disease must be established. As experience has shown, the examination of the peripheral vitreous, the so-called vitreous base, can yield important information in this respect. All painstaking efforts to perfect the visualization of the most peripheral parts of the fundus are, therefore, justified.

Why are the most peripheral parts of the fundus invisible? At first thought, the iris might be made responsible for impeding the view. However, even in colobomatous and aniridic eyes the fundus periphery remains invisible. In fact, the *lens edge* with its poor optical properties is responsible for the invisibility of the peripheral fundus. The most peripheral parts of the fundus can, therefore, be examined only if the lens border either has a rounder shape or if it does not interfere at all with the observation beam. The latter condition is fulfilled either when the observation beam passes outside the lens (aphakia, ectopia lentis posterior), or when it passes through sectors of the lens nearer to the optical axis, i.e. sectors with better optical properties (in ectopia lentis anterior, or in the displacement of the peripheral sectors of the fundus towards the optical axis, e.g. in choroidal detachment). Consequently, the most peripheral parts of the fundus have long remained unexplored. Biomicroscopically, only scanty reports are available concerning abnormal, predominantly aphakic eyes [20, 21, 92, 190, 191].

In a normal eye with a normal position of the lens, the periphery of the fundus can be seen only by producing an artificial choroidal detachment, i.e. by deforming the eyeball through indentation, thus displacing the peripheral sectors of the fundus centripetally (Fig. 2). As early as 1900, A. Trantas [220] proceeded in just this fashion in order to examine the ciliary processes. While indenting the sclera with his fingernail he viewed the fundus with the direct ophthalmoscope. This form of examination with scleral depression became popular after Schepens [180] had introduced a method which provides a more comfortable working distance, a larger visual field, better illumination, and stereoscopic observation. By means of a special

1

depressor and the binocular indirect ophthalmoscope of Schepens, the peripheral fundus has become accessible for routine examination [100, 101, 108]. Many reports, principally by Schepens and his co-workers, emphasize the significance of indirect indentation ophthalmoscopy.

Via the ophthalmoscope, however, the *normal vitreous* is poorly seen or completely invisible. Only conspicuous opacifications can be observed clearly, but even then their exact localization is not demonstrable. A detailed examination of the vitreous base, one of the most important indications for an indentation examination, is quite impossible.

The vitreous, like other transparent structures (such as the lens or the zonule), can be rendered visible by focal illumination; this is based on the separation of the beam of observation from the beam of illumination. This is the principle of the *slit lamp*. Furthermore, in the slit lamp, the optical section permits an exact spatial localization. The high magnification is an additional advantage which, however, causes a decrease in the visual field. This disadvantage can be overcome by an appropriate examination technique.

The intermediate and posterior parts of the fundus have long been accessible to the slit lamp with the help of various accessory lenses [21, 74, 110, 219, 126], primarily Goldmann's mirror contact glass. In order to examine the most peripheral parts of the fundus, these must be combined with scleral depressors (indenters). As a result, all interior parts of the eye (the reverse side of the iris, admittedly, only diaphanoscopically) are now open to biomicroscopic examination.

The purpose of the present book is to acquaint the reader with the use of these indentation contact glasses, thus helping to overcome the initial difficulties, and to give instructions on making full use of the technical possibilities of the method. This includes not only the mastery of the examination technique, but also a knowledge of the anatomy and pathology of the area concerned. It is not the purpose of this book to repeat generally well-known facts. The chapter on anatomy, therefore, is merely a brief survey, and details are included only if they are necessary for the understanding of the biomicroscopic findings. The description of the biomicroscopic findings is limited topographically to the region which is visible only by indentation. For additional information about all the remaining areas the reader is referred to the well-known textbooks of Vogt [224], Berliner [11], Busacca [20], and to the report of the French Ophthalmological Society by Busacca, Goldmann and Schiff-Wertheimer [21].

I. The Principles of Indentation

1. The Optical Phenomena of Indentation

The methodical difficulties facing the beginner may be overcome through a better understanding of the fundamentals of the method; thus the novice will learn to minimize the ever-present, unavoidable disadvantages.

In biomicroscopy, a major drawback is the *limited visual field*. Those proficient in indirect ophthalmoscopy will quickly become aware of this disadvantage when using an indentation contact glass for the first time. The usual, extended movements of the depressor must be avoided, otherwise the indented area immediately disappears from view. Because the interpretation of many findings is substantially improved by these movements, this decreased mobility seems initially to be of a definite disadvantage. But, as a closer analysis shows, more extensive movements are unnecessary, and slight displacements (readily possible with a contact glass) are quite sufficient. The analysis of the physical and geometrical principles of indentation is therefore essential in order to establish an appropriate technique of examination, providing optimal information and avoiding misinterpretations. In addition, important knowledge about the construction of indentation contact glasses is provided by this analysis.

The optical effect created by indentation may be attributed to *two angular changes* [58] (Fig. 1):

1. A change in the *angle of eccentricity*, i.e. the angle between the observation beam and the optical axis;

2. A change in the *angle of acceptance*, i.e. the angle between the observation beam and the object observed (more precisely, between the observation beam and the tangent at the curvature of the wall of the eye at the site of the object observed).

Let us first examine the change in the **angle of eccentricity**. This angle is reduced by displacement towards the optical axis of the fundus area to be examined. The conditions of observation are affected in three ways:

(a) *Lens sectors* which are nearer to the axis, hence *optically more favourable*, are now used for observation [43]. The peripheral areas to be examined emerge from the shadow of the "opaque" border of the lens and thereby become visible (Fig. 2).

(b) The *visual field* becomes larger (Fig. 4). The perspective deformation of the pupil (through the contact-glass mirror) is reduced because of the smaller angle of eccentricity [58]. The aperture for the observation of the peripheral fundus thereby becomes enlarged, the visual field widens, and viewing conditions improve [95]. In addition, the stereoscopic field becomes larger in the lateral parts.

(c) The *magnification* changes. When the angle of eccentricity becomes smaller, the magnification decreases (Fig. 3). According to Lotmar [132], with a Goldmann's three-mirror contact glass the magnification for the ora serrata is 1.5. If this area is indented by 2.5 mm, the magnification is reduced to 1.0.

This change in magnification is to be distinguished from that which occurs when examining the same peripheral sectors, now extralentally (through the iridolenticular space), then translentally (Fig. 92a).

The change in the **angle of acceptance** is produced by deformation of the globe via indentation (Fig. 1, Fig. 37). Anatomic structures are then observed from different angles whereby their appearance is altered in two respects:

(a) The *perspective deformation* is changed. The anatomic structures take on an altered *shape* (Fig. 5, Fig. 108).

(b) The *transparency of the tissues* seemingly changes, since, the smaller the angle of acceptance, the longer becomes the path of the rays through a semi-opaque layer; semi-transparent media therefore appear more opaque (Fig. 6). For example, the normal retina appears completely transparent on the anterior side of the indentation protuberance; it turns greyish near the summit, and almost white in silhouette. Accordingly, through the alteration of the angle of acceptance, the anatomic structures appear in different *colours*.

From this change of colour, another feature should be distinguished, which is also dependent on indentation, but is independent of angles. The bloodless protuberance appears brighter and can be made nearly white by very deep indentation, because the blood is expelled from the vessels of the choroid. This effect is useful in therapy [56]. Indentation during light- and cryo-coagulation prevents loss of energy through the blood flow, thus improving the effect of coagulation.

The optical phenomena produced by the change in the angle of acceptance can make the interpretation of findings difficult. The biomicroscopic findings can only be transferred mentally to a normal anatomical (i.e. non-indented) condition if the examiner can recognize all optical phenomena resulting from indentation. A special technique of examination is used for this purpose, which, in contrast to the above described *static* technique (i.e., with an immobile depressor), is termed "*kinetic* indentation".

In the **kinetic** technique, the depressor is constantly shifted, causing continual changes in the angle of acceptance and, consequently, in all the resultant phenomena. Their interrelation is thus demonstrated. However, kinetic indentation not only prevents misinterpretations but also serves as a source of additional information concerning morphology and differences in level [182, 100]. This technique is clinically essential, especially in cases of precarious conditions of observation.

The recognition of shapes and their interpretation is considerably helped by kinetic indentation, for the constant change of the angle of acceptance produces *parallactic displacements*. Instead of the observer moving, as is the case in ophthalmoscopic examination of the posterior segment of the eye, the object observed is now moved. The structures are examined at various angles and from different sides (Fig. 5). A special case of parallaxis is the examination "in silhouette" (in profile): the indenter is shifted into a position which brings the area to be examined to the summit of the protuberance. It is now observed with tangential incidence, i.e. the angle of acceptance is 0°. Differences in level and the true distance between superposed objects can now be judged exactly and without perspective distortion.

Another advantage of kinetic indentation is the shifting of the structures against *different backgrounds*. New contrasts are thereby produced. These are particularly important for the interpretation of so-called transparent media, which are visible only by their scattered light against a dark background. Vitreous structures near the retina, for instance, can be examined only in this way.

Finally, diagnosis can be improved by the use of the *transparency change* (Fig. 6). In order to detect structures under semi-transparent layers of tissue (e. g. the pigment epithelium or the choroid under the retina), the corresponding areas should be positioned on the anterior side of the protuberance, i. e. the angle of acceptance should be as large as possible. Similarly, if the visibility of the retina and the layers beneath it is obstructed by preretinal opacities, it can be improved by an examination on the anterior side of the protuberance. Conversely, differences in the thickness of layers are best detected by examining the summit of the protuberance. This position is sought for when thinning and thickening of the retina, extremely thin epiretinal deposits, or subretinal accumulations of fluid are to be detected.

In conclusion, indentation can be used in two ways: **Static indentation** reveals the most peripheral parts of the fundus. It is based on a diminution of the angle of eccentricity. The depth of indentation necessary depends on the position and form of the lens in the individual patient. **Kinetic indentation** improves the interpretation of findings. It is based on a constant changing of the angle of acceptance and is in no way confined to the peripheral fundus. How far should the depressor be shifted? Every possible change of angle is produced by displacing the depressor by *half its diameter*.

2. The Effects of Indentation on the Eyeball

Scleral depression deforms not only the immediate area of indentation, but also the adjacent area, thus creating **corneal astigmatism,** which varies with the distance from the limbus and with the depth of indentation. The astigmatism itself presents no technical problem, since the contact glass is corrective. But the deformation makes a pathway through which air bubbles can enter between the cornea and the contact glass. To prevent this, the indentation contact glass should be designed in such a fashion that the deformed area remains covered, e. g. by an extension of the scleral cone (Fig. 7 and Fig. 13).

Obviously the indentation **increases intra-ocular pressure** by diminution of intra-ocular volume. As experiments show (Eisner, unpublished data), intra-ocular pressure during indentation may rise above the diastolic, and even above the systolic pressure of the central arteries; however, it decreases quickly, levelling off to the initial value after one minute. Hence, a deeper indentation may safely be performed if sufficient time is taken. These experiments demonstrate that the episcleral veins are not compressed by the rim of the indentation funnel and that aqueous drainage is, therefore, not impeded.

Extended clinical experience reveals that neither deformation nor the increase of pressure produce any harmful effects in the *healthy* eye. In the *diseased* eye, however, there are some exceptions (see contra-indications, p. 11).

3. Instruments for Indentation Biomicroscopy

Once interested in this field, the examiner may begin by combining indentation and biomicroscopy, at first attempting to use a normal three-mirror contact glass for observation and a simple blunt instrument for indentation. Such an attempt is usually not successful, but it will demonstrate some of the many problems connected with the combination of a contact glass with a depressor.

Air bubbles will enter between the contact glass and the cornea. In an attempt to avoid this, Liesenhoff [128] has covered the sclera with a cuff made of flexible plastic, which can be affixed to the three-mirror contact glass (Fig. 7). The problem of air bubbles solved, other difficulties arise. If the depressor is not attached to the contact glass, both hands are needed for manipulation, which prevents the simultaneous use of the slit lamp. Liesenhoff, therefore, fixed the slit lamp to his head by means of a special attachment. Liesenhoff's instrument is quite simple with regard to the apparatus, but its manipulation is difficult, requiring much practice to synchronize the movements of the depressor and the contact glass. At the beginning of the examination, it is difficult to align the indented protuberance with the contact glass mirror, and thereafter it is even more difficult to maintain the correct position while rotating the contact glass. Obviously, unlimited freedom of movement is a disadvantage with a small visual field (in contrast to the large visual field in indirect ophthalmoscopy). Nevertheless, Liesenhoff's technique is indicated in cases where a *previously determined* area is to be given an intensive kinetic examination.

Fankhauser [57] has, therefore, firmly attached the depressor to a contact glass (Fig. 8). This indenter can be shifted in various directions by means of a mechanical device. However, the apparatus is quite awkward considering the little space within the orbital margin. Fankhauser therefore uses a special, very small, contact glass. Consequently, the mirror and the visual field become smaller, too. Additional difficulties arise with the manipulation of multiple knobs. This type of indenting contact glass is too complicated for routine examination, but may be used when a *predetermined retinal area* must be presented in various depths of indentation, e.g. in light coagulation through the contact glass.

Goldmann and Schmidt [93] have completely sacrificed the mobility of the indenter to avoid such difficulties. They have designed a simple, easily manageable instrument, which, nevertheless, owing to the proper ratio of mirror size to indenter, permits a kinetic examination. This is accomplished by the use of a special contact glass with a mirror inclination of 59° specifically for examination of the ora serrata (Fig. 9). The front plate of the contact glass is reinforced by a metal disc to which the indenter is affixed. The button of the indenter is broad enough to produce a sufficiently large indented area, yet narrow enough for the lateral parts of the indented protuberance to remain visible. The whole contact glass must be rotated for a kinetic examination. The indentation protuberance is thereby shifted laterally. The area to be examined is thus seen from different angles of acceptance; its position in the visual field, however, is decentered (Fig.17). If the indenter is to be moved in an anteroposterior direction, the whole contact glass must be shifted (Fig. 18). The principal advantage of Goldmann and Schmidt's indentation contact glass is its simple manipulation. Its small size makes its application within the palpebral fissure quite easy. The indented area always appears in the centre of the mirror. The possibilities for kinetic examination are sufficient in most cases. There is, in fact, only one major disadvantage. An exchange of the contact glass being necessary, the periphery of the fundus cannot be examined simultaneously with the other remaining segments of the fundus. This increases the difficulty of interpretation of many findings. Goldmann and Schmidt's contact glass is thus best suited for the *examination of changes confined to the ora serrata area*.

The examples described above suggest that an ideal contact glass, an all-purpose model, cannot easily be designed. Each type has advantages as well as disadvantages, and each is reserved for a specific use. What features are indispensable for an **indentation contact glass in routine examinations?** The essential requirements include:

(a) The contact glass must be *operable with one hand*, as the other hand is needed for slit lamp adjustments.

(b) The examination of the entire fundus must be accomplished in a *single operation*, i.e., with a contact glass also suited for all the other areas of the fundus. The Goldmann three-mirror contact glass has three mirrors, each of different inclination. With each one it is possible to survey an area of the fundus corresponding to the angle of inclination (Fig. 10). The indented ora serrata region can be made visible by either the middle or the gonioscopic mirror. The two areas of the mirrors overlap each other. According to the situation, one of these mirrors will prove more favourable than the other one. For this reason, the mirror in position opposite the button must be easily interchangeable.

(c) *Size of the indenter:* The volume of global content which can be shifted (which in turn depends on the intra-ocular pressure) limits the size of the indenter. The *depth* to be attained by indentation is determined by the position of the lens border, the usual depth being 2.5 mm. The *breadth* of the indenter is limited by the visual field: it is useless to indent areas outside the visual field. Broad indenters provide a good view of the area indented; a kinetic examination, however, can be performed only if they are movable.

(d) The *mobility* of the indenter must be minimal, since otherwise the instrument becomes too complicated for single-handed manipulation. The *radius of movement* may reasonably be restricted to the visual field available. Among the many *directions of movement* only those will be chosen which are absolutely important. Which are they? For the *static* examination it is sufficient to set the correct limbus distance and the right depth of indentation, i.e. the indenter need not necessarily be movable. For the *kinetic* examination, only the changing angle of acceptance is essential. It is immaterial in which direction the indenter is moved in order to change this angle. Unidirectional movement is sufficient.

Of all possible directions, the one which is helpful also for other reasons may be selected: the movement around the axis of the contact glass, by which the mirrors opposite the indenter are interchanged. The indenter is shifted laterally by this movement, i.e. in a direction parallel to the limbus. This is sufficient to bring the anatomical structures into all the various angles of acceptance (Fig. 17); they are thus first observed at the summit of the protuberance, then at its lateral slopes, and finally in a state free from indentation. Therefore only a free *lateral* mobility of the indenter is necessary for an indentation contact glass intended for routine use. Small displace-

7

ments are sufficient in an anteroposterior direction, and the depth of depression may remain constant.

The necessary criteria are provided by *indentation funnels* consisting of thin open cones in which the three-mirror contact glass is inserted. An indenter is fixed to the funnel. At the present time two types of funnels are available: one has an immobile [42], the other one an adjustable indenter [51].

4. Indentation Funnel with Immobile Indenter

A plastic or metal funnel surrounds the contact glass (Fig. 12). Methocel placed between the funnel and the contact glass supplies lubrication as well as adhesion. Both parts are thus fixed to each other, yet can easily be counter-rotated. The funnel has a "scleral brim" forming a narrow groove upon which the edges of the eyelids may rest. This prevents their being wedged under the border of the funnel during the examination. By a local broadening of the brim a "*scleral plate*" is formed, covering the indenter and preventing the entry of air. The edge of the funnel is broader on the upper side and is slightly recessed in comparison with the frontal plate of the contact glass. A *step* is thus formed (Fig. 14), thanks to which the fingertips, which counter-rotate the funnel and the contact glass, are not hampered. A notch on the upper edge of the funnel indicates the place of the indenter. In order to simplify the methodology of examination for the novice, the counter-rotating movement of funnel and contact glass can be blocked by a fixing mechanism, e. g. a screw-ring.

By means of this funnel, the three-mirror contact glass can be converted into an indentation contact glass with free lateral mobility of the indenter. The indenter can also be displaced posteriorly or anteriorly by tilting the contact glass over the surface of the eyeball or by having the patient gaze in specific directions (Fig. 18). Practice shows that, with a suitable choice of indenter length, the entire periphery can be adequately examined in almost every case. It is only rarely, e. g. in advanced myopia, that another funnel with a longer indenter is needed.

5. Funnel with Variable Indenter Length

If the indentation contact glass is tilted over the surface of the eyeball in order to move the indenter anteriorly or posteriorly, disturbing optical effects appear. They are eliminated in a routine examination by short, corrective movements. These movements, however, are disturbing in many situations, such as during photography or in light coagulation through the contact glass [56]. An indenter with variable length is desirable in such situations, even if its manipulation will inevitably be more cumbersome.

The indenter is attached to the end of a pliable flat spring (Fig. 13). The flat spring is inserted into a track on the funnel and can be drawn backwards and forwards therein. The corneal end of the track extends beyond the funnel aperture, curving according to the scleral surface. This way the inserted indenter is manoeuvered in the proper direction, moving along the ocular surface at a constant depth of depression. A special fixing mechanism for maintaining a predetermined limbus distance is unnecessary, since the spring tilts in its groove and is therefore locked in position as soon as the funnel is rotated. Indenters of various shapes and sizes are interchangeable. Three shapes of funnel are available: for normal eyes, for narrow palpebral fissures, and for long myopic eyes.

The funnel with an indenter of variable length has some disadvantages. The greater freedom of movement involves a more complicated manipulation. It is not possible to manipulate spring and funnel single-handedly in all situations. The fact that the other hand is needed, however, is of little disadvantage in practice, as the meridional displacement need seldom be continuous, and occasional changes of the limbus distance are sufficient. A further difficulty arises with the funnel for myopic eyes, which has a long scleral plate, allowing the indenter to be pushed farther posteriorly. This long plate may occasionally cause pain during the examination, especially in the area of the caruncle.

This description of the various instruments is not chronological. The first prototype was designed by Goldmann and Favre [60, 94], who fixed the indenter to the upper border of a three-mirror contact glass by means of a hinge connected to a ring. In order to depress the indenter, this ring, acting like a lever, could be pulled from all sides. Yet, even in the smallest possible size, such a ring takes up too much space; therefore this ingenious solution was abandoned.

The next model was the indentation contact glass of Goldmann and Schmidt [93] described above. It was followed by the indentation funnels of Eisner [42, 51]. A prototype of this funnel, produced by Haag-Streit, was published by Slezak [194], who at that time was not aware of its true origin. In Linder's [129] variation of the funnel, the indenter was fixed with screws, so that heads of different sizes could be interchanged. The funnels were followed by the contact glass of Fankhauser and Lotmar [57] and by the indentation cuff of Liesenhoff [128]. Gloor [83] fixed the indenter into a track directly on the contact glass, allowing anteroposterior mobility but no rotation of the indenter on the contact glass. Belmonte [10] designed an indenter consisting of two levers, fixed by hinges onto the contact glass. By depressing one of the levers, the depth of indentation can be changed.

6. Practical Application of the Indentation Funnel

As the success of the examination depends entirely on whether it can be carried out painlessly and without inconvenience, a detailed explanation of the practical procedure during the examination follows.

The portion of the contact glass to be inserted into the palpebral fissure has become enlarged because of the additional funnel. This problem, however, is easily overcome by paying attention to a few practical rules, and examination is painless if one follows the correct technique. The author has examined four-year-old children without difficulty. There are, however, some patients in whom the palpebral fissure is so narrow that an indentation contact glass cannot be employed.

6.1. Insertion of the Indentation Contact Glass into the Palpebral Fissure

The conjunctiva is anaesthetized, as in the usual contact glass examination, with a few drops of a *surface anaesthetic*, e.g. 0.4% oxybuprocaine (in both eyes, to avoid blinking reflexes). Surface anaesthesia of the conjunctiva is sufficient, no deeper anaesthesia being necessary. It appears that the examination causes pain only when cilia or lid structures are pinched or pulled by the rotation of the funnel. Therefore precautions must be taken to see that the funnel lies free within the conjunctival sac. Nevertheless, many patients describe a feeling different from that of the routine examination with a contact glass. As a calming measure, the patient should be advised that there will be no pain during the examination, but a certain sensation of pressure.

Special care should be used in the insertion of the funnel into the palpebral fissure (Fig. 15). *Full retraction of the eyelids* is necessary but may present difficulty, owing to lack of space. It is best to use cotton-tip applicators (Fig. 16) which are placed upon the skin below the eyebrow, followed by moderate pressure upward towards the bony orbital rim. If the cotton-tip applicator is then rotated (not pulled), the skin of the eyelid, together with the musc. orbicularis oculi, is drawn back by friction. This is a very effective method of preventing eyelid closure.

First, the *empty funnel* is inserted in order to be sure that no lid tissues are caught within the funnel opening. The proper fit of the funnel is also controlled from without. Care must be taken to see that the depressor button is positioned within the palpebral fissure. The contact glass is then inserted, Methocel having previously been applied. As soon as the contact glass touches the cornea, excess Methocel will be pressed into the space between funnel and contact glass, thus acting as a lubricant. The examination may now begin.

6.2. Course of the Examination

During the examination, the indenter and the position of the mirror must constantly be synchronized by delicate finger movements. This is only possible if the examiner assumes a *comfortable position*. The comfort of the patient, as well as one's own, should be established before beginning. It is essential that the elbow of the examiner be comfortably supported. With most slit lamps, the table is too low, and a suitable support must be placed beneath the elbow.

First, the *anterior and posterior sections* of the eye are examined in the usual manner. For this purpose, the funnel is held firmly between the thumb and the middle finger and is left in a constant, fixed position (Fig. 14b). The contact glass must be held at its anterior edge with the index finger, so that it may be rotated within the funnel, which at this stage only acts as a lid retractor. For the *examination of the periphery*, the middle or the gonioscopy mirror is placed opposite the indenter. The contact glass and the funnel are then rotated co-axially, while the upper edges of both instruments are held firmly together (Fig. 14a). A slight displacement of the finger tips is sufficient for this. At positions where one wishes to examine *kinetically*, the index finger is again brought to the edge of the contact glass, which is then rotated within the funnel (Fig. 14b).

To *shift* the indenter *posteriorly* or *anteriorly*, either the entire indentation contact glass is tilted over the surface of the eyeball or the patient is asked to look in the desired direction (Fig. 18). When using the mobile indenter, the spring is pushed backwards and forwards with the other hand until the protuberance is seen in the correct position in the contact glass mirror.

10

The *depth of depression* can be increased by pressing the funnel in the direction of the observation mirror.

7. Contra-Indications

The eye may be traumatized by the increase of intra-ocular pressure and also by the displacement and deformation of indented tissues, as previously described in the chapter on side effects of indentation, p. 5. In order to evaluate the consequences of increased pressure during the examination, the *optic disc* should be checked occasionally through the central part of the contact glass. Pressure on the contact glass should be decreased if the central artery pulsates or is closed.

In certain situations, however, special care is needed. For example, *after surgical or traumatic perforations*, the increased pressure or the deformation of the eyeball may lead to a rupture of the wound. We have, therefore, made it a rule not to examine by indentation until eight weeks after a perforation. *After blunt traumata* or *spontaneous haemorrhages*, too, deformations could cause additional damage through laceration of the tissues, so that we do not indent until six weeks after these events. These rules have been observed, unless more urgent reasons led one to suspect that proper and significant therapy might be called for, rendering examination by indentation unavoidable. Probably because of the observance of these precautionary measures, no complications have been noted in the ten years that indentation has been used at the University Eye Hospital in Berne. There have been no vascular occlusions or haemorrhages and, most important, no retinal detachments have occurred or been aggravated.

However, cases of vitreous haemorrhage have been reported after ophthalmoscopy which may have employed deeper indentation. For this reason, Schepens [184] has warned against unnecessarily deep indentation.

II. The Anatomy of the Extreme Periphery of the Fundus

The term "*extreme periphery of the fundus*" involves a clinical concept rather than an anatomical one, since its boundaries are not anatomically defined. Depending on the motivation and the methodology, every author partitions the periphery of the fundus into specific zones. Within the scope of this book, the term covers those regions of the eyeball which, in normal eyes, are not visible without indentation: *the most peripheral zones of the retina, the ora serrata, the posterior ciliary body and the vitreous base.* The remaining sections of the eye will be dealt with only insofar as they are necessary for an understanding of the peripheral structures.

Knowledge of the macroscopic and microscopic anatomy of this area has not changed essentially since Salzmann's [172] classic work (see also the textbooks by Kolmer [123], Lauber [125], Rohen [156], and Duke-Elder [37]). Only in recent years has newer knowledge appeared, on the one hand through the development of electronmicroscopy [107], and on the other through examination of the peripheral fundus in the living eye.

Electron-microscopic examinations deal with dimensions which are far below those of biomicroscopy. They are, therefore, of little significance for the biomicroscopist in so far as they concern details of the intracellular structures. However, the differential behaviour of various tissue layers under the effect of traction can be to some extent explained by recent discoveries concerning the nature of the intercellular connections.

The *micro-examination of the living eye* enables one to decide whether histological findings come about in vivo or are artefactitious; in addition, it can reveal temporal changes, thus providing information about the development and the frequency of variations and of senescent and degenerative morphology [44–50, 169 to 171]. Conversely, many findings in the living eye have stimulated new anatomical investigations [139–141, 215–217, 67–72, 144–145, 202–206, 208–210]. Daicker's monograph [32] summarizes the present state of this research.

In the following survey of topographical relations and of the fine structure of ocular tissues in the extreme periphery of the fundus, the author has limited himself to those aspects relevant to biomicroscopy. For details, the reader is referred to the sources quoted above.

1. Topography of the Extreme Periphery of the Fundus

The three-dimensional structure of the anterior sections of the eyeball may be subdivided into three characteristic patterns: (a) limbus-concentric belts, (b) meridional segmentation ("orange slice"), (c) a layered arrangement ("onion peel").

By the **limbus-concentric** arrangement belts are formed as a result of the anterior-posterior sequence of the organs (Fig. 19). The *ciliary body*, e.g. can be subdivided into three belts: the anterior belt is the *pars plicata* (or corona ciliaris) with the ciliary processes. Behind that, there is the flat portion, the *pars plana* (or orbiculus ciliaris), which is again divisible into an *anterior* (light-coloured) section and a *posterior* (dark-coloured) section. Between these, the boundary is formed by a scalloped line, the *linea serrata of the pars plana*. Posteriorly, the retina commences at a distinct boundary, the *ora serrata*. The interior structures of the eyeball also follow the limbus-concentric arrangement. The *zonular fibres* form a dense fibrillar layer above the pars plana, ending at the linea serrata (Fig. 21). They are overlaid by three narrow belts of *circular zonular fibres* (Fig. 22). The stronger intravitreal tracts are inserted into these (Fig. 28). The *vitreous base*, the zone of the firmest connections of the vitreous with the internal retinal layer, extends in a ring-shaped belt, the anterior boundary lying at the linea serrata, the posterior boundary behind the ora serrata. Thus, the anterior pars plana is related to the zonule (Fig. 20), the posterior pars plana to the vitreous. All the ring-shaped belts which are connected to the zonule have the same limbus distance. The remaining belts are more distant from the limbus on the temporal side than on the nasal side and for this reason they are somewhat excentric to the anatomical axis.

The **meridional segmentation** subdivides each belt into individual, adjoining compartments. This is evident in the ray-like formation of the *ciliary processes* (Fig. 19). It is repeated in the *serrations* of the linea serrata, from which dark stripes (*striae ciliares*) extend from the posterior pars plana into the ciliary valleys. There is a narrow elevation (*crista ciliaris*) in the middle of the striae. The cristae ciliares represent, in fact, the axes of the meridional segmentation. Most of the typical variations are related to them. At the *ora serrata*, the meridional segmentation is apparent in the characteristic serration. The formation is, however, no longer so regular, for serrations are formed only at some of the cristae. They are most abundant and longest on the nasal side; temporally, the serrations are rarely present and the ora serrata is only slightly scalloped.

The anterior portions of the eyeball have, in principle, a central symmetry. A deviation results from the well-known *temporal expansion* of the eyeball. The intervals increase temporally between the limbus-concentric belts as well as between the individual meridional compartments. Because of this, an axial symmetry is formed with the axis nearly horizontal, although a slight rotation may occur from the nasal superior quadrant towards the temporal inferior quadrant (i.e., nearly perpendicular to the meridian of the fetal eye-cup fissure).

The meridional segmentation creates multiple histologic misinterpretations. With the methods usually employed in histological slides, only *one* section per eyeball can

Table 1. Distance of the ora serrata from the limbus (after Duke-Elder [37])

	Hypermetropia	Emmetropia	Myopia
Nasal	6.2	6.6	7.0 mm.
Temporal	6.7	7.9	8.4 mm.
Superior	7.0	7.4	8.1 mm.
Inferior	6.5	6.9	8.0 mm.

be precisely in a meridional direction. In all other sections the meridionally arranged structures will be cut obliquely. In addition, many other confusions of the anatomical picture are attributable to the meridional segmentation. Owing to the recession and protrusion of tissue layers at ora bays and teeth, the histological picture varies from one section to the next.

The **layered arrangement** stems from the superposition of layers from the outside towards the centre of the globe. From the sclera to the centre of the vitreous, the tissues are arranged in **concentric layers** (*"onion peel"*) (Fig. 27). First, the layers of the wall of the eye, the retina and the ciliary body will be discussed; secondly, the layers of the interior of the eye, the zonule and the vitreous.

2. Retina and Ciliary Body

At the ora serrata the multilayered retina merges into the single-layered ciliary epithelium (Fig. 20). The latter covers the entire ciliary body, contains pigment in its most anterior parts, and forms the posterior pigmented layer of the iris. At the pupillary margin it turns into the pigment epithelium. As a consequence of the inversion of the optic cup, the cells of the two neuro-ectodermal layers meet at their apex. The cell base is on the external side and has—like all epithelial tissue—a *basal membrane* visible only via electron microscopy. On the inner surface, this basal membrane is part of the *"internal limiting membrane"* [77] which covers the retina and the ciliary epithelium. On the outer surface, the basal membrane forms the inner lamella of *Bruch's membrane*. With light microscopy this appears double-layered and consists of a lamina cuticularis and a lamina elastica. These layers diverge near the ora serrata; an additional stratum, consisting of collagen fibres, appears between the two, forming an irregular reticulum (*Müller's reticulum*) at the pars plana [172, 207]. Its meshes are relatively large (40–50 μm) in the posterior pars plana; in the anterior pars plana, they are fine (10–20 μm). The exterior lamella of Bruch's membrane is part of the choroid.

The *choriocapillaris* terminates at the scalloped border of the ora serrata. The larger uveal vessels, however, do not change their course, but continue directly from the choroid into the ciliary body. The ora serrata derives its *arterial supply* from branches of the recurrent arteries from the circulus iridis major. They anastomose with the short, posterior ciliary arteries. The arteria ciliaris longa occasionally gives off branches at the ora. The *veins* in the region of the pars plana run in a straight meridional direction. Only when they are posterior to the ora serrata do they converge and pass over into the venae vorticosae. In the vicinity of the A. ciliaris longa the veins diverge, thus forming an intervascular *raphe* at the horizontal meridian [32]. Some vessels perforate the lamina elastica near the ora serrata [152, 153] and pass anteriorly within the interlaminar connective tissues, forming, so to speak, the skeleton of the cristae ciliares [32].

Histological sections of the **marginal retina** demonstrate that the different retinal layers are poorly defined there. The *sensory cells* and the connected nerve elements become scarcer; glial cells predominate. The *basal membrane*, which is thick in the central region of the retina, filling all the irregularities of the cell surfaces, there narrows with multiple folds, following the cell surfaces into all depressions and crypts. The fibrillae of the vitreous then follow, strongly interdigitating with the cells [81, 103, 80]. This probably explains the firm attachment of the vitreous at its base. The pattern of the *pigment epithelium* becomes irregular towards the periphery and the pigment content of each cell diminishes.

At the **ora serrata** there is a narrow transitional zone. Normal *retinal cells* are replaced first by immature and finally by undifferentiated cells [150]. The *retro-retinal interstice* ("virtual ventricle") ends here, and the first firm connections between the two retinal layers appear in the form of desmosomes. The retina then passes over abruptly into the single-layered *ciliary epithelium*. The pigment content increases suddenly in the *pigment epithelium*, and the cells become taller. The *choriocapillaris* terminates here.

In the **posterior pars plana** the cells of the *ciliary epithelium* are tall and columnar, closely apposed, and slightly inclined anteriorly. There are fine intercellular spaces which, according to Fine and Zimmermann [65], contain acid mucopolysaccharides. The *pigment epithelium* is firmly connected with the ciliary epithelium by desmo-somes and junctional zonules. Thus, a *retroretinal adhesion* is formed in which the two layers can scarcely be separated. The pigment epithelium dips with its basal membrane into all the folds and meshes of *Müller's reticulum*. The surface appears granular because the meshes are relatively coarse here; and in histological section the pigment epithelium appears hyperplastic, with proliferations into the layers beneath (Fig. 20).

In the **anterior pars plana** the cells of the *ciliary epithelium* are slightly flatter. The *pigment epithelium* between the striae ciliares runs evenly hardly deforming the surface, as Müller's reticulum shows only fine meshes here (10–20 μm). The *lamina elastica of Bruch's membrane* disappears between the walls of the vessels and the fibres of the ciliary muscle.

3. The Zonule

Zonular fibres are visible even at low magnification. In microscopic examination, they appear to be fascicles composed of numerous individual fibrillae. They originate from various parts of the ciliary body, some also from the vitreous, uniting to form thicker strands which proceed toward the lens [133]. Approaching the lens the fibres fan out before attaching to the lens capsule. However, individual fibrillae may branch off before reaching the lens, thereby forming other fibre systems. Thus there is a polymorphic, fine fibrillar network in which the coarser zonular strands form regular, strictly-ordered systems with *meridional main layers* and three *circular belts* [201] (Fig. 22).

The **meridional fibres** may be divided into an *orbiculociliary system* extending evenly over the pars plana into the ciliary valleys, and a *ciliocapsular system* linking the corona ciliaris with the lens (Fig. 20). Neither autoptic nor biomicro-scopic examinations demonstrate clearly how these fibrous systems are connected [37, 157]. For the purpose of biomicroscopic description it is reasonable to designate all the fibres running over the pars plana as the *epiciliary leaf*, and to term the coarser, biomicroscopically visible fibres extending from the ciliary body to the lens the *anterior and posterior (ciliocapsular) leaves.*

The **epiciliary leaf** begins near the linea serrata of the pars plana. The fibres mostly originate from the "basal membrane fibril complex" of the ciliary epithelium in the anterior pars plana. The striae ciliares, being extensions of the posterior pars plana, are free of zonules. The fibres form a dense carpet over the pars plana and then cluster together in the ciliary valleys. The **anterior and posterior** (ciliocapsular) **leaves** pass through the circumlental space to the lens and are there attached to the zonular lamella, anteriorly at about 1 mm, posteriorly at a distance of 1.5 mm from the equator. In a sagittal section, they circumscribe a triangle whose base is at the edge of the lens, its apex at the corona ciliaris.

The **circular fibres** form three fine bands; the most posterior above the middle of the pars plana (*ligamentum medianum of the pars plana*), the second one above the posterior third of the corona ciliaris (*ligamentum coronarium*), and the anterior one just behind the edge of the lens (*fasciculus retrolentalis*). Both posterior zonular bands are connected to the ciliary body by fibres which branch out from the belt. In addition, there are numerous finer fibrillar systems, which connect the main fibres to the ciliary body, bridge adjoining ciliary processes, or penetrate the vitreous.

In freshly enucleated, unfixed eyes the **space between the fibres** is filled with a transparent viscous fluid which is not apparent in the usual histological preparations [37]. It is difficult to answer the clinically important question as to whether the fibrous systems of the zonule comprise self-contained areas. Air injections [9] prove nothing, as artefacts may be formed in the gel. Membraneous boundaries are not detectable. As a topographical designation, both the concept of a **previtreal space** (between the anterior hyaloid membrane and the ciliary body), as well as the concept of an **intrazonular space** (between the anterior and the posterior zonular leaves) are, however, useful (Fig. 20).

4. The Vitreous Body

Unlike other ocular areas, little is known about the nature and structure of the vitreous body, primarily because artefacts occur with most of the methods related to histological examination. Currently, there are few observations and interpretations which have not been questioned by other observers. This is apparent from the textbook by Lauber [125] and the comprehensive survey of Brini and his co-workers [12, 13].

The vitreous, macroscopically a transparent gel, in its free state assumes a spherical shape, yet becomes deformed within the eye by its bordering structures. The vitreous gel consists of a dilute solution of salts, plasma proteins and hyaluronic acid, contained within a fine meshwork of insoluble collagen fibrils [6, 7, 8, 63].

Most important for the biomicroscopist is the anatomical base of the optical phenomena observed. Histological interpretation is difficult since the vitreous body consists of approximately 99% water. For this reason, dehydration occurring during fixation creates artefacts and misinterpretations of the stained structures. A correlation with biomicroscopic findings has therefore been rejected by many examiners.

Through experiments with artificial gels, it has been suggested that the structures visible in the vitreous gel are formed purely accidentally (cf. Lauber [125]). This theory, however, is disproved by examination of the living eye. The structures visible in the living eye have a typical, specific arrangement, as well as a characteristic evolution and involution [20, 86, 89, 91]. Moreover, the same structures are observed also in unfixed autopsy eyes with the slit lamp [52, 54]. Since the latter findings correspond with those in fixed histological specimens (provided that an appropriate technique is used, such as that of Szent-Giyörgy [212]), they cannot possibly be fortuitous. The structures with a higher optical density demonstrate in experiments their increased mechanical strength, i.e. their capability of transmitting traction, or of acting as a barrier to prevent the passage of substances.

The vitreous gel is surrounded by a membrane-like condensation, the so-called **vitreous, or hyaloid, membrane** [8, 77, 81, 103]. When this membrane is injured, holes develop through which semi-fluid central vitreous may herniate [52] (Fig. 34).

Whether the surface of the vitreous may be considered a membrane, is still a controversial question. The interpretation obviously depends on the definition of the term "membrane". In biomicroscopic studies, as in its behaviour in pathological conditions, it may be interpreted as a membrane insofar as it represents an extremely thin layer surrounded by media of lesser density. This is also true of the intravitreal membranules, and it is in this sense that the "membrane concept" is here retained.

The intravitreal structures have the same limbus-concentric, meridional and layered arrangement characteristic of the ocular parts previously described. Membranules in the form of funnels fitted into one another ("onion peel", Figs. 26, 27) originate at the posterior pole. Diverging anteriorly, these membranules insert at ring-shaped belts of the anterior parts of the eyeball, the meridional segmentation ("orange slice") of which extends to the sections of the vitreous with which they come into contact (Fig. 29).

The vitreous may be divided into **three zones** on the basis of structural density [52, 212], (Fig. 24):

(a) The *posterior vitreous cortex*, existing wherever the vitreous body adjoins the retina, terminating at the ora serrata.

(b) The *central vitreous*, which anteriorly comes into contact with the ciliary body and the anterior hyaloid membrane.

(c) The *central canal*, which is the part of the central vitreous limited anteriorly by the lens (more exactly, by the retrolental patellar portion of the anterior hyaloid membrane).

The **posterior vitreous cortex** is relatively thick (2–3 mm). It consists of dense, fine membranules parallel to the surface and closely united by radial "fibres" (Figs. 30, 35). Thus, a uniform cover is formed, relatively resistant to mechanical stress. In this dense cortex, there are zones of lower density (mechanical as well as optical), which are clinically important as "weak points". Such *"holes" in the cortex* exist at characteristic sites: (a) at the papilla (the *prepapillary hole*, Fig. 31), (b) at the fovea centralis (the *prefoveal hole*, Fig. 31), (c) over anomalies at the ora serrata (above meridional ridges, very deep ora serrata bays, etc. Fig. 33), (d) over the retinal vessels (*prevascular fissures*, Fig. 32). These holes have a characteristic appearance, suggesting "shadows" cast through the vitreous cortex by structures which interrupt the normal retinal surface. In addition to these constitutional holes of the cortex, there are *secondary holes* above retinal lesions, e. g. above choroiditic scars (Fig. 35) or at equatorial degenerations [52] (Fig. 53).

Anteriorly, the vitreous is bounded by the **anterior vitreous cortex** (Fig. 20). The latter is so narrow and dense behind the lens that with a low magnification it could be interpreted as a cuticular membrane (biomicroscopically: the **"anterior hyaloid membrane"**). With higher magnification, however, it is found to consist of several lamellae which can be separated individually. During its course from the edge of the lens towards the ciliary body, the cortex, by the apposition of vitreous tracts on its posterior face, becomes broader, yet also looser. Above the posterior pars plana the cortex is crossed by dense clusters of very fine vitreous fibrils which are attached to the ciliary epithelium. The anterior vitreous cortex disintegrates in the region of the ora serrata.

The **central vitreous** is semi-fluid. It consists predominantly of optically empty spaces containing the tractus vitreales which determine the biomicroscopic picture of the vitreous. The tracts form fine, funnel-shaped membranule systems which begin at the edge of the papilla and diverge anteriorly towards the anterior hyaloid membrane (Figs. 25–28). Bordering the vitreous cortex internally is the most peripheral tract, the **tractus praeretinalis** (Figs. 27b, 28, 30), which is inserted at the ora serrata. The innermost tract, the **tractus hyaloideus,** is inserted at the edge of the lens. Between these there are several finer membranules. Two of these, more prominent, are inserted at the belts of the circular zonular fibres, the **tractus medianus** at the ligamentum medianum of the pars plana, the **tractus coronarius** at the ligamentum coronarium (Fig. 28). Within these membranules, there are densified meridional striae, which correspond to the axes of the ora bays [52] (Fig. 29).

The **central canal** is the space within the tractus hyaloideus, optically empty and free of further membranule systems. Only a few single fibres—among them rudiments of Cloquet's canal—are arranged there in a random manner.

In humans, the regularity of the pattern described above is disturbed by the presence of the prefoveal cavity. The general picture becomes further complicated as a result of the deformation of the funnel system by elongation, occurring with growth and senescence. The funnels thus are forced to deviate from their straight course into an S-shaped curve or into Z-shaped folds (Fig. 25). When folded, the tractus first run almost rectilinearly in the posterior sections; directly posterior to the lens they are arranged in *Z-shaped folds* (Fig. 27c). In the case of the *S-shaped course*, the membranules drop behind the lens, rise steeply in the centre of the vitreous space towards the temporal superior quadrant and then extend on towards the papilla (Fig. 27b). In addition, the individual fibrils are twisted around the funnel axis (Fig. 25a). Thus, the course of the tractus vitreales in three-dimensional space, though basically simple, in section appears extremely complicated [52].

The **connections of the vitreous** to the adjoining tissues are of great clinical importance. In the region of the retina, as electron-microscopic examinations show, its fibrils merge with the basal membrane of Müller's cells, forming the so-called "*membrana limitans interna*" [77, 81, 103]. The vitreous is more strongly adherent in some areas: viz. at the edge of the *papilla*, at the edge of the *prefoveal cortex hole* [103], as well as at the surfaces of *blood vessels* [76]. Anteriorly, the hyaloid membrane is attached to the *edge of the lens*. It is connected to the ciliary body by *zonular fibres* of the circular belts (lig. coronarium and lig. medianum). The firmest connection is found in the so-called *vitreous base*, which extends from the posterior pars plana for 2–3 mm behind the ora serrata.

5. Growth and Ageing

Throughout the life span, from the embryonic stage until old age, the eye undergoes constant change. The phenomena of growth and senescence are closely inter-related. In a transitional zone, such as the extreme periphery of the fundus, many variations may be anticipated which are comprehensible only through a knowledge of embryology and postnatal development [136, 32]. The course of development obviously varies with each individual. For this reason, the different descriptions of embryonic development may disagree.

5.1. The Retina and the Ciliary Body

The border between the retina and the ciliary epithelium is indistinct in early **embryonic stages.** The presence of the *ora serrata* is anticipated at the site where the retina turns into the single-layered epithelium. At first, it is very anterior: near the limbus, approximately in the middle of the primordium of the ciliary body (50-mm stage). It then moves posteriorly: on the one hand by a posterior displacement of the entire ciliary body, on the other hand by the ora serrata shifting over the ciliary body towards its posterior end. Even at birth, these movements are not complete [125]. In the newborn child, the ciliary processes are still on the posterior face of the iris, the ora serrata is behind the processes; the pars plana is thus narrow.

The *meridional segmentation* is already established before birth: cristae ciliares are found as early as the thirty-eighth week of pregnancy, striae ciliares at this point are already recognizable as zones with a taller ciliary epithelium [32]. The dentate processes of the ora serrata are already formed, lying between the ciliary processes. At this stage also primordia of the meridional variations (ciliary epithelium ectopies) are already visible [32]. The asymmetry of the nasal and temporal sides may be observed as early as the twentieth week of pregnancy [32].

Shortly **after birth,** the ciliary processes move away from the posterior face of the iris. The pars plana broadens, especially on the temporal side, keeping pace with the general enlargement of the eyeball.

The development is usually complete by the seventh year. Subsequent changes primarily involve *increase of connective tissue.* The originally thin, smooth ciliary processes (Fig. 19) become thicker and irregularly nodulated. Accessory or intermediate processes arise between them (Fig. 22). Müller's reticulum develops. The cells of the ciliary epithelium in the posterior pars plana become taller and are inclined anteriorly. In the intercellular space small cavities appear, filled with some granular material [238]; in the peripheral retina, cystoid cavities containing hyaluronic acid are formed.

In **old age,** the heads of the ciliary processes (Fig. 19) may become depigmented, appearing whitishgrey. The stroma of the processes becomes hyalinized. The basal membrane of the ciliary epithelium thickens. Vessels penetrate into the interlaminar connective tissue of Bruch's membrane [152, 153].

5.2. The Vitreous Body

The **embryonic development** of the vitreous [116, 151] occurs in two phases; the *primary vitreous body* contains the vasa hyaloidea running from disc to lens and is completely formed at the 13 mm stage. From the 44 mm stage on, the vessels begin to regress and have disappeared by the time of birth, except for remnants of the hyaloid artery. These usually disappear in the first few years of life, leaving residues only at the posterior surface of the lens and at the papilla. The primary vitreous becomes enveloped by the *secondary vitreous*, which develops between the 13- and 65-mm stages. Increasing in volume, the secondary vitreous finally fills almost the entire vitreous cavity.

At birth (Fig. 27a) there remains only a small canal containing primary vitreous (*Cloquet's canal*), which runs straight from the papilla towards the lens. This canal disappears in early childhood [54, 212]. Residues remain at the posterior surface of the lens, enveloping the remnants of the hyaloid artery (arcuate line of Vogt) [224], and probably in front of the papilla. In the newborn child [54, 212] the vitreous body has a regular pattern composed of *radial striations* emerging perpendicularly from the retina. The typical holes of the vitreous cortex (which is not yet formed at this stage) are already present in this radial pattern: the prevascular holes in the form of the typical fissures; the prepapillary hole as part of Cloquet's canal; and at the fovea there is even a complete channel running straight through the vitreous space [54]. This channel disappears in the first few months of life, its only residue being the prefoveal hole.

The *vitreous tracts* develop only later, in the **first years of life,** beginning in the anterior sections, at their typical insertion lines [54]. During adolescence they extend slowly posteriorly, reaching the posterior pole only in old age. Thus for a long period the anterior sections of the eye show the adult vitreous structure with vitreal tracts, whereas the posterior sections retain their infantile radial pattern. This regular arrangement of vitreous structures is, however, disrupted by the formation of cavities and fibrillar condensations (Fig. 27d), a process called vitreous destruction, which begins already in childhood.

With **advancing age** the attachments of the vitreous to the papilla, the retina and the lens become weaker. On the other hand the vitreoretinal adhesions at the vitreous base increase in strength and expand posteriorly [103, 32, 80]. In infancy no vitreo-retinal adhesions exist posterior to the ora serrata, and the posterior vitreous base is formed only with advancing age.

In **old age** the fibrillar part of the internal limiting membrane of the retina may split [78]. The vitreous may then detach from the retina and collapse.

5.3. The Zonule

The genesis of the apparatus suspensorius lentis, i.e. the zonule, is not clearly understood. Probably it develops from an anterior and lateral part of the embryonic vitreous, the so-called tertiary vitreous, at the 65 to 110 mm stage [37, 125]. Subsequently the zonule separates from the vitreous by development of the anterior hyaloid membrane. A division of the zonule into the meridional leaves and the three circular belts may be detected even prior to birth [32]. The fibres are then extremely fine and closely juxtaposed. They become coarser and form thicker strands with age.

In conclusion, embryology provides important information for the interpretation of peripheral variations, since the normal variants are established early in the embryonic stage [32]. They apparently do not develop, as is often asserted, because of zonular traction during accommodation, for they may be observed long before the latter occurs. They are probably not the result of vitreous traction, either, since they appear when the vitreous body is still homogeneous and local traction unlikely. It is possible that variations are produced by developmental disturbances. A limbus-concentric arrangement of anomalies indicates a general disturbance of growth. A meridional arrangement of anomalies is connected with the cristae ciliares and thus probably with the primordium of the vascular system.

III. The Examination of the Normal Periphery of the Fundus

During the examination of the living eye it is not possible to proceed in the same manner as when examining an anatomical specimen. Since the view is limited, the individual structures of interest can neither be surveyed nor followed in a continuous way. First, orientation must be obtained, and hence the morphologically most striking structure must first be sought out. In this chapter a schematic survey of the picture of a normal fundus in the mirror of an indentation contact glass will be given (Fig. 36). Details will be discussed later in the chapter on variations.

The structures of the peripheral fundus are biomicroscopically accessible in two ways. One view is through the *iridolenticular space*, i.e. the space between the iris and the edge of the lens upon maximal mydriasis. The second picture is obtained *through the lens*, i.e. on the indented protuberance. The position and form of the lens determines how far posteriorly the peripheral fundus can be examined through the iridolenticular space, and conversely, how far anteriorly it can be examined translentally. It must be emphasized that the magnification differs in each of these views (Fig. 92).

The examination begins with a survey of the *anterior chamber*, including the angle where the most anterior part of the ciliary body forms the ciliary-body band. The examination could then be continued without a break posteriorly into the iridolenticular space. In practice, however, a rapid survey of the area suffices at first, since only the most anterior parts, i.e. the heads of the ciliary processes and the zonular fibres, are clearly visible in the iridolenticular space. No details are demonstrable in its depth. It is, therefore, practical to continue the examination posteriorly—translentally with indentation—and to localize the ora serrata first. This is by far the most striking landmark in the peripheral fundus; it can be used as a point of orientation and as a point of reference for the description of all findings. This procedure also yields information concerning the meridional segmentation, which subsequently may be correlated.

At the **ora serrata,** the retina slopes steeply toward the ciliary body. A step is thus created which can best be appreciated in the optical section. The difference in the layer thickness becomes evident when the ora serrata is examined at the summit of the protuberance, where the retina appears white and stands out clearly behind the dark pars plana. If, however, the ora serrata is examined on the anterior surface of the indented protuberance, the retina and the ciliary epithelium appear to be of equal transparency. Nevertheless, the ora serrata border is still recognizable as a dark line, produced by the abrupt increase of pigmentation in the pigment epithelium (Fig. 42c).

Anterior to the ora serrata the **pars plana of the ciliary body** is very dark. The difference between the anterior and posterior pars plana is less prominent biomicroscopically than ophthalmoscopically or histologically. The contrast in colour is less pronounced under the optical conditions of slit-lamp microscopy, i.e. with a small visual field and high magnification. On the other hand, the surface structure can thus be evaluated more easily. The posterior pars plana has a granular surface; the anterior pars plana is striated. This structural difference is most evident when examined on the summit of the protuberance; the differences in colour are most pronounced on its anterior face. The **granular zone** is broader temporally; nasally it is only a narrow band. This zone has peak-like anterior extensions, the so-called striae ciliares. A fine meridional striation is observed in the anterior pars plana, in the so-called **striated zone**. It is produced partly by changes in the pigment epithelium, partly by the fibres of the epiciliary zonule. The former are observed best at the anterior face of the protuberance, the latter by examination at the summit or in silhouette.

The anterior and posterior leaves of the **zonule** appear in the iridolenticular space. The fibres emerge from the ciliary valleys in separate fascicles, spread out towards the lens and reach the line of insertion on the lens almost equidistantly. They are inserted at the anterior and posterior borders of the lens and in zones parallel to the equator. On the posterior face of the lens, a bright, *dentate reflex* appears, with serrations corresponding to the zonular fascicles. Single zonule fibres may pass centripetally beyond the dentate reflex line. Insofar as the zonule fibres appear in the iridolenticular space, they are most readily seen focally with the wide slit beam as grey striae against a black background. Behind the edge of the lens, they are best observed in the reflected light as black striae against a red background.

From the lens, the **anterior hyaloid membrane** extends along the ciliary body posteriorly. It is helpful first to examine the membrane anteriorly, since it is most readily visible there: at the border of the lens and in the iridolenticular space. In the fossa patellaris, the anterior hyaloid membrane is visible only in pathological cases, i.e. when it is detached [228, 229]. Even the *ligamentum hyaloideocapsulare*, the attachment of the hyaloid membrane to the edge of the lens, can be localized only in exceptional cases. After the anterior hyaloid membrane has left the lens, it can be seen for a short distance translentally, subsequently in the iridolenticular space. It differs from intravitreal membranules in its thickness and stiffness; the fine folds are lacking. In the optical section, it appears as a homogeneous membrane, being much thicker than the zonular fibres anterior to it. In the wide slit beam it appears as a diffusely reflecting surface. A dullwhite band appears at the curves in the silhouette (silhouette reflex). The *silhouette reflexes* change if the incidence of illumination is altered. They differ, therefore, from the true structural densifications, e.g. from the circular zonular fibres. The anterior hyaloid membrane forms an anteriorly convex curve. A silhouette reflex is usually produced above the ciliary processes.

The *connections to the corona ciliaris* are difficult to examine. In the iridolenticular space, illumination is generally so weak that no details can be recognized. For a translental observation of this part of the anterior hyaloid membrane, indentation must be so deep as to cause the ciliary body to become greatly deformed. It is pressed tightly against the anterior hyaloid membrane, which is thus stretched and folded upon the processes. The plicae and peaks observed there are thus probably all indentation artefacts (Fig. 37).

The anterior hyaloid membrane comes into contact with the ciliary body only at the middle of the pars plana. A whitishgrey line, the **"white midline"**, is found at this point. Above the posterior pars plana, i.e. between the white midline and the ora serrata, the anterior hyaloid membrane can be discerned only with great difficulty. Its distance from the ciliary body is minimal, so care must be taken during the examination to keep this distance as great as possible. For this purpose, either the light beam is placed obliquely to the surface of the protuberance (whereby, for geometric reasons, this distance becomes greater), or the examination is carried out at the lateral slopes of the protuberance. The depth of indentation should be kept at a minimum so as to compress the tissues as little as possible. Under favourable optical conditions a fine, light band may then be detected passing posteriorly over the pars plana and disappearing at the ora serrata. Whether this is the anterior hyaloid membrane can be ascertained only with difficulty, because of the risk of confusion with perspective superpositions of the midline and accessory lines, of the epiciliary zonule and the intravitreal membranules.

Within the vitreous body, the **circular zonular belts** are seen directly behind the anterior hyaloid membrane. The *retrolental fascicle* is seldom visible but may appear as a fine, greyish fibrillar band where the anterior hyaloid membrane leaves the lens. Because of the afore-mentioned unfavourable conditions of observation, the *ligamentum coronarium* is identifiable only if the lens has been displaced (Fig. 92). The *ligamentum medianum* of the pars plana is the most distinct of the three circular belts and is part of the white midline.

The **tractus vitreales** form finely pleated, reflecting membranules in the wide slit beam. In optical section, they appear as delicate "fibres". The *tractus hyaloideus* is inserted at the anterior hyaloid membrane near the border of the lens. The *tractus coronarius* is drawn towards the posterior third of the ciliary processes. The *tractus medianus* is inserted in the region of the white midline. Other fine membranules may sometimes be found in the interstices between the tractus vitreales. They are inserted at fine lines, structured similar to the white midline, and called *accessory lines*. These are usually present in some segments only and do not involve the whole circumference.

The tractus vitreales are extremely mobile, undulating at the slightest movement of the eye and only gradually resuming their normal position. The *tractus praeretinalis* alone does not move. It extends anteriorly at some distance from the retina and is inserted at the ora serrata. Details of the insertion are difficult to determine because of light reflected from the retina. For the same reason the **vitreous cortex** can only be evaluated in silhouette against a black background. In biomicroscopic examination the cortex appears structureless and "optically empty". The typical pattern present in slit-lamp examinations of autopsy eyes [52] is not visible because the angle of illumination is too small in biomicroscopic examination. Only occasionally a very fine pattern can be dimly seen; coarser opacities within the cortex are of pathological nature.

IV. Variations in the Periphery of the Fundus

Development and involution differ in each individual, which explains why no periphery of the fundus is identical with another. Developmental variations are present in every eye in differing numbers, shapes and sizes, but most of them have no clinical significance. In the differential diagnosis of pathological conditions, however, a sound knowledge of these variants is indispensable. In the following chapters, the peripheral retina, the ciliary body and the vitreous base will first be presented separately. Subsequently, the transitional zone of the ora serrata, in which all three formations are involved, will be described.

1. The Peripheral Retina

Peripheral retinal lesions "per se" do not directly cause visual disturbances. They may, however, be the source of complications which later on may affect the central retina. The main complication is, without doubt, *detachment of the retina*. Therefore the relation of peripheral lesions to the development of an amotio retinae is our main clinical concern. From this point of view peripheral lesions may be grouped, according to their location within the retinal lamina, in three categories:

– Changes **within the retinal lamina** have scarcely any clinical importance.

– Changes on the **internal surface** of the retina are connected with the vitreous. Vitreoretinal adhesions can transmit vitreal traction to the retina. Such changes are therefore clinically significant.

– Changes on the **external surface** of the retina are connected with changes in the pigment epithelium. The retroretinal interstice is usually obliterated here. An adhesion to the pigment epithelium suggests increased clinical safety.

1.1. Changes within the Retinal Lamina

1.1.1. Cystoid Degeneration

Cystoid changes in the peripheral retina have been known for a long time. Following reports by Blessig and Iwanoff [118, 119], numerous authors have emphasized them in histological studies [66, 216, 218]. They are not easily recognized in the living eye because of difficulty of observation. Pau [147] defended the view that cystoid degeneration is a post-mortem artefact.

More recent examinations by indentation show, however, that the cystoid spaces are present in the living eye [45, 169, 170]; they are, indeed, not infrequent [145].

In a histological examination—in the usual meridional sections—or in an ophthalmo-scopic examination of the living eye there seems to be an agglomeration of cysts. For this reason, the changes have been included under the term "cystoid degenera-tion".

In fact, there are two varieties of cystoid degeneration, one affecting the *middle* retinal layers ("typical", or external, cystoid degeneration), the other affecting the *innermost* retinal layers only ("reticular", or inner, cystoid degeneration). Both have a characteristic appearance and distribution.

In **external cystoid degeneration** (Fig. 43b), there is a sequence of *marginal cysts, coarse cystoid spaces and fine cystoid spaces* from the retinal border on posteriorly [45]. The term marginal **"cyst"**, although anatomically incorrect, may be used in connection with cystoid degeneration, as there is one single cavity entirely delineated by a wall. If the diameter of the "cyst" exceeds the thickness of the retina, the interior surface of the retina curves inwards (Fig. 41). This inner wall is not always readily visible, and the differentiation between a very thin wall and a partial-thickness defect may be made only in optical section.

Conversely, in **cystoid spaces** there are large, flat cavities crossed by strands of tissue (Fig. 43a). The strands resemble pillars connecting the outer with the inner cavity wall. They are spaced at almost regular intervals so that the configura-tion resembles a colonnade. The pillars broaden when inserting at the interior cavity wall; between them, this wall is thin and almost transparent. Thus a regular pattern of tissue opacifications and attenuations is produced, which may, at a superficial observation, give the impression of cysts closely juxtaposed (Fig. 49). However, when seen in optical section, the interior wall of the cavity is not, as in regular "cysts", curved towards the vitreous space, but forms a straight line (Fig. 47).

In **coarse cystoid spaces** the pillars are relatively thick and the intervals fairly broad; nevertheless, they are not easily identifiable in biomicroscopy. Owing to the deformation of the wall of the globe through indentation, they face in different directions and are scarcely identifiable individually because of perspective defor-mations and superpositions. Transparent pillars behave as light conductors: they reflect on the side opposite the incident slit beam. Opaque pillars reflect on the same side as the incident slit beam. The *individual pillars* are best recognizable by an exami-nation in silhouette (Fig. 37a). Their *topographic distribution* can best be seen by indirect or retro-illumination, which reveals the distribution of opacifications and attenuations on the inner layer (Fig. 49).

In **fine cystoid spaces** the pillars are very thin and the intervals very small. In focal illumination the retinal surface appears normal so that fine cystoid spaces are easily overlooked. They are observed best in retro-illumination, when they reveal a fine, meridional parallel striation, with finely granulated individual striae. It is only by an examination in silhouette that the actual pillars and their intervals become recognizable (Fig. 49).

In the **distribution** of external cystoid degeneration there is a striking bilateral sym-metry [145] and a characteristic regularity. The marginal *"cysts"* occur at the retinal edge in one or two rows. Behind them are *coarse cystoid spaces*. In the nasal quadrants (Fig. 46) they form circumscribed areas which are situated predominantly behind the ora serrations, almost symmetrical to the axis of the latter. Temporally (Fig. 47) the coarse cystoid spaces are oval, with their longer diameter parallel to the ora serrata.

Such areas may merge to form broad belts, finally encompassing the entire circumference. Islands of intact retina may occasionally remain. *Fine cystoid spaces* succeed the coarse cystoid ones. They are found almost exclusively in the temporal quadrants. If they are observed at other sites, reticular cystoid degeneration must be suspected. Anteriorly the fine cystoid areas may change imperceptibly into coarse cystoid ones or may be delineated by sharp borders. Posteriorly a sharp boundary is not detectable, and the fine cystoid areas appear to merge gradually into the intact retina. However, with biomicroscopic light incidence a sharp delimitation, though present, can easily be overlooked, and indentation, which would perhaps make it visible, is difficult so far posteriorly.

Occurrence. Cystoid degeneration has been observed in nearly all eyes both histologically and biomicroscopically [32, 45, 145, 170]. Marginal cysts have been found even in earliest childhood. Coarse cystoid spaces appear in early adolescence, becoming more frequent and more extensive with increasing age. Fine cystoid spaces are observed only in later years. In conclusion, cystoid degeneration is to be considered as a *manifestation of normal age involution*. It is not related to any specific pathological condition, and there are no reports of cases where cystoid spaces have been the cause of serious complications.

Deviations from these involution processes can, on the other hand, be pathological [45]. For example, edges of the retina completely free of cysts have been observed in members of two families with hereditary retinal detachment.

These patients were all highly myopic with marked destruction of the vitreous body. The posterior hyaloid membrane was rigid, appearing like a cuticular membrane. In each case retinal detachment was produced by giant, rapidly expanding retinal dialyses.

The absence of cysts is obviously, in certain cases, an indication of an abnormal retinal condition. On the other hand, broad belts of real "cysts", though extremely rare, are probably also pathological (Fig. 41). In a case where the cyst belt was present in only one eye, a large retinal defect was found, which—for lack of any other known cause—was suspected to be of degenerative nature (Fig. 42).

Histologically, the *distribution* of cystoid spaces and their connecting pillars can be recognized only in flat preparations of the retina (Fig. 43). In meridional sections the cavities appear as round holes, resembling cysts (Fig. 45). They may be found in the middle retinal layers, especially in the outer plexiform layer, and less frequently in the inner granular layer. The outer retinal layers with the sensory epithelium remain intact and are not affected by cystoid degeneration. The *cavities* contain hyaluronidase-sensitive mucopolysaccharides according to Zimmermann and Spencer [239]. They are often crossed by a membrane in the outer plexiform layer, which seems to be more resistant and is termed *"membrana limitans media"* by Fine [64]. Biomicroscopically, it is not visible. The *supporting pillars* consist of fibres and nuclei. They were for a long time interpreted as Müller's supporting fibres. Fine and Zimmermann [64], however, postulate exactly the opposite, viz. that Müller's supporting fibres (their outer parts) have degenerated and that the persisting pillars consist of nerve elements. Because of their dense synaptic connections they may readily form strands. This theory is sustained by Vrabec [225] who, using special staining methods, successfully demonstrated nerve fibres, and by Yanoff and Tsou [237], who detected characteristic mitochondrial enzymes. In some areas the pillars become hyalinized so that no cell elements can be detected.

Table 2. Cystoid degeneration and schisis retinae (in biomicroscopic examinations)

Age	4–20	21–40	41–60	> 60
Number of patients (eyes)	26 (44)	35 (52)	27 (49)	25 (45)
Marginal cysts and coarse cystoid spaces	26 (44)	35 (52)	27 (49)	25 (45)
Fine-cystoid spaces	0	1 (2)	9 (17)	13 (23)
Schisis retinae without holes	0	1 (1)	5 (8)	8 (14)
Schisis retinae with holes in one of the two laminae	0	0	3 (3)	2 (4)

Schisis retinae in autopsy eyes (after Foos *et al.* [71])

	Number	Schisis	%
Patients	430	16	4
Eyes	845	22	3

"**Reticular cystoid degeneration**" has been described by Foos and Feman [72]. In contrast to the cystoid spaces described above, the cavities are situated in the *innermost* retinal layers (Fig. 45). At the junction of reticular and external cystoid degeneration, the cavities are separated by a membrane consisting of the inner plexiform layer. Morphologically, reticular cystoid degeneration resembles the previously described fine cystoid spaces. It differs from external cystoid degeneration in that *no particular meridian* is preferred, it is sharply *delineated by branching vessels*, and the *normal pattern* of the *overlying vessels* is *preserved* (Fig. 44). Reticular cystoid degeneration has been observed by Foos and Feman in 17% of 200 autopsies. In the *living eye*, however, reticular cystoid degeneration is seldom detected. The fine pattern of the pillars may be seen only with a small angle of acceptance, i.e. only via examination at the summit of the indentation protuberance. In this position, however, the characteristic arrangement, especially the delineation by vascular branches, is hard to make out. Biomicroscopic differentiation between a reticular and the external fine cystoid degeneration is therefore difficult. In addition, reticular cystoid degeneration is situated so far posteriorly that indentation usually causes pain. Therefore the whole circumference of the fundus cannot be scrutinized for reticular cystoid degeneration.

The **etiology** of both types of cystoid degeneration is unknown. Biomicroscopy refutes the often-asserted relationship of cystoid degeneration with structures of the vitreous base or with pathological vitreoretinal adhesions: the delimitation of cystoid degenerative areas is in no way identical with the configuration of the vitreous base. Abnormal vitreoretinal adhesions occur no more frequently there than elsewhere. A nutritive disturbance of the peripheral retina may be presumed [242] but has not been proved so far.

In several cases, coarse cystoid spaces were found in areas where an *external stimulus* was operative. Fig. 48 depicts an intra-ocular foreign body in the region of the ciliary body. Nearby, in less than one year, coarse cystoid spaces have developed. Cystoid areas have also been observed developing in the adjacent retina in cases of an inflammatory focus of the pars plana. These are, however, exceptions. Usually, eyes with cystoid degeneration show no signs of present or previous pathological disturbances. It is still uncertain whether an external stimulus is responsible for the appearance of cystoid degeneration in *normal* eyes. It has been suggested that the traction of the zonule is responsible for this. In fact, cystoid areas begin at sites where an insertion of zonule fibres even beyond the ora serrata has been described [133], i.e. at dentate processes. Daicker [32], however, describes cystoid spaces in the fetus, where zonular traction is unlikely.

While the pathogenesis is not fully understood, one thing is certain. Cystoid degeneration is primarily a *sign of senescence* and is, in general, neither the cause nor the consequence of any pathological processes in the eye. According to the anatomical substratum, this process of involution occurs in various forms, as marginal cysts, as coarse cystoid spaces, or as fine cystoid spaces. The latter may eventually lead to a large splitting of the retina, the so-called schisis retinae.

1.1.2. Senile Retinoschisis

Retinoschisis is the term used for the splitting of the retina into two layers. The rare *hereditary* and *juvenile* forms are primarily the consequence of a widespread disturbance of the vitreoretinal relationships. They may assume bizarre forms and must be distinguished from the more frequent *senile* schisis which will be discussed below.

Senile schisis seems to be the result of atrophy of the pillars in fine cystoid spaces [68, 120, 187, 241]. It shows the same frequency and age distribution, is located for the most part temporally, bilateral, and occurs only in older persons [24, 187]. Schisis retinae has been biomicroscopically observed in those over forty in 31% of our cases [45], i.e. somewhat more frequently than by other researchers [187, 68] using different methods of observation. This is probably due to the fact that in our figures even the slightest changes have been included.

In its *early stages,* when only a few pillars are lacking, a schisis forms merely a flat fissure in fine cystoid spaces. At this stage, diagnosis is difficult, since at first there seems to be only a slight thickening of the retina in a fine cystoid area (examination in silhouette). The residual fragments of the supporting pillars still remain, forming nodular excrescences towards the cavity on the inner layer. Thus the striated pattern in retro-illumination, characteristic of fine cystoid spaces, is at first still present. The beginning of the schisis can only be diagnosed in optical section [49]. In the case of a *large schisis,* however, the picture changes. There is a large "cyst" whose inner layer protrudes towards the vitreous; it is thin-walled, and the nodules are absent. The vessels disappear, leaving only single, mostly sheathed, larger branches. In extremely large vesicles, the interior layer is almost completely transparent. Diagnosis becomes difficult, yet may still be made ophthalmoscopically if the parallax of the vessels is observed against choroidal irregularities or against the indentation protuberance. Occasionally, though, diagnosis can be made only with the slit lamp in the optical section.

The cavities of typical senile schisis do not usually extend quite to the retinal edge but are separated from it by a narrow belt of "normal" coarse cystoid spaces. At the retinal edge sometimes another variety of schisis is observed. The **marginal schisis** extends along the ora serrata (Fig. 50). In contrast to the pre-equatorial vesicular schisis the cavity is flat and does not protrude from the retinal level. Rudimentary pillars are present only upon the outer layer, whereas the inner layer is completely transparent. Detection is thus difficult, since the picture may be confused with an anomaly of the pars plana, i.e. with proliferations of the ciliary epithelium. Suspicion of a marginal schisis arises, however, on account of the regular intervals of the "proliferations", which are similar to the intervals of the pillars in the adjacent coarse cystoid spaces. Careful examination in optical section and in silhouette will then reveal the inner layer. Examination of the lateral ends of the marginal schisis will determine the true position of the ora serrata in comparison with the normal retinal edge. The marginal schisis is often overlooked, owing to the difficulties in diagnosis. Its clinical significance is therefore unknown.

Conversely, **pre-equatorial schisis** has been the object of investigations by many authors. Let us first describe its biomicroscopic appearance: The *vitreal side* of the **inner layer** is, in general, normal. If there are any retinal glistening dots on the inner layer, their distribution and number is similar to that in other retinal areas. The vitreoretinal relations show no pecularities: in a posterior detachment of the vitreous, the line of insertion of the posterior hyaloid membrane is at the same distance from the ora serrata as in the still intact surroundings. Thus it passes over the schisis and does not coincide with its posterior border. There are neither vitreoretinal anomalies nor intravitreal findings which could be considered characteristic of a schisis. The *side of the wall facing the cavity* shows the nodular excrescences already mentioned. *Holes* in the inner wall are not infrequent. They are normally very small, round and so fine that they are discovered only with difficulty. The location of the suspect areas may be seen best in retro-illumination, when the somewhat thickened edges of the holes become evident. Only the optical section differentiates an attenuation from a real defect.

The **outer layer** of a schisis is more difficult to examine since details are scarcely recognizable because the nodules of the interior layer obstruct the view. Improvement may be obtained by increasing the angle between the beam of observation and the beam of illumination. Yet this approach is restricted when examining the peripheral regions. Another solution is provided by indentation, which improves the view by approaching the outer layer to the inner one, thereby diminishing the obstructive effect of the nodules, which depends on distance. Under these conditions of observation, the outer layer appears dull grey. Shallow depressions of variable depth are found at irregular intervals. There are also *holes*. They are difficult to detect, since, as long as the outer schisis layer remains attached to the pigment epithelium, a contrast is hardly noticeable between the areas where the thin outer schisis layer is still present and where it is lacking. Such defects therefore have to be sought by examination at the summit of the indentation protuberance. Conversely, larger defects are more easily detected for, as their edges thicken, they appear greyish, thus forming a clear contrast to the reddish background of the hole.

Because the diagnosis of holes in the outer layer is often difficult, *indicative signs* must be looked for (Fig. 52). These signs result from the fact that holes may appear in connection with localized adhesions between the two schisis layers. Portions of the outer layer remain attached to the inner layer, so that there are connecting strands which either remain intact or are torn apart. The diagnosis of a hole is facilitated when the outer layer is detached from the pigment epithelium, i.e. in places where a schisis has developed into a retinal detachment (Fig. 52b).

One portion of the cavity is then outlined as a "schisis" by the two retinal layers, the second portion by the pigment epithelium and the full-thickness retina. The two parts of the cavity are separated from each other by the membraneous outer schisis layer. A hole is more readily recognized in this membrane, since the contrast becomes greater as the distance from the pigment epithelium increases.

In **histological sections** a schisis differs from cystoid spaces only by its size [241, 143]. The splitting occurs in the same layers. The receptor cells remain intact and are part of the outer layer. The inner layer is formed by the ganglion cells and the nerve fibres. This layer, however, becomes atrophic in advanced stages and no retinal tissue may be identified. The same mucopolysaccharides have been found in schisis cavities and in cystoid spaces [239].

There is another type of vesicular splitting, affecting the inner retinal layers only (Fig. 51). On the base of this topography it might be related to the "reticular cystoid degeneration". There are no pillars in this type of schisis. Underneath the cavity, in the outer layer, cystoid spaces may still be present [96]. For this form of "inner" schisis the term **"retinal cyst"** may be used. Simultaneous occurrence of both types, i.e. an "inner" schisis separated by a lamella from an "external" one, has not been reported.

Differentiation of schisis from retinal detachment is most important in practice. It is not too difficult in a retinal detachment of recent origin, but where the detachment is of long standing, the detached retina atrophies and becomes transparent. Its appearance cannot be distinguished from that of the inner layer of a schisis. One possibility of differentiation is by examination of the *visual field* [211]. In a schisis absolute scotomata occur in the affected area, caused by a complete break in the nervous connections, whereas in a retinal detachment there is a relative scotoma at the margins. Through perimetry, however, the process is only detectable when it has already extended far posteriorly, because the areas affected by an incipient schisis or retinal detachment are situated outside the visual field. Yet for appropriate prophylaxis and treatment, diagnosis of a retinal detachment should be made early.

Is there any possibility of differential diagnosis based on *morphological signs*? A most important sign is observed on examination of the marginal areas. In a retinal detachment which has remained localized for a long time, scars with fibrous and pigment proliferations develop at the borders. These *demarcation lines* form a characteristic marginal area which may appear triangular in optical section. On the other hand, a schisis blends gradually into the surrounding cystoid degenerations, from the thin, structureless layer into zones with nodules, thence into zones with elongated pillars, and finally into simple cystoid areas. The pillars at the edges around the cavity, laterally or anteriorly and posteriorly, are characteristic of a schisis (Fig. 51). This sign, however, is not present in the case of an "inner" schisis, i.e. of a *retinal cyst*. Its differentiation from a retinal detachment is then based upon the presence of a relatively thick outer layer which covers the pigment epithelium underneath and is clearly recognizable on the summit of the protuberance.

Observation of the *pigment epithelium* provides additional information for a differential diagnosis. If, as in the case of an amotio, the pigment epithelium has been exposed for a long time, the familiar proliferations and drusen are formed. However, in the case of a schisis where the pigment epithelium remains covered by the outer retinal layer, there are no reactive changes. The *shape of the holes* can only be used with great

31

caution in the differentiation, although horseshoe tears should arouse suspicion of retinal detachment. Similarly, *bilateral symmetry* can be taken as an indicative sign only. A schisis usually occurs in both eyes, often symmetrically. This symmetry is quite rare in retinal detachments.

What is the **prognosis** of a schisis? A schisis may be considered the final stage in the involutional process which begins in early childhood with the formation of marginal cysts and extends posteriorly in the form of cystoid spaces. But many questions remain unanswered. How does the atrophy of the fine pillars occur? Why do large cysts occur so seldom, considering the marked frequency of the flat schisis? No explanation has been found for the extremely slow evolution. Long-term follow-ups (up to seven years) do not demonstrate any progression in many cases of schisis, even with very large vesicles (including cases where the intraretinal cavity communicated with the retroretinal space through a hole in the external layer). For this reason, it seems possible that a schisis may develop, not continuously but in a single, more or less acute process or through several intermittent stages.

From the clinical point of view, the main problem is whether a *progredient retinal detachment* will develop from a pre-existing schisis. It is generally assumed that there is no danger if holes are found in only one of the two layers of the schisis [187]. On the other hand, if holes exist in *both* layers, the criteria for the development of a retinal detachment are fulfilled although a progredient retinal detachment does not occur in all such cases. It has not been decided so far whether the state of the vitreous (posterior vitreal detachment) plays a role similar to that encountered in the "normal" rhegmatogenous retinal detachment.

What is the proper **therapeutic approach** at this point? It is obvious that in the case of a disease which is not, or no longer progressive, no measures should be taken that involve even the slightest risk. It is advisable to make an occasional check of spontaneous progression. The frequency of schisis and its usually benign course, however, necessitate a selection of the patients to be observed. What are the criteria which establish the prognosis? As the cause of the origin and progression of a schisis is still unknown, one must rely on practical experience according to which the flat schisis is evidently harmless and requires no treatment. A bullous, dome-shaped elevation without holes should be observed for some time in order to evaluate possible progression. If holes are found in both layers, frequent checks are necessary, especially if the vitreous is destroyed. Prophylactic and therapeutic measures [143, 181] should be related to the rate of progression.

1.2. Changes on the Inner Retinal Surface

1.2.1. Equatorial Vitreoretinal Degenerations

This subdivision may be applied to a group of polymorphic changes in the peripheral retina which share the following characteristics. They are primarily lesions of the internal retinal surface and affect vitreoretinal relations; the vitreous cortex is split (Fig. 53), allowing communication with the semi-fluid central vitreous [52]. The membrana limitans interna is eroded, as well as the nerve-fibre layer, and even the ganglion-cell layer. In later stages, there is glial degeneration at the edges and glial proliferation into the vitreous, atrophy of deeper retinal layers with the formation of partial-thickness or full-thickness defects, pigment proliferation, and characteristic sclerosis of the vascular walls.

Equatorial degenerations can already be seen in children and adolescents. With advancing age, their number does not seem to increase [32] but their appearance is altered by secondary changes.

Characteristically, the lesions are at the equator or anterior to it. Only rarely are they seen in the posterior sections of the fundus or directly at the ora serrata. They are round, oval or band-shaped, the longer axis always being parallel to the equator.

Owing to their morphologic aspect, these lesions have been referred to as "snail tracks", "lattice degenerations", etc. As they occur in areas accessible without indentation, they have long been known and have been studied exhaustively [22, 25, 202, 208]. Yet for the examination of details, indentation is helpful. Recognition of attenuations on the inner side of the retina, differential diagnosis between partial-thickness and full-thickness defects, or the diagnosis of subretinal fluid pockets are often possible only by kinetic indentation. The diagnosis of a *split in the vitreous cortex,* however, is always difficult. Under biomicroscopic conditions the normal vitreous cortex appears optically empty, even when examined against a dark background, and holes in it produce no contrast. Only if, by a suitable incidence of light, reflexions can be produced on their border surfaces can cortex holes be visualized. "Reactive" alterations, e.g. vitreous condensations, fibrous or glial proliferations, however, are recognizable as greyish-opaque strands or networks.

Equatorial degenerations are of great clinical importance, since retinal holes, if present there, may induce *retinal detachment.* How great is this danger? We have, in fact, a situation predisposing to retinal detachments since the split in the vitreous cortex may provide a free passage from the liquid central vitreous through the underlying retinal hole into the retro-retinal space. The presence of this passage is demonstrated by the not infrequent pockets of retro-retinal fluid. However, these may remain stationary for years. A progredient retinal detachment usually develops only after a posterior vitreous detachment.

1.2.2. Paravascular Vitreoretinal Attachments

Paravascular attachments represent another form of vitreoretinal degeneration. They have been described in autopsy eyes by Spencer and Foos [206]. Lacunae appear in the innermost layers of the retina, immediately beneath the inner limiting membrane (*paravascular retinal rarefactions*). If the posterior hyaloid membrane is detached, partial-thickness tears are formed (*paravascular retinal tears*). The paravascular attachments are found adjacent to blood vessels [29], usually at bifurcations or crossings; frequently they form groups circumscribed by branches of blood vessels (Fig. 54a). In the case of paravascular retinal tears (i.e. after a vitreous detachment), the groups are delimited anteriorly by the posterior vitreous base. In some cases, a posterior vitreous detachment may lead to *full-thickness tears* at paravascular attachments.

In *autopsy eyes*, paravascular rarefactions or tears are frequently observed in patients over fifty years of age. Spencer and Foos [206] found paravascular retinal rarefactions in 25% of 252 eyes; 38% of these had a posterior vitreous detachment and 29% paravascular tears. There was no correlation with the patients' sex or the size of the eyeball.

In the *living eye*, on the other hand, paravascular attachments are rarely observed. In order to make rarefactions and partial-thickness defects visible, the affected area must be examined at the summit of the protuberance, requiring thus a very posterior indentation. Their location may, however, be suspected from indicative signs: If the posterior hyaloid membrane detaches above a paravascular attachment, the inner layers of the lacunae may detach, too, appearing as circumscribed thickenings of the hyaloid membrane (Fig. 54b). If such opacifications are found near the posterior vitreous base, kinetic indentation will reveal the characteristic groups of paravascular retinal tears.

1.2.3. Angioids

Various cone-shaped proliferations may be observed in the periphery of the retina, between the equator and the ora serrata, singly or in groups. Vitreous condensations are attached at their tops. Most of these proliferations are so minute that further differentiation is not possible with biomicroscopic magnification. For this reason, they are termed "micro-adhesions" and will be discussed in detail in a special chapter (see p. 58). Conversely, there are larger cones appearing as small, sharply-defined nodular protuberances or as oblong cones of greyish white tissue (Fig. 55). Characteristically, they are connected with *vascular anomalies*, since abnormally large, tortuous or anastomosing vessels penetrate the cones at their bases. A vitreous strand branches off from the peak of these cones; it is relatively broad and may strongly reflect the light beam. This strand may be followed for a short distance in a radial direction towards the centre of the eyeball, where it disappears from view.

Studies in *autopsy eyes* [52] demonstrate that the adhering vitreous strands run within a round defect in the vitreous cortex. These strands are relatively broad, sharply defined, and occasionally tubular. They appear not unlike the vascular residua of the arteria hyaloidea of the central canal. They cross the vitreous cortex radially, either splitting off at the border of the central vitreous into several branches which follow the surface of the tractus praeretinalis, or piercing the tractus prae-retinalis, bending sharply at its edge, and following the generally tortuous pattern of the fibres in the central vitreous (Fig. 56).

Resembling rudimentary vitreous vessels, they are termed as "angioids", not meaning to anticipate their actual genesis. At present, nothing specific is known about their origin or nature [79, 148, 149]. Their clinical importance is questionable. In a posterior detachment of the vitreous, retinal tears may arise at angioids, as at all places of vitreoretinal adhesions.

1.2.4. Retinal Glistening Dots

Retinal glistening dots are frequently found in the peripheral fundus, diffusely dispersed or in circumscribed groups. The yellow-white dots are strongly reflective.

Depending on the incidence of light, they may sparkle like crystals. In focal illumination, they appear as bright dots; in retro-illumination, as opacifications. They are situated on the inner retinal surface. In coarse cystoid spaces, they are found at the insertion points of supporting pillars. In other areas, they are evenly dispersed at regular intervals. In zones of equatorial vitreoretinal adhesions their distribution is more irregular, with the glistening dots closely packed in patches, occasionally forming oblong, bright "snail tracks" parallel to the equator. The retinal glistening dots are frequently the only sign of a retinal change, with the surrounding retina appearing biomicroscopically normal. Stronger vitreoretinal adhesions are not evident, since the vitreous detaches there without complication. Glistening dots may also be found near pathological retinal changes, especially at equatorial vitreoretinal degenerations or posterior to meridional ridges. Glistening dots may disappear following a posterior vitreous detachment.

According to Daicker's **histological examinations** [33] the glistening dots are microglia cells containing lipoid or lipoprotein material. Primary or secondary retinal degeneration is always present histologically in this area: senile atrophy of the inner retinal layers, cystoid degenerations, schisis retinae, or vitreoretinal adhesions.

Clinical and histological examinations reveal that retinal glistening dots are a non-specific phenomenon [33]. They merely indicate *chronic retinal atrophy* and do not tell us anything about the quality of the tissue. Foci composed solely of glistening dots are not likely to tear. Prophylactic or therapeutic measures are unnecessary.

1.2.5. The Problem of Vitreoretinal Adhesions

The importance of vitreoretinal adhesions in the origin of retinal tears is generally accepted and thus requires no further discussion. Another problem, however, is still open to question: Are there any *morphological signs* permitting diagnosis of vitreo-retinal adhesions and evaluation of their dangers? This question is very important in practice, since the indication for prophylactic coagulation depends upon it. All sorts of retinal "degenerations" have been labelled dangerous adhesions and various classifications of their dangers have been proposed [4]. Clinical experience, however, has demonstrated that a prognosis based on such classifications is not very reliable.

This is, indeed, not surprising. What are vitreoretinal adhesions? As long as the vitreous is still *attached*, it is adherent everywhere. There is a "*total vitreoretinal adhesion*", and it is of no practical consequence whether there are areas of stronger connection in it.

In a *posterior vitreous detachment* the *fibrillar part of the "inner limiting membrane"* is split [78], one part remaining adherent to the retina, the other becoming the posterior hyaloid membrane. Areas where this splitting is impeded are from the clinical point of view to be considered vitreoretinal adhesions. These alterations have submicroscopical dimensions and are therefore not in any way visible in the living eye. But their location may be suspected, as they presumably are present wherever the regular pattern of the vitreous cortex is disturbed. This is the case at all *scars* and *degenerations* of the inner retinal layers [52]. Irregularities of the vitreous cortex, however, are to be expected also at the *constitutional cortex holes*, i.e. at the papilla, at the posterior pole, and at the vessels, all of which present no visible intravitreal alterations.

Vitreovascular adhesions illustrate this nicely. They are easily demonstrated in histological examinations [76], as well as in anatomical specimens of unfixed autopsy eyes [52]. In the living eye, however, no pathological changes are visible and there are no vitreous strands attached to the vessels. It is only *after* a vitreous detachment that complications arise: either a vessel is stripped from the intact retina, or the retina is torn, the horseshoe tear characteristically being crossed by the vessel at its apex. Even in a vitreous detachment without complications, alterations may be observed which may be attributed to vitreo-vascular adhesions. On the posterior hyaloid membrane, condensations are visible resembling the casts of retinal vessels and continuing into vessels where the vitreous is not yet detached.

In *conclusion*, vitreoretinal adhesions must be expected even at places where there are no visible alterations—at least not visible with our present methods of examination. On the other hand, vitreoretinal adhesions connected with visible alterations may be weak and clinically insignificant. Vitreoretinal adhesions are only of interest *in relation to tractions already effective*, in other words, they are clinically relevant only after a vitreous detachment. For this reason, Goldmann [88] has suggested that prophylactic coagulations *should not be performed prior to a vitreous detachment*. With the vitreous still attached, it cannot reasonably be predicted whether, and where, the retina will be torn. Coagulations should not be made unnecessarily [26] since this form of prophylaxis is certainly not without risk.

1.2.6. "White with Pressure"

The term "white with pressure" has been retained to describe an area of whiteness in the retina which results from pressure caused by the indenter [171, 177, 227]. Upon removal of the indenter the area re-assumes its normal colour. Vitreoretinal condensations, subclinical retinal detachments, etc., have been made responsible for this phenomenon.

In principle, all areas with slight opacifications above the pigment epithelium, whether situated pre-, intra-, or retroretinally, may turn white with indentation (see p. 4). In indirect ophthalmoscopy this discoloration is all the more striking because of the low magnification and the large visual field. Biomicroscopically it is less obvious; instead, the nature of the process responsible for this phenomenon can be diagnosed directly, as well as its location within the different layers: slight pre-retinal vitreous opacifications, subretinal fluid accumulations or intraretinal oedema can easily be distinguished in the optical section.

There is, on the other hand, a **pseudophenomenon** that may be described as "white with pressure", but which is visible even *without* indentation. It is characterized by sharply defined zones of the peripheral fundus reflecting more strongly than usual. For no known reason, a sharply delineated area may gleam brightly, according to the incidence of light; only in this respect is this "pseudo-white with pressure" phenomenon influenced, but not caused, by indentation. The *reflecting layer* is extremely difficult to localize exactly. The retina is completely transparent in these areas; its surface structure is unchanged. Even the pigment epithelium appears completely intact, its fine granulation is preserved, and there is no sign of a reaction. The layer affected must therefore be deeper than the pigment epithelium and might be Bruch's membrane, perhaps its *interlaminar connective tissue*.

At present, no definitive conclusion can be drawn about the *nature of the change*. In several cases, these reflex zones were observed in connection with relatively mild inflammatory conditions involving the anterior segments of the eye (uveitis anterior) (Fig. 91). First "true" areas of "white with pressure" were formed by slight subretinal fluid accumulations in the pre-equatorial retina. After the absorption of the fluid, only the "pseudo-white with pressure" reflex zones remained. The above findings are, however, exceptional. In general, no signs of a previous disease can be found. These reflex zones are quite common in the strongly pigmented fundus of dark races.

1.3. Changes in the External Layers

Deep-seated changes are most easily observed on the front of the indentation protuberance. Pigmentation also may be seen via transillumination.

The gradual disintegration of the pigment epithelium in the peripheral fundus, which begins in childhood, appears as a fine granulation or a tigroid reticular pattern. With advancing age it becomes less visible, for the overlying cystoid degeneration tends to obscure the view. The variations of the pigment epithelium pattern have no clinical significance.

1.3.1. Senile Choriatrophy (Paving-Stone Degeneration)

After the age of forty, paving-stone lesions are not infrequently found in the pre-equatorial fundus, usually with bilateral symmetry and occurring mainly in the lower periphery. Small foci appear in the form of round, sharply defined, bright areas of depigmentation. The larger lesions are pigmented irregularly. They may become confluent, coalescing to form bands, yet their circinate delimitation indicates their origin from individual round foci. The process frequently ends at the ora serrata, but may extend beyond it anteriorly.

Histologically, atrophic changes appear in the external retinal layers, in the pigment epithelium, and the choriocapillaris [71, 144, 140, 210, 236]. Characteristically, Bruch's membrane is preserved, so that a histological differentiation is possible between choriatrophic foci and chorioretinal scars.

The **etiology** of paving-stone degeneration is unknown. It is agreed by most authors that it is unrelated to the length of the eyeball, to refraction, or to any eye diseases.

There seems to be no relation to the local vascular condition. Daicker [32] presumes that paving-stone lesions result from the progredient disintegration of the peripheral pigment epithelium in old age. Characteristically, only the most external retinal layers are affected by senile chorioatrophy. The inner layers are not involved and are either quite normal or show a typical cystoid degeneration above the chorioatrophical foci.

Conversely, in *inflammatory scars* there are also alterations in the inner retinal layers and even in the vitreous. A **differential diagnosis** may thus be made by an examination in silhouette. In chorio-atrophic foci the retina has usually retained its thickness.

Table 3. Paving-stone degeneration in biomicroscopic examinations

Age	4–20	21–40	41–60	>60
Number of patients (eyes)	26 (44)	35 (52)	27 (49)	25 (45)
Paving-stone lesions	0	4 (7)	13 (23)	10 (18)

Paving-stone degeneration in autopsy eyes (after Foos *et al.* [71])

	Number	Lesions	%
Patients	614	134	22
Eyes	1 223	185	17

In chorioretinitic scars, however, there is an attenuation of the retina and often a condensation of the vitreous cortex at the margins (Fig. 34) (visible in silhouette against a dark background).

Paving-stone lesions are *clinically relevant*, since they may form chorioretinal adhesions. Examinations of autopsy eyes by Daicker [32] reveal that the retina and the pigment epithelium can still be separated from one another at small white depigmented patches. This is not possible in the larger paving-stone lesions with marked pigmentary disturbance. Clinical observation of retinal detachments shows, however, that even large chorioatrophic foci are not an insurmountable obstacle. The retina may detach, and on the detached lamina an attenuation, corresponding to the lesion and occasionally infiltrated with pigment, may be observed via retro-illumination.

2. The Pars Plana Corporis Ciliaris

The pars plana may be examined either through the iridolenticular space or translentally by means of indentation. When observed through the *iridolenticular space*, the pars plana appears as a brown band (Fig. 36). Details are not visible; nevertheless, gross changes, particularly inflammatory foci, may be detected (Figs. 92, 97). Fine variations are only recognizable by a *translental* examination. The pars plana may be observed translentally without indentation, if either the lens is displaced anteriorly, or the pars plana is detached from the sclera (choroidal detachment, tumour).

The pars plana appears darker than the retina posterior to the ora serrata (Fig. 77). The *dark colour* is produced by the greater amount of pigment within the pigment-epithelium cells. The increase in pigmentation at the ora serrata begins abruptly. A pigmented fine borderline may be seen occasionally even in the albino (Fig. 40). In the pars plana, there are individual differences in pigmentation as elsewhere in the body. In a generally dark fundus, the pars plana is of brown colour; in negroes it is almost black (Fig. 39). In a light fundus, where there is little pigmentation, the choroidal vessels are readily perceived even in the pars plana (Figs. 37, 38). Pigmentation is usually denser in adolescents; with advancing age it becomes granular and patchy, especially in the anterior pars plana.

The **posterior pars plana** and the striae ciliares always seem more pigmented than the anterior pars plana. This is due to an optical artefact produced by *Müller's* *reticulum*, in which, though the pigment epithelium is single-layered, several pigment cells can be seen one behind another at the lateral slopes of the individual meshes. The irregularity of the *ciliary epithelium* in the posterior pars plana may be best seen when examining at the summit of the indented protuberance. The surface is slightly *granular* and may even present wartlike protrusions, formed by proliferations of ciliary epithelium. These occur spontaneously in old age, but may also appear following trauma or inflammation [32].

Conversely, in the **anterior pars plana** the surface is smooth. The fine pattern of the *striate zone* is produced in part by the *epiciliary zonula leaf* and is seen as a microscopic striation in retro-illumination or as striated reflexes in focal illumination (Fig. 37). The individual epiciliary zonula fibres can best be identified in silhouette on the indented protuberance. There is another type of striation: fine *pigmented lines* running in a meridional direction (Fig. 40) in the pigment epithelium. They are best seen in adolescents, since with advancing age they become indistinct owing to the general disintegration of the pigmentation.

The fact that in the pars plana the pigmented epithelium and ciliary epithelium are closely linked (*retroretinal adhesion*) is *clinically* highly important. These connections act as a barrier at which detachments (amotio retinae, pars plana cysts) usually stop. This retroretinal adhesion seems stronger at the interdigitations of Müller's reticulum, the barrier being obviously more effective in the granular zone. In the course of time, however, connections loosen even in this area. Consequently, detachments can expand further beyond the granular zone.

2.1. The Detachment of the Ciliary Epithelium (Pars-Plana Cysts)

Bullous cavities, formed by a separation of the ciliary epithelium from the pigment epithelium, have been of great interest since they are an analogon to retinal detachment. Although they do not represent real cysts, this term has been generally accepted and is therefore retained here. The cysts are found in all quadrants, but predominantly in the temporal inferior periphery, and are often bilaterally symmetrical [2, 98, 142].

The size of the cysts seems to be related to their position upon the pars plana. In the *posterior* pars plana, they appear as **microcysts**, numerous small vesicles often closely juxtaposed (Fig. 57). They are of different sizes. Many of them are scarcely visible, others are quite prominent. As their inner layer has the same structure as the still attached surroundings, small cysts can be diagnosed only if they can be shown to be transparent via retro-illumination or by examination in silhouette. In the *anterior* pars plana, they may be observed as well-rounded **macrocysts** which, singly, fill the entire space between two striae ciliares. Neighbouring cysts are separated at the striae ciliares by a deep sulcus (Fig. 58).

The anatomical relation of the vitreous and of the zonule to the vesicular wall shows no abnormalities. The zonular fibres are inserted at the usual places on the anterior side of the macrocysts. The anterior hyaloid membrane extends over them at some distance, bridging the intervals between neighbouring cysts. Pathological adhesions or extensions of the vesicular wall, which might be a sign of traction, have not been observed biomicroscopically.

Table 4. Pars-plana cysts in biomicroscopic examinations

Age	4–21	21–40	41–60	>60
Number of patients (eyes)	26 (44)	35 (52)	27 (49)	25 (45)
Microcysts	0	1 (1)	2 (4)	3 (5)
Macrocysts	0	0	1 (2)	1 (2)
Macro- and microcysts in the same eye	1 (2)	0	3 (4)	2 (4)
Total of pars-plana cysts	1 (2)	1 (1)	6 (10)	6 (11)

Pars-plana cysts in autopsy eyes (after Okun [142])

Age	1–20	21–40	41–60	>60
Number of autopsies	62	19	66	104
Pars-plana cysts	0	0	8	32

The **evolution** of "pars-plana cysts" can be followed biomicroscopically. Macro-cysts are initially a flat elevation in the anterior pars plana slowly extending laterally up to the adjacent striae and posteriorly to the linea serrata where their expansion is at first obstructed. It is not until a large cyst has developed that the barrier is crossed. However, even then, continued extension into the posterior pars plana seems to be impeded, for initially the cyst is visibly narrower there than in its anterior parts, with a *neck-like constriction* beyond the transition, i.e. the linea serrata. The cyst wall facing the vitreous, i.e. the *detached lamina*, is of the same texture as the adjacent ciliary epithelium. In the anterior pars plana it is thin and finely striated; in the posterior pars plana it is thicker, granular and sometimes finely pigmented. Within the detached lamina frequently there are very fine vesicles, which are probably enlarged intercellular spaces. In the course of time, the neck-like constriction disappears and the cyst assumes a regular oval shape. The detached lamina loses its texture, becoming homogeneous and transparent. The *pigment epithelium* may disappear, so that the uveal vessels and the sclera become visible. The cysts can extend posteriorly as far as the ora serrata, laterally beyond the striae ciliares, and coalesce with the neighbouring cysts (Fig. 61). In microcysts, the progression is more difficult to observe, owing to their abundance.

The extension of cysts beyond the ora serrata has, in contrast to the histological examinations of Adam [1], not yet been observed in the living eye. It should be remembered, however, that the nearly ever-present cystoid spaces may obstruct the view of extensions lying beneath the retina. Therefore, detachments would have to be fairly large to be visible behind the ora serrata.

Reports on the **frequency** of cysts vary. This may be due to the fact that large transparent cysts can easily be overlooked in an examination of the *living* eye, particularly if the edge of the lens is somewhat opaque. For this reason, they have been reported more frequently in *autopsy* eyes [2, 142, 30]. They occur in greater numbers only after the fortieth year of age, being rather exceptional in adolescents [46].

Histological examinations reveal a detachment of the ciliary from the pigment epithelium, in fact, a "retinal detachment" (Figs. 59, 60). Three varieties of cysts are at present distinguishable by their *contents*. Most cysts contain hyaluronic acid [240]. The cysts formed in connection with uveitis contain protein [32]. Cysts of patients with paraproteinemia contain paraproteins [5, 70, 114, 115, 174, 188].

The **etiology** of the senile detachment of the ciliary epithelium is unknown. Many different hypotheses have been suggested. A degenerative mechanism is suspected in most cases, on account of its occurrence in old age, its bilateral symmetry, and the absence of other pathological signs [142, 2]. The suggestion that vitreous traction might produce the detachment [98] seems unlikely, since biomicroscopic observation has never revealed a pathological adhesion or any signs of traction. Zonular traction is not a likely cause either, since cysts occur also in the posterior pars plana where the zonule does not attach. Daicker [30] has ruled out a vascular etiology, since the areas in question are no more prone to angiofibrosis or hyalinosis than others. Slezak [197] suggests, on the basis of observations made following intravenous fluorescein injection, that there is a pathological permeability in the outer walls of the cysts. This is supported by Gärtner's observations of capillaries piercing Bruch's membrane and penetrating into the cysts [82]. Zimmermann and Fine's theory [240] is of interest for, in their opinion, the basal membrane of unpigmented ciliary epithelium becomes thickened with advancing age. The hyaluronic acid secreted at the apex of the ciliary epithelium cells into the "retroretinal interstice" can no longer reach the vitreous via the intercellular spaces. It is thus retained between the two layers of epithelium, causing a detachment. It is not known how secondary pars plana cysts (with protein content) are formed.

One conclusion may be drawn from clinical observation: cysts may develop simultaneously at different sites. According to their topographical position, they may expand more or less rapidly. Their expansion is restricted in the posterior pars plana, where they remain small and do not coalesce. In the anterior pars plana, on the other hand, large vesicles may develop, which may spread as far as the linea serrata and the striae ciliares. The marked tendency of the cysts to expand within the anterior pars plana may be due to various causes. Perhaps the connections of the two epithelial laminae may loosen more easily in the finely meshed zone of Müller's reticulum than in the coarsely meshed zone. Secondly, the formation of large vesicles might be facilitated by the vitreous-free space above the anterior pars plana. Finally, it is also conceivable that zonular traction is involved in the expansion, if not in the genesis, of the cysts.

In the evaluation of their **clinical significance,** we may agree with Grignolo [98] and Rutnin [170] that there is no connection between pars-plana cysts and any pathological changes in the eye, at least where *senile* cysts are concerned. However, cysts connected temporally and topographically with inflammatory processes have been observed in *adolescents* [50]. They have also been observed in a case with a general malformation of the ciliary body and a pathological permeability for fluorescein [48].

What is the **prognosis?** The possibility of pars-plana cysts producing ocular complications is the clinician's main concern. Can pars-plana cysts cause a *retinal detachment?* This possibility might be anticipated as a consequence of a posterior extension of a ciliary epithelium detachment, since in both processes there is a separation of the two retinal laminae. However, clinical experience demonstrates the contrary: in their statistics, Schepens *et al.* [182] could find no relation between retinal detachment and pars-plana cysts. So far, no cases have been reported in which pars-plana cysts have developed into a retinal detachment by mere expansion.

Despite Adam's histological findings [1], the ora serrata evidently forms an insurmountable barrier preventing the expansion of a detachment of the ciliary epithelium. This is paradoxical, since in the opposite direction the barrier is less effective; it can only temporarily halt the anterior expansion of a retinal detachment and does not prevent the coalescence of a retinal detachment with pre-existing pars-plana cysts, as described by Grignolo [98].

There is, however, another mechanism by which pars-plana cysts can induce retinal detachments. Goldmann [91] reported the development of a giant tear at the ora serrata (Fig. 105) in the area of coalescence of large pars-plana cysts. The tear "secondarily" caused the retinal detachment.

In the light of present knowledge, *senile* pars-plana cysts are obviously harmless and require no treatment. On the other hand, cysts in *adolescents* are more serious. Their genesis must be investigated. In case of bilateral cysts, paraproteinemia is to be suspected, whereas unilateral cysts may be related to a local disease process. Follow-up may reveal large epithelial detachments which could lead to complications.

2.2. The Detachment of the Pars Plana

As opposed to the detachment of the ciliary epithelium, a *choroidal detachment* also involving the ciliary body is termed "detachment of the pars plana" (Fig. 60b). It occurs most frequently after surgical or traumatic perforations of the eye, sometimes after a blunt trauma, and occasionally without any apparent cause (uveal effusion) [55, 124, 146, 168, 185].

In a detachment of the pars plana, the lens becomes displaced anteriorly; the pars plana itself is displaced towards the optical axis. As a result, viewing conditions for minute structures in the pars plana are excellent, even without indentation.

The **differential diagnosis** of a retinal detachment presents no problems when viewed in the optical section, since the prominent choroid is clearly visible. The exclusion of a choroidal tumour is more difficult. If, in retro-illumination, a reddish glow is visible behind the choroid, a retrochoroidal effusion is suspected. However, even then the possibility of a tumour cannot be excluded, as effusions may be a concomitant sign of tumours. Diaphanoscopy is of considerable help [186]; even the finest local shading can be detected if this technique is used in combination with a contact glass (Fig. 12c).

3. The Vitreous in the Periphery of the Fundus

3.1. Definition of the Vitreous Base

The sections of the vitreous in the most extreme periphery of the fundus are part of the vitreous base [179]. This is the portion of the vitreous that is strongly connected to the inner retinal lamina. The area in which corresponding anatomical connections are developed forms the *anatomical vitreous base*. This is not identical with the *functional base*, the zone in which the vitreous cannot be detached from the retina by applied force.

The form of the **functional base** is determined not only by the nature of the anatomical vitreoretinal connections but also by the strength, direction, and movement of *tractional forces*. The border of the *anatomical* base may assume various shapes with anterior and posterior prolongations corresponding to the meridional division of the ora serrata region. The border of the *functional* base, on the other hand, usually is rectilinear, since the detached hyaloid membranes form rectilinear folds between the respective points of anatomical fixation.

Clinically, only the *functional base* is significant. Its boundary is situated where the vitreous body detached, i.e. anteriorly at the *insertion of the anterior hyaloid membrane* and posteriorly at the *insertion of the posterior hyaloid membrane* (Fig. 62). The overall extension of the functional vitreous base varies in different eyes. The factors determining the individual dimensions, the variations of the anterior and posterior hyaloid membranes, will be described below.

3.2. The Anterior Hyaloid Membrane

The most anterior section of the anterior hyaloid membrane can be examined without a contact glass by having the patient gaze in an extreme direction.

The head is usually held at an angle of 60–70 degrees towards the floor. As opposed to contact-glass examination, stronger magnification is obtained via *microzonuloscopy*, as described by Rosen [159–167]. The main advantage is the possibility of observing vitreous phenomena during eye movements. Unfortunately, with this method it is possible to examine only the inferior area, approximately 160–180 degrees.

In its most *usual formation* the anterior hyaloid membrane closely approximates the bordering structures (Fig. 63). It extends from the lens beyond the ciliary processes to the middle of the pars plana. There are, however, numerous situations in which the hyaloid membrane is separated in specific sectors from the adjacent structures and undulates freely.

In its *most anterior section* the anterior hyaloid membrane is seen to undulate during forced accommodation in all eyes [8, 166]. In the case of constitutional variations, though, it undulates even in accommodative paresis, i.e. in cycloplegia. This is usually connected with destruction of the vitreous framework, particularly in cases of high myopia.

Slezak described two variations as "retrozonular" and "anterior ciliary" vitreous detachment [190, 191], in analogy to posterior vitreous detachment. The term "detachment", however, implies former attachment of the vitreous. This is not the case in the constitutional variations with undulating hyaloid membrane. The concept "detachment" should be reserved for cases of secondary (i.e. inflammatory or traumatic) detachment.

When floating, the anterior hyaloid membrane leaves its insertion at the posterior border of the lens centripetally, thereafter curving back towards the ciliary body. It meets the ciliary body either at the posterior end of the processes, i.e. *near the ligamentum coronarium*, or near the *white midline*, at *accessory lines* or at the *ora serrata* (Fig. 63). This anterior hyaloid flotation is probably caused by the partial absence of the normal connecting systems.

The **connecting systems** are normally invisible, since the anterior hyaloid membrane is too close to the adjacent tissues. The connecting fibres become visible only when stretched, i.e. when the anterior hyaloid is semi-detached. This is the case with a floating anterior hyaloid membrane. The position of the *ligamentum hyaloideocapsulare* can only be determined if the anterior hyaloid membrane leaves the lens at a large angle (Fig. 65). Normally, this circular insertion line is 1–2 mm distant from the edge of the lens [228, 224]. If the anterior hyaloid membrane is not floating, this line is visible only when pathological deposits (blood, pigment) have collected there, in the hyalocapsular sinus [173, 160].

The same is true of the *zonula fibres* which insert at the anterior hyaloid membrane [164]. They, too, are visible only when the membrane floats. They are found either singly or in groups, producing peaked extensions of the anterior hyaloid membrane (Fig. 65). In the *aphakic eye* they may be observed as an entire circular corona of fibres tautening the anterior hyaloid membrane (Fig. 64). The individual fibres are singly and regularly spaced, not in groups like the fibres inserting at the lens. Where the fibres are deficient the anterior hyaloid membrane is no longer under tension, allowing mushroom-like protrusion into the anterior chamber.

The *ligamentum coronarium* and its connections are usually difficult to evaluate (Fig. 92). Only in exceptional circumstances is the greyish fibrous band above the posterior third of the ciliary processes visible i.e. with an anterior displacement of the lens. Coarser fibres branch off it and disappear from sight into the ciliary valleys.

The anterior hyaloid membrane then passes freely to the *white midline*, where it finally comes into contact with the pars plana. The biomicroscopic aspect of the white midline stems from a combination of the fibrous condensations of the ligamentum medianum with the fine folds of the hyaloid membrane (Figs. 38, 39).

A whitish band present above the posterior ciliary body has been described by several authors [179, 180, 169]. It is not clear from the many descriptions whether this is a silhouette reflex or the white midline. Generally, with indirect ophthalmoscopy only the silhouette reflexes are visible; the white midline is visible only with the high magnification of the slit-lamp microscope.

The *ligamentum medianum* appears as a fine greyish band in both wide and narrow slit beam. Connecting fibres branch off it to the ciliary epithelium. However, they cannot be detected biomicroscopically in the normal eye, since a dense mass of fibres appears there, among which only the coarse, parallel clusters of the epiciliary zonular lamina can be identified (Fig. 37). The connecting fibres can be seen distinctly only in a partial detachment of the ligamentum medianum (Fig. 119), in which case rather coarse fibrous strands appear at fairly wide intervals. Probably there are also finer, more densely packed fibres in between, for particles from the previtreal space are retained there, accumulating in lines of blood or exudates (epiciliary hyphema or hypopyon) (Fig. 67).

In the case of *traumatic* detachments of the anterior hyaloid membrane, the greyish ligamentum medianum remains in its proper position upon the detached anterior hyaloid membrane (Fig. 107). On the other hand, it is absent in the *constitutional* floating anterior hyaloid membrane. Upon the ciliary epithelium, the insertion of the ligamentum medianum is not characterized by any morphological peculiarities. Only exceptionally are there any proliferations of the ciliary epithelium (Fig. 66).

From the vitreous space, the membranules of the *tractus medianus* approach the white midline. Traction of the membranules and counter-traction of the ligamentum medianum are probably responsible for the formation of fine circular folds upon the anterior hyaloid membrane at the white midline (Figs. 37, 38).

The examination of the vitreous boundary *between the white midline and the ora serrata* is difficult, as mentioned above. Nevertheless, in optical section a continuation of the anterior hyaloid membrane is usually visible, extending along the pars plana towards the ora serrata (Fig. 37).

These biomicroscopic observations disagree with anatomical reports suggesting that there is a zonular fissure (Salzmann) but no true anterior hyaloid membrane above the posterior pars plana [172]. The contradiction may be explained by optical phenomena. The anterior vitreous cortex, so narrow and so dense in its anterior sections as to suggest a membrane, becomes looser posteriorly while its layers retain their direction towards the ora serrata. Viewed biomicroscopically from a very narrow angle of acceptance it nevertheless may appear quite bright owing to the apparent decrease in transparency (see p. 4).

Observations made in aphakic eyes, where the posterior pars plana is visible without indentation, strengthen this view. An "anterior hyaloid membrane" above the posterior pars plana cannot be seen here unless the angle of acceptance is reduced by kinetic indentation.

But also in cases of a floating anterior hyaloid membrane inserting at the ora serrata no zonular fissure is seen. Here a constitutional anomaly must be presumed, i.e. an abnormal configuration of the anterior vitreous cortex.

The insertion of the anterior hyaloid membrane at the *ora serrata* cannot easily be evaluated, owing to the bright light reflected by the retina. No case of insertion *posterior* to the ora serrata has been reported so far.

3.3. The Posterior Hyaloid Membrane

As long as the vitreous is attached to the retina, the posterior hyaloid membrane is not visible. Histological studies suggest it may not exist prior to posterior vitreous detachment [103, 238]. At any rate it becomes evident, histologically or biomicroscopically, only after the vitreous is detached.

In fact, there is no real "vitreous detachment", since the separation does not occur between the retina and the vitreous. It is the *fibrillar part of the internal limiting membrane* that becomes split; consequently, a very thin fibrillar layer always remains upon the retina [78]. The other part covers the detached vitreous and is called the *posterior hyaloid membrane*. Its traction determines the extent and the form of the posterior vitreous base. The traction varies according to the type of posterior vitreous detachment.

Vitreous detachment, of course, is a well-known clinical entity [154, 155], the biomicroscopic aspects of which have been described exhaustively by both Hruby [110] and Goldmann [87, 89, 90, 61]. Numerous classifications have been suggested for its various forms. It is probably most practical to divide them into rhegmatogenous and arrhegmatogenous forms, according to the nature of the volume transfer from the vitreal into the retrovitreal space [52].

In **rhegmatogenous detachment** there is a hole in the posterior hyaloid membrane through which the destroyed, liquefied vitreous can pass abruptly into the newly formed retrovitreal space (Fig. 69). Large quantities can flow quickly through the hole. The *rapidity* of this process promotes complications: *disruption of vitreoretinal adhesions* and, if the latter remain intact, of *parts of the retina*. The hole through which the passage occurs is nearly always the prefoveal hole. Hence, this hole always being in the same position, rhegmatogenous vitreous detachments practically all have the same configuration, with a characteristic biomicroscopic appearance. The main mass of vitreous substance rests in the inferior half of the eyeball

45

Table 5. Forms of vitreous detachment

Posterior vitreous detachment	Rhegmatogenous detachment	Arrhegmatogenous detachment
Occurrence	Vitreous destruction and liquefaction	Concomitant sign of pathologic condition of adjoining tissues
		Vitreous shrinkage
Mode of volume transfer	Through a hole in the posterior hyaloid membrane	Through an "intact" posterior hyaloid membrane
Morphological aspect:		
General configuration	Typical	Atypical
Course of the tractus vitreales	Stretched towards the hole in the posterior hyaloid membrane	Normally curved, occasionally slightly deformed in direction of traction
Posterior hyaloid membrane	Loose, plicated	Taut, with occasional tractional folds
Holes in posterior hyaloid membrane	Cause of the detachment	If present, formed by secondary processes
Prefoveal and prepapillary holes	At typical position; initially vertical, later horizontal	Moved to atypical positions, deformed by traction
Course of the vitreous detachment	Rapid and sudden	Slow and steady
Complications:		
Traction	Rapid and irregular	Slow and steady
Effect of traction on − vitreoretinal adhesions	Vitreous ripped off from the retina	Vitreous peeled off even at points of strong vitreoretinal adhesions
	Tearing of the retina	Formation of retinal folds
− posterior hyaloid membrane	Remains intact as a relatively thick membrane	Is split into several lamellae
Type of induced retinal detachment	Rhegmatogenous	Arrhegmatogenous

(Fig. 68). The *course of the vitreal tracts* is altered since they run, as in all perforations of the vitreous body (Fig. 35b), straight towards the hole in the cortex. Frequently, the tracts are seen indistinctly, owing to marked destruction of the vitreous framework. If, however, they are impregnated by blood cells, their course may be followed easily.

In an **arrhegmatogenous posterior vitreous detachment,** volume transfer is effected through the "intact" posterior hyaloid membrane. Complex physical and chemical processes are at work here, the detailed nature of which is unknown. The process is slow. It may be confined to small isolated sections or it may eventually develop into a complete detachment (Fig. 70). The *vitreoretinal connections* dissolve slowly. Where the vitreous remains adherent, the retina is drawn into folds rather than torn. The *posterior hyaloid membrane* may split into several lamellae, the evaluation of the vitreous boundaries thus becoming extremely difficult. The *vitreal tracts* maintain their typical shape—at least in those parts of the vitreous which are not affected by shrinkage—owing to the fact that the vitreous body is not perforated and has remained intact. The clinical picture *varies* according to the extent and the location of the detachment, depending also on the concomitant processes.

The posterior detachment of the vitreous is a very *important clinical condition,* since the retina is no longer protected by the broad, stable vitreous cortex shielding it from the vigorous movements of the central vitreous. The main **complications,** however, derive from the fact that there is now vitreous traction directly affecting the retina. It is only after posterior vitreous detachment that a dense "membrane" is formed, inserting *at the retina itself.* Prior to vitreous detachment, no membranules are inserted there, since all the normal vitreal tracts reach the inner wall of the globe *anterior* to the ora serrata (Fig. 28) in a region protected against tractional forces by retroretinal adhesion. After vitreous detachment, the traction of the posterior hyaloid membrane works on the retina, i.e. above the retroretinal interstice, leading to the numerous and well-known complications [111–113, 214].

As regards **prognosis,** it is important to determine precisely whether vitreous detachment is complete, since no further complications are to be expected once the detachment process has come to a standstill. No further tearing is likely and if no retinal lesions have been produced by the detachment the patient may be dismissed from observation.

A *rhegmatogenous* vitreous detachment may be considered completed when the "vitreous bag" is emptied as much as possible, the posterior hyaloid membrane falling down *perpendicularly* from its insertion onto the gap (the prefoveal hole of the membrane), the main mass of the vitreous having settled in the lower half of the globe (Fig. 68). The *prepapillary* and the *prefoveal holes* are now lying horizontally (and are quite difficult to recognize). The *posterior hyaloid membrane* is finely plicated and has no tractional folds. The *insertion line* is rectilinear and equidistant from the ora serrata.

Conversely, in an *arrhegmatogenous* vitreous detachment the process may continue indefinitely, so that it is impossible to determine when it is complete. The *slow* and *continuous* traction in case of vitreous shrinkage will detach the posterior hyaloid membrane even from very strong adhesions that do not usually come apart, e.g. the ora serrata. On the other hand, if the adhesions remain, the retina will be drawn into *folds* instead of being torn. Since the arrhegmatogenous detachment may never be completed, the possibility of further complications cannot be excluded. The patient should be checked regularly. Fortunately, any ensuing retinal detachment will expand *slowly,* being of the arrhegmatogenous, tractional type, so that the patient need not be followed too frequently.

The intervals between checks will be determined rather by the evolution of the underlying process (uveitis, diabetic retinopathy etc.) than by the appearance of the arrhegmatogenous vitreous detachment.

For the prognosis, the *examination of the insertion line* of the posterior hyaloid membrane provides valuable information. It is mainly here that retinal lesions caused by the vitreous detachment will be detected. It is here, also, that the signs indicating further complications in case of a progredient detachment have to be sought. In fact, an *irregular course* of the insertion line is caused by vitreoretinal adhesions which exist wherever it is extended posteriorly. Consequently, there is an irregular distribution of traction forces. Thus tractional folds of the posterior hyaloid membrane are a common finding at such posterior extensions of the insertion. Tearing of the retina eventually may occur there, so that the patient must be followed up. Conversely, with a *rectilinear course* traction is evenly distributed along the insertion line and no further tearing of the retina is likely to occur.

There is another reason why the examination of the insertion of the posterior hyaloid membrane is important in clinical practice: it offers a further possibility for *diagnosing* a posterior vitreous detachment. This diagnosis is, as is wellknown, often not easy, the posterior hyaloid membrane being very fine and scarcely recognizable. Thus other signs have to be sought, for instance, the presence of a prepapillar opacity or a prefoveal hole. An additional sign is the presence of the insertion of *a membrane posterior to the ora serrata*. As mentioned above, all normal vitreous tracts are inserted either at the ora (tractus praeretinalis) or anterior to it. Thus, a membrane inserted behind the ora serrata is to be interpreted as the posterior hyaloid membrane (if there are no retinal lesions, such as scars or degenerations, showing vitreal condensations around cortex holes).

In children, if posterior vitreous detachment is complete, the insertion line of the posterior hyaloid membrane is situated as far anteriorly as the ora serrata; later, it comes to lie farther posteriorly, corresponding to the posterior expansion of the vitreous base with advancing age.

3.4. The Extent of the Vitreous Base

The biomicroscopic examination of the insertion lines of the anterior and posterior hyaloid membranes reveals an extremely variable extent of the functional vitreous base. Its maximum width, in analogy to histological findings, comprises a zone between 1–2 mm anterior and 2–3 mm posterior to the ora serrata (Fig. 62). The boundaries may vary according to the strength of the effective forces. In the individual case the insertion of the hyaloid membranes may be situated anywhere within the anatomical vitreous base. At the ora serrata, however, the cohesions are so firm that they cannot be disrupted by the forces usually effective within the eye. The boundary formed by the ora serrata is therefore never crossed by an anterior or posterior detachment. It is only in severely pathologic states, i.e. under very extreme tractional forces, that the vitreous becomes detached from this particular adherence. The ora serrata accordingly represents the *"absolute"* vitreous base.

The **connecting systems** differ fundamentally anterior and posterior to the ora serrata. *Anterior to the ora serrata* the anterior hyaloid membrane is fixed by means of well-defined fibre systems which are already present in the fetus [32]. They are arranged in belts so that only a few specific types of detachment can possibly occur in this area (Fig. 63).

No such specific structures can be detected *posterior to the ora serrata;* rather, there seem to be a multitude of diffusely dispersed, connective spots, comparable to a Velcro band, whose opening depends on the degree of traction exerted. This kind of connection might possibly be caused by collagenous fibrous proliferations, the so-called "spider-like bodies" [32], which, emerging from the vitreous, run into the retina and branch off into the middle layers. They are absent in adolescents, increase in number with advancing age and ultimately form broad areas which extend from the ora serrata in the direction of the equator, with an irregular posterior delimitation.

3.5. The Vitreal Structures within the Vitreous Base

The epiretinal layer of the vitreous posterior to the ora serrata, i.e. the **vitreous cortex,** appears almost "optically empty" in the normal eye. The finely flecked, almost homogeneous pattern seen in autopsy eyes is seldom visible in the living eye (see p. 24). Coarse opacifications are only seen near vitreoretinal scars or degenerations.

The first distinct membranular structure appears at the ora serrata, where the **preretinal tract** is inserted. This tract, which is separated from the retina by the homogeneous vitreous cortex, may consist of several lamellae converging on the ora serrata and inserting there together (Figs. 38, 64). Details of the insertion are difficult to evaluate owing to the reflected retinal light, yet may be seen quite easily in a densely-pigmented negroid fundus (Fig. 39). With the wide beam, the lamellae appear as finely folded, plicata-like, thin membranules, or as a fluffy, loose, fibrous material. In the optical section, the preretinal tract forms a wedge pointing towards the ora serrata, sometimes displaying in its middle portion a structure similar to the lamellar separation in cataracts [85, 87].

The preretinal tract may be so narrow and membranoid that it cannot be distinguished from the posterior hyaloid membrane. Differentiation is then possible only by the determination of the points of insertion. A membrane inserted at the retina *posterior* to the ora serrata cannot be the preretinal tract, but rather is the posterior hyaloid membrane.

The preretinal tract is present in the entire circumference of all normal eyes. It remains also in cases of senile or myopic vitreous destruction, even when the centre of the vitreous is devoid of any distinct normal structures. Only in cases of asteroid hyalitis and other severe vitreous anomalies, such as hereditary vitreoretinopathies, will the preretinal tract sometimes be unrecognizable.

Anterior to the preretinal tract, almost parallel to it, the finer lamellae of the **other tractus vitreales** reach the ciliary body (Figs. 28, 37). These tracts are narrower, barely apparent in the wide slit beam and visible only in optical section as fine lines which disappear towards the centre of the eye. They are extremely mobile, but with the eye steadied by means of the contact glass, they may nevertheless be examined easily. The *tractus medianus* and the *tractus coronarius* are inserted on the anterior hyaloid membrane, at the white midline, and above the posterior third of the ciliary processes, respectively.

3.6. The Previtreal Space

The space between the anterior hyaloid membrane and the ciliary body may be subdivided into different compartments which have been classified in various ways, reflecting the respective author's approach [37, 25]. In biomicroscopy, a subdivision of this space is not practical, and therefore the entire space is termed "previtreal space" (Fig. 20). It is bounded exteriorly by the ciliary epithelium, anteriorly by the posterior (ciliocapsular) zonula leaf, interiorly by the anterior hyaloid membrane and posteriorly by the anterior edge of the anatomical vitreous base (at the linea serrata). It encompasses the epiciliary zonular layer, the connections of the anterior hyaloid membrane to the ciliary body, as well as optically empty spaces which become visible only when the anterior hyaloid membrane floats.

It is doubtful whether the space is closed off by a membrane anteriorly, i.e. towards the posterior chamber. At any rate, no *morphological demarcation* is detectable in the normal eye.

In aphakic eyes, however, a very thin membrane is sometimes visible (Fig. 65); it is stretched out between those zonula fibres which connect the anterior hyaloid membrane with the ciliary body. It might be termed, as it were, the "*posterior limiting membrane of the posterior zonula leaf*". The membrane is extremely fine and not very refractile. The fact that it is not a border surface between two media is suggested by the clearly definable "holes" which may appear in it. It is seldom observed since the ideal viewing conditions are rarely fulfilled.

It can only be identified when isolated, i.e. when the anteriorly situated zonula leaf is absent (in the aphakic eye) and when the hyaloid membrane is detached from it. Besides, it is seldom visible in the whole circumference because of numerous holes. The insertion of this membrane at the ciliary body is not recognizable because a fluffy, fibrous net covers the ciliary valleys there, thus obstructing the view. In histological examinations this membrane has not been observed. Examination of freshly enucleated eyes has suggested the presence of such a membrane [9], but the methods employed do not rule out artefacts.

In any case, from a practical point of view only the question of a *functional boundary* is of interest. Is there a barrier preventing the passage of certain substances at the anterior boundary of the previtreal space? There seems to be no such boundary for pigment and for dandruff-like flakes in pseudo-exfoliation of the lens, as these substances are deposited in both the previtreal space and the posterior chamber [173]. This, however, does not prove that there is free circulation, or rule out a barrier, as nothing is known about the origin of the deposits. On the other hand, observations made in aphakic eyes support a demarcation. Blood residues are occasionally detected in the previtreal space of aphakic eyes that are sharply delineated anteriorly, i.e. in the area of the "limiting zonular membrane" described above. These hemorrhagic deposits may persist for a long time after blood residues elsewhere have been resorbed. A functional barrier was actually detected by means of fluorescein dye injection [48] in a patient with a slight deformation of the ciliary body.

Another important question regards the presence of a functional boundary of the previtreal space interiorly, i.e. towards the vitreous. Many clinical as well as histological observations in cases of inflammation or haemorrhage indicate an effective barrier at the anterior hyaloid membrane.

The *posterior border* of the previtreal space extends along the linea serrata. Hyphema-like sediments are therefore scalloped, in contrast to those at the ligamentum medianum. Whether the deposits appear at the linea serrata or at the ligamentum medianum probably depends in each case upon the size of the particles, or on the density of the fibrous net which connects the ligamentum medianum with the ciliary epithelium.

4. The Transitional Zone of the Ora Serrata

4.1. Transitional Structures

At the ora serrata there is a boundary, not only between the retina and the ciliary epithelium but also in the other tissue layers. The *pigment epithelium* exhibits an abrupt increase in pigmentation. In the *vitreous* there is a separation between the cortex and the looser central vitreous, formed by the preretinal tract. Thus, we find several **morphological boundaries,** important as points of orientation during an examination. True, they do not always coincide precisely, e.g. the pigment epithelium boundary may be slightly posterior to the retinal ora serrata. This is of little practical importance and, if pathological changes obscure one of the boundaries, the remaining ones may be used to locate the ora serrata.

In addition, the ora serrata is also a **functional boundary**, where the strength of adherence between superposed tissue layers changes. The *retroretinal interstice* ends here and the firmly connected zone (i.e. the *retroretinal adhesion*) between the ciliary epithelium and the pigment epithelium begins. Furthermore, the absolute vitreous base is situated here, where the vitreous always remains attached even in the case of a detachment. These functional boundaries are of clinical importance because they confine pathological processes and can halt them temporarily. The functional boundaries in the different layers probably do not exactly coincide either, which may explain certain differences in the clinical picture of processes dependent on these boundaries. *Clinically*, the ora serrata is to be considered, not as a boundary-line between the ciliary epithelium and the retina alone, but as a *transitional zone affecting all layers*. However, in biomicroscopic examination the *retinal* ora serrata boundary is by far the most striking of all and therefore usually chosen for reference.

The ora serrata being also a transitional zone of developmental differentiation, there are numerous individual **variations of shapes** and, in fact, no one ora is similar to the other. There is however a certain regularity in so far as the developmental variants are related to the meridional segments of the linea serrata. Apart from the characteristic serrations, there are many very fine transitional form variants. Biomicroscopic examination provides no information regarding their histological nature. Findings in autopsy eyes, however, provide means of interpreting the biomicroscopic findings [32, 67, 69, 141, 202–205, 209, 215, 217]. A classification for the purpose of biomicroscopy will, however, always involve a certain simplification which, though it meets practical needs, will not satisfy the pathologist.

The variations of the ora serrata are due to a variable *intermingling of adjacent tissues*. The resulting tissue formations are already partially present in the embryonic stage. Examiners of both living and autopsy eyes [32] agree that the frequency of these variations apparently does not increase with advancing age. However, their appearance changes because of secondary tissue transformations during growth and ageing. The course of the ora serrata is generally bilaterally symmetrical. Particularly striking form variants, including many bizarre formations, are found predominantly in the horizontal meridian. The anatomical relation of these variations to the cristae ciliares, as well as their agglomeration near the horizontal ciliary vascular raphe, suggest a developmental connection with the vessels. There is no correlation with any pathological condition, refraction, or length of the globe. Neither is there an explanation for the predominance of the male sex in certain forms, as mentioned by some authors [202–204].

The transitional variations at the ora serrata may be attributed to two different developmental processes. On the one hand, they are formed by an *irregular course of intact ora serrata boundary*, i.e. of the three layers when unchanged in their mutual relationship: pigment epithelium, retina, and vitreous cortex. On the other hand, variants are due to *ectopia of the tissues*, whereby portions of one layer are displaced into extraneous zones.

The **irregularities of the border course** lead to serrations and bays characteristic of the human ora serrata. Some of the bays may be cut off from the ora serrata, thus forming enclosed ora bays or pars-plana islands within the retina [205]. The typical pars-plana structure is preserved in them, their edges having the characteristics of the ora serrata borders (see p. 55).

The **ectopies** are caused by the displacement of either retinal tissue onto the pars plana or ciliary epithelium onto the retina. These ectopies may include the adjacent structures connected with them; thus, the retina takes the vitreous along with it, and the ciliary epithelium takes the zonular fibres. Other ectopies seem to consist of the adherent tissues, i.e. vitreous and zonula, alone.

4.1.1. Retinal Ectopies above the Pars Plana

Retinal ectopies may be difficult to differentiate from an anterior extension of the intact ora serrata boundary. In both formations *ora teeth* may result. In an ora serrata extension, however, normal cystoid spaces with a regular distribution of pillars are anticipated, whereas in retinal ectopies irregularly arranged microcysts and glial proliferations occur. Besides, an ora tooth consisting of a retinal ectopy is not connected with its whole surface to the pigment epithelium, but only with a narrow zone at a crista ciliaris. At either side of the crista, this type of ora tooth forms a pterygium-like cover suspended above the pars plana. It has no direct contact with the pigment epithelium but is separated from it by a hollow space and by the ciliary epithelium. At the bottom of a defect which might occur in one of these "side wings" (Fig. 71o), intact pars plana is exposed and not pigment epithelium. Other retinal ectopies form isolated ora teeth, i.e. "islands" of retinal tissue upon the pars plana (Fig. 71f) having lost contact with the retinal edge.

4.1.2. Ectopies of Ciliary Epithelium

Ectopic ciliary epithelium [75] may be apposed both on the retinal surface posterior to the ora serrata, as well as on retinal ectopies anterior to it. The ectopies either occur as apposed epiretinal ridges and patches, or they have become detached, partially or completely, from the surface.

In *infancy* they form single-layered accretions, consisting of cubocylindrical epithelium of the unpigmented ciliary epithelium type, in different degrees of differentiation (Fig. 75a). When detached, they are frequently tube- or rosette-shaped and arranged around a central cavity [215, 217]. *In the course of time*, glia proliferations and vesicles develop under the epiretinal ectopies, the latter being covered by the characteristic epithelial cap [32] (Fig. 75b). Typically, the normal vitreoretinal boundary is interrupted here and vitreous fibres may penetrate into the interior of the vesicular tufts, intermingling there with the glial fibres. Zonular attachment is observed on some of the protrusions of ciliary epithelium [67], which might indicate that the ectopies originated from the anterior pars plana. No such zonular attachment will be expected in ectopies from the posterior pars plana, since there the ciliary epithelium is connected to the vitreous.

The various shapes of ciliary epithelial ectopies have been described as meridional folds, granular tissue, zonular traction tufts, rosettes, clubs, pyramids, pillars, etc. [170]. Classification on a morphological basis alone is not satisfactory, for the shape is obviously fortuitous, depending on the traction and the firmness of the tissues. From the clinical point of view, it is practical to classify the ectopies of the ciliary epithelium according to the *changes they cause within the vitreous body*.

Thus, a group of relatively *coarse changes* may be distinguished from *micro-variations*. The coarser changes are characteristically arranged at the meridional axis of ora serrations or bays. They are so large as to deform the vitreous cortex. Their appearance varies according to their position and extent. Secondary changes, such as pigment infiltration, effects of traction or atrophy, produce a great variety of forms. For the purpose of biomicroscopic description, the coarse ectopies as a whole are classified as *meridional ridges*. The micro-variations, on the other hand, are so minute as to produce no changes in the vitreous cortex that are detectable with the slit-lamp microscope.

4.1.3. Ectopies of Vitreous and Zonula Fibres

In histological studies vitreous strands departing from the anterior hyaloid membrane towards the ciliary body on the one hand, and zonular fibres entering the vitreous on the other hand, have been described [32]. They may be interpreted as a special kind of vitreal or zonular ectopies. It cannot be excluded, however, that such ectopies are in fact connected to epithelial ectopies which, not being in the same plane, are not visible in the histological section or might have atrophied altogether. Biomicroscopically, such minute translucent structures will anyhow not be visible.

The anterior extensions of the "intact ora serrata" and the ectopies create a multitude of variations whose biomicroscopic appearance will be described in greater detail in the following paragraphs.

4.2. The Form of the Retinal Edge

The sharp ora serrata boundary is formed by the abrupt transition of the relatively thick retina into the single-layered ciliary epithelium. The step thus formed can best be evaluated in the optical section. Its form changes in the course of the individual's lifetime. In a child, the step is still rounded, gradually growing taller and more sharp-cornered, and, if marginal cysts develop, even protruding (Fig. 59). In the aged, the internal (vitreal) surface is drawn anteriorly by fine, peaked proliferations of glial tissue, the so-called "spiculae of the ora serrata" (Daicker [32]), which form a fringe at the retinal border (Fig. 57).

4.3. The Course of the Boundary Line

The **ora serrations** differ in size and shape [135, 209, 218, 226]. All variations, from an almost straight ora serrata to processes which reach the pars plicata, can be found

Table 6. Shape of the ora serrata in biomicroscopic examinations

Age	4–20	21–40	41–60	>60
Number of patients (eyes)	26 (44)	35 (52)	27 (49)	25 (45)
Smooth edged ora serrata without teeth	3 (6)	3 (7)	4 (8)	2 (3)
Ora with teeth	23 (38)	32 (45)	23 (41)	23 (42)
Interrupted ora teeth	0	4 (6)	1 (2)	0
Teeth infiltrated with pigment	7 (12)	4 (5)	10 (17)	8 (14)
Drusen in ora teeth	8 (10)	8 (9)	5 (8)	2 (3)

in the same eye (Figs. 71, 78). There are numerous, sometimes bizarre deviations from the simple dentate form: branched processes, extremely broad processes caused by coalescence, processes cut off the ora serrata, rudiments floating freely in the vitreous, etc.

Some dentate processes are avascular, others contain vessels. In short teeth, the *vessels* may either extend from the retina into the process and then branch off there, or they may border one edge, turn round at the tip, and, recurrently, branch off into the equatorial retina. Long dentate processes often contain one single vessel which is sometimes difficult to distinguish from reddish-brown pigment proliferations.

Other processes may be covered with *pigment*. They are difficult to detect, owing to the poor contrast offered by the dark pars plana. These processes form irregular, deep brown ridges, often containing gleaming crystalline particles. The smallest "crystals" are barely recognizable, the largest are broader than the whole ora tooth (Fig. 83). Histologically, the crystals are layered *drusen* and have no clinical significance [34, 131].

Bays between the serrations vary in width and depth. *Abnormally deep bays* may extend far posteriorly. Such extremely deep bays are not immediately apparent in a rapid examination with the contact glass, the comparison with neighbouring bays being difficult with the small visual field. Thus, extremely deep ora bays are discovered with a contact glass only if they are diligently searched for.

In general, the serrations are most pronounced nasally; temporally, the ora serrata is only slightly scalloped or smooth-edged, with only occasional serrations. The abnormal dentate processes and extremely deep bays are found most frequently in the horizontal meridian.

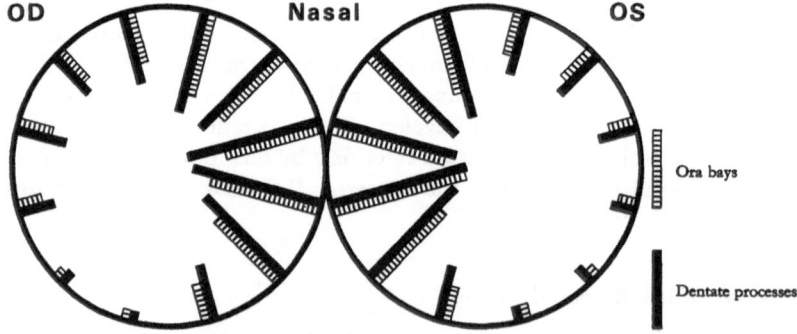

Diagram I. The meridional incidence of dentate processes and ora bays in 200 adult human eyes. (After Straatsma *et al.* [209])

The various forms of the ora serrata are primarily of theoretical importance in connection with developmental processes. However, knowledge of these is also important in clinical practice, since forms occur which are easily confused with retinal holes.

Pseudo-holes result either from the *coalescence of processes* into rings (Fig. 71 n) or by *defects in the "side wings"* of abnormally broad processes (Fig. 71 o). They can be easily distinguished from true retinal holes because of their *location anterior to the ora serrata*.

Other pseudo-holes are formed by the isolation of deep bays (Fig. 71 i and k). These *enclosed ora bays* are situated *posterior* to the ora serrata. They differ from retinal holes in the colour and the structure of the *bottom* of the hole, which is actually normal pars plana tissue (Fig. 72). The bottom of the hole, consequently, appears brown and not red, as opposed to retinal holes. The bottom surface is granular, not smooth as in retinal holes. Issuing from this granular structure, lines of traction are sometimes found, which are produced, as demonstrated histologically, by the insertion of zonula fibres [32]. The *borders* of the enclosed ora bays are, in fact, ora serrata borders. Thus, the preretinal tract is inserted around the borders of these "pars-plana islands" (Fig. 73).

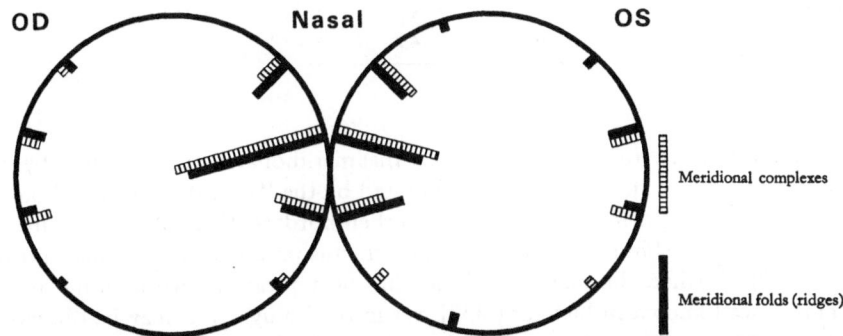

Diagram II. The meridional incidence of meridional ridges and meridional complexes in 400 adult human eyes. (After Spencer *et al.* [204])

4.4. Meridional Ridges ("Folds")

Meridional ridges are usually described in the literature under the name meridional folds [172, 182, 169]. Contrary to our policy not to change generally accepted terms, we prefer the designation meridional ridges here, in order to permit a differentiation from genuine folds.

Meridional ridges are oblong *retinal protuberances* with their longer axis running in a meridional direction (Fig. 76). They are usually situated at dentate processes (Fig. 77) or, less frequently, in the centre of bays (Fig. 78). They may extend posteriorly some millimetres beyond the ora serrata into the pre-equatorial retina and anteriorly, forming abnormally long dentate processes as far as the corona ciliaris. The ridges have an irregularly nodulated surface and consist of transparent or whitish tissue with small, densely juxtaposed cavities (Fig. 77). At first glance, they appear to be mere protrusions of a cystoid retina, but more careful examination reveals, not supporting pillars, but clearly circumscribed vesicles.

Table 7. Meridional ridges in biomicroscopic examinations

Age	4–20	21–40	41–60	>60
Number of patients (eyes)	26 (44)	25 (52)	27 (49)	25 (45)
Number of patients (eyes) with meridional ridges	9 (13)	15 (23)	12 (21)	13 (24)
Meridional ridges				
– situated at ora teeth	8 (12)	11 (16)	8 (15)	7 (13)
– situated at ora bays	5 (8)	7 (10)	8 (13)	3 (5)
– with partial thickness defects of the retina	3 (5)	6 (7)	8 (14)	7 (12)
– interrupted by normal retina	2 (3)	6 (10)	6 (9)	6 (11)
Rudimentary meridional ridges	14 (21)	16 (24)	15 (27)	19 (34)
Vessels passing over the meridional ridge	0	0	0	1 (2)
Vessels passing underneath	4 (6)	2 (4)	3 (5)	2 (4)

Meridional ridges and meridional complexes
in autopsy eyes (after Spencer *et al.* [203])

	Number	Meridional ridges	Meridional complexes
Patients	200	51	31
Eyes	400	79	49

The **relation to the vitreous** indicates that meridional ridges are formed by ectopies of pre-ora tissue. In fact, they are delineated by the "vitreal ora serrata boundary", since the tractus praeretinalis is inserted at their borders (Fig. 76). Where a meridional ridge extends behind the ora serrata, the tractus praeretinalis also turns posteriorly (Fig. 80). Further, the meridional ridge has no typical internal limiting membrane. This is well known in histology [32], yet in the living eye it may be observed only in a posterior vitreous detachment by a defect in the posterior hyaloid membrane, corresponding to the ridge (Fig. 81).

Such observations are exceptional, since only in the case of vitreous shrinkage will a detachment extend so far anteriorly as to sever even the vitreoretinal connections at the margins of a meridional ridge which, being an "ora serrata border", is part of the absolute vitreous base.

A pre-ora origin is also indicated by the insertion of zonula fibres upon the ridges which, however, are scarcely visible biomicroscopically on account of the reflected retinal light.

There are different **vascular patterns** of meridional ridge vessels. The vessels either pierce a ridge or pass over it. When running *through*, the exiting vascular branches are either visibly a continuation of the entering vessels (Fig. 77a), or they have no direct connection at all; calibre and direction do not coincide so that other hidden drainage channels must be suspected (Fig. 77b). Daicker [31] has actually detected *chorioretinal anastomoses* under such meridional ridges. In case of vessels running *over* a ridge, the presence of a true retinal fold may justly be discussed (Fig. 78).

Meridional ridges may also show other forms than those described above; they may be partially or completely *detached* from the retina (Fig. 76). In a semi-detached ridge usually the posterior end is raised and drawn anteriorly. Zonular fibres inserted there may be visible in kinetic indentation against a dark background. The under-lying retina is often attenuated, and occasionally even full-thickness defects may occur (Fig. 79) [67]. The complete detachments may occur in the middle of the ridges, thereby interrupting them, or at the posterior edge, or they may even in some cases involve the whole ridge (Fig. 76). A floating "operculum" is thus formed which has no corresponding retinal defect.

Small patches of protrusions of the retinal surface are interpreted as **rudimentary meridional ridges**, provided their diameter corresponds approximately to the width of ordinary meridional ridges. They may be differentiated from protrusions of other origin by the characteristics of meridional ridges, i. e. by their *location at the meridional axis of ora teeth or bays* and by their *connection to recessions of the preretinal tract*. The course of adjoining vessels may sometimes suggest Daicker's chorioretinal anastomoses (Fig. 76 c).

Spencer *et al.* [203] described a special type of meridional ridge on the basis of their autopsy examinations, calling them **meridional complexes**. These meridional ridges are exceptionally long, extending anteriorly, not into ciliary valleys as is usual, but onto ciliary processes which, too, are outstandingly large. An oval attenuation of the retina is usually situated somewhat posteriorly to them. Meridional complexes are found more frequently in the horizontal meridian. A meridional complex is not easy to differentiate *biomicroscopically* from a simple meridional ridge, because its connection to a ciliary process—the most indicative differential diagnostic sign available—is difficult to recognize. Occasionally, though, the abnormally prominent ciliary process may be seen in the iridolenticular space.

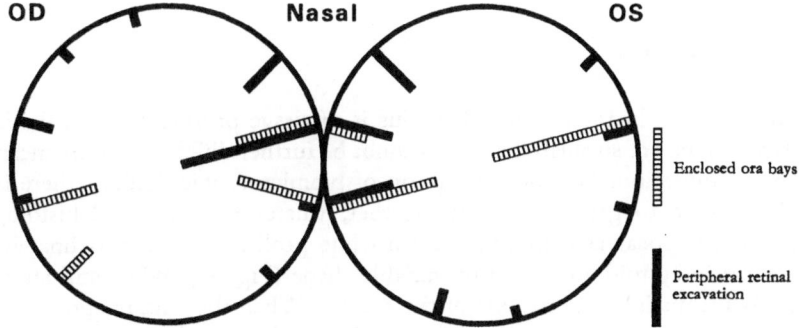

Diagram III. The meridional incidence of enclosed ora bays and localized retinal attenuations (peripheral retinal excavations) in 400 adult human eyes. (After Spencer *et al.* [204])

From the clinical point of view, it is important to know whether meridional ridges lead to any **complications**. Are patients with meridional ridges more likely to develop a retinal detachment? Schepens [177] believes that no predisposition to a retinal detachment derives from meridional ridges, even if there is a small full-thickness defect behind them. This may seem surprising at first, since vitreous conden-sations are inserted at the borders of meridional ridges. It confirms, however, general clinical experience, viz. that the traction of *intravitreal* densifications does not induce retinal detachment. In fact, long-term observations of meridional ridges lead to the conclusion that, as long as the vitreous is still attached to the retina, there is no danger of a detachment. The situation, however, is different in the case of a *posterior vitreous detachment* when the retina may tear posterior to meridional ridges, as in all places of vitreoretinal adhesions (Fig. 76f). The relative infrequency of horse-shoe tears immediately posterior to meridional ridges may be attributed to the fact that a posterior vitreous detachment seldom extends so far anteriorly, viz. into the region of the posterior border of meridional ridges.

In conclusion, meridional ridges are not dangerous, so that prophylactic coagulation is unnecessary.

Differential diagnosis of similar-looking lesions which are capable of inducing retinal detachment is therefore important. Meridional ridges are easily confused with horseshoe tears of the retina. Even the "normal" adherent meridional ridges may resemble elevated opercula since they appear in the contact-glass mirror as white cystic, tongue-like protrusions with vitreous strands inserting at their edges. When kinetic indentation is employed, differential diagnosis presents no problems in such cases (Fig. 78). Evaluation is more difficult, however, in the case of a semi-detached meridional ridge with a full-thickness defect beneath its posterior end, which may look exactly like a horseshoe tear at the posterior edge of the vitreous base (Fig. 79). The examination of the *vitreous* will provide the clue for differential diagnosis: At the edge of a *meridional ridge* the *preretinal tract* is inserted, and intravitreal fibres similar in appearance to zonula fibres adhere to the end of the detached ridge (Fig. 76d). In the case of a true horseshoe tear (Fig. 76f), on the other hand, the posterior border of the hole is usually free of vitreous structures, and the *posterior hyaloid membrane* inserts at the semi-detached operculum.

4.5. Micro-Adhesions

A common finding in the peripheral fundus is of tissue proliferations at the inner retinal layer which are so small that they cannot be further differentiated by means of slit-lamp magnification. For the description of biomicroscopic findings there is no other choice than to group them all together, whatever their actual histological structure. They appear as compact, greyish-white proliferations approximately the size of pillars in cystoid areas, and of variable shape (Fig. 82). While still attached, they merely form slight protrusions of the surface. When they occur upon the pars plana they appear as very fine, greyish elevations, whereas on the retina they are scarcely visible, because of the reflected light on the one hand, and because they do not offer a sufficient contrast in the irregular pattern of cystoid spaces on the other hand. They are therefore seen best in silhouette. Many of these micro-adhesions are elongated—evidently owing to traction—forming pillars or clubs. Others float within the vitreous, forming minute round "opercula" anterior or posterior to the ora serrata. Usually no related defect of the inner retinal layer can be detected. Since at their peaks these small proliferations are *characteristically adherent to vitreous strands,* they are termed *micro-adhesions.*

The **connection to the vitreous** occurs in two forms. In the first a taut, tense, relatively *coarse fibre* (resembling a zonula fibre) is inserted at the micro-adhesion. If the latter is elongated it becomes inclined anteriorly. In a floating intravitreal micro-adhesion, the fibre does not remain taut but becomes twisted like a corkscrew, suggesting previous traction. Such "*zonular*" *micro-adhesions* are usually seen in the most anterior sections of the retina, even anterior to the ora serrata. In the second form, a *fine, loose fibre* is inserted, leaving the retinal surface perpendicularly and bending posteriorly at the border of the vitreous cortex. Such *"vitreal" micro-adhesions* are usually found somewhat posterior to the ora serrata. When elongated, they are inclined posteriorly. A clearcut difference may exist between the two forms. However, a definite evaluation is not always possible, so that the division into "zonular" and "vitreal" micro-adhesions is of limited importance clinically.

Micro-adhesions are found throughout the entire circumference, but predominantly nasally. There is no relation to the meridional segmentation nor to dentate processes or bays. They are extremely frequent, being observed in all eyes, including children's, if viewing conditions permit. Because of the difficulties involved in recording, it cannot be ascertained whether they become more numerous with advancing age.

The biomicroscopic aspect provides no information regarding the **histological nature** of micro-adhesions. The fact that they are situated in a narrow zone both anterior and posterior to the ora serrata indicates ectopic tissue. In fact, there are histological reports concerning smaller ectopies of the ciliary epithelium in exactly the same localization and with the same forms as micro-adhesions [217]. They describe flat deposits, elongated cones, and freely floating flocculi (rosettes). Probably at least the *"zonular" micro-adhesions* are ectopies of the ciliary epithelium.

Clinically it is important to know whether micro-adhesions may lead to complications. Can the traction of this variety of vitreoretinal adhesion possibly detach the retina? Are holes following the tearing of micro-adhesions dangerous? General experience rules out this possibility, at least where phakic eyes are concerned. In aphakic eyes, however, there is a special form of retinal detachment [39, 176]. Very small holes in the ora serrata region seem to be responsible for the genesis of this detachment, for the retina attaches again as soon as the micro-holes have been closed surgically. These very small holes might be related to micro-adhesions. Why an aphakic eye should differ in this respect from a phakic one remains unanswered so far.

Should such microlesions be *coagulated prophylactically?* This is in fact seldom necessary as shown by the frequency of lesions and the rarity of complications. However, in suspicious cases it is advisable to check occasionally the natural course of events. Only the future will show whether during systematic follow-ups of aphakic eyes special symptoms will be discovered which can lead to a more exact prognosis.

There is another question of practical relevance. Can micro-holes *complicate the healing process* of a retinal detachment which was caused by other factors? As they form a connection to the retro-retinal space, which remains open even after the causal retinal tear has been closed, we are justified in asking whether they may prevent the re-attachment of the retina. Our experience shows this to be rare, probably because the intact vitreous cortex above such defects prevents the passage of liquefied vitreous into the retro-retinal interstice. As there might be cases, though, where peripheral micro-defects could endanger the success of an operation, it seems advisable to include the small holes in the operation plan, especially where it is doubtful whether the covering vitreous cortex is intact.

V. The Pathology of the Peripheral Fundus

1. Intravitreal Changes Accompanying the Spreading
of Pathological Processes into the Vitreous Space

In diseases of the inner retinal layers and of the retinal vessels, pathologic exudations infiltrate the vitreous. Responding to gravity, these exudates float or settle inferiorly. If the content of the vitreous cavity was entirely *fluid*, the particles would accumulate at the bottom with a strictly horizontal surface. This happens, indeed, in the free *retrovitreal space* following a posterior vitreous detachment. *Within the vitreous body* however, sedimentation is obstructed by the meshes of the *vitreous framework*. Knowledge of the general arrangement of the vitreous framework will provide clues for the location of such pathological sediments. Infiltrating substances originating from pathological changes at *cortex holes* seem to penetrate more easily than exudates derived from locations covered by a dense vitreous cortex.

This is exemplified by products from the posterior pole (through the prefoveal and prepapillary holes) as well as those from the large vessels (through the prevascular fissures).

Soluble material, such as soluble proteins, creates Tyndall's phenomenon. When this reaches a certain intensity, the zones of discontinuity disappear, since the difference in indices of refraction is reduced and the reflection of light in the previously transparent space now equals that of the vitreous structures. The tractus vitreales and minute floating particles may thus become invisible, so that the entire space appears in part or in toto homogeneously blurred by the intensity of Tyndall's phenomenon. As the soluble substances are resorbed, the zones of discontinuity become visible again. Therefore, paradoxically, the "increase" of circumscribed opacifications in the vitreous may signify an improvement in the condition.

If the proteins are of high specific gravity, they sink downwards with the vitreous proper floating above them. This causes the well-known ascension of the vitreous structures **(ascension phenomenon)** [19] in diffuse inflammatory processes (Figs. 84, 85). The tractus vitreales change their course and, instead of sinking behind the lens, they ascend immediately and pass upward through the superior half of the vitreous cavity to the papilla. Even without a contact glass this can be seen behind the lens, as the tractus hyaloideus now runs inversely to the normal pattern (Fig. 86). The inferior plicata rises steeply, the superior plicata turns upward shortly beyond its insertion at the lens. Examination with a contact glass shows the remaining tractus vitreales also affected [50] for the tractus coronarius and the tractus medianus also run straight upwards from their inferior insertion. The tractus vitreales return to their original position as the pathological process improves. Knowledge of the "ascension phenomenon" is important in practice because it provides information concerning activity in diffuse inflammatory processes which have no other morphological guidelines, such as exudates or scars. The fact that the "ascension phenomenon" is actually caused by the subsidence of heavier, soluble products has been established in autopsy eyes [52].

Insoluble protein particles and cells are usually unable to pass through the denser vitreous structures. At first, they are intercepted by the cortex and remain in the vicinity of the places of entry. It is only after they have penetrated the cortex that they sink downwards into the central vitreous. As the tractus vitreales are impermeable to blood cells, these must follow the course of the respective vitreous layers [52]. Thus the well-known onion-peel arrangement of sediments is produced (Fig. 87). Further their distribution is uneven within each tract, reflecting the meridional segmentation of the tractus vitreales. As the latter are funnel-shaped, the particles, wherever their point of entry, always accumulate at the same place, the *lowest point* of the funnel. Particles *between the preretinal tract* and the *tractus medianus* may travel as far as the inner surface of the globe and be deposited upon the pars plana between the ora serrata and the white midline (Figs. 88, 96). Theoretically, particles in the inner tractus vitreales—*between the tractus medianus* and the *tractus hyaloideus*—might reach the anterior hyaloid membrane, but this seldom happens since sedimentation occurs at the lowest part of the tracts, which lies farther posteriorly. The particles thus do not reach the most anterior region of the tracts, where re-ascension begins. The sediments therefore float in the ora serrata region, in superposed layers within the vitreous. Anteriorly, their delimitation is relatively sharp; posteriorly, the number of particles decreases gradually.

The most posterior line of sedimentation is the insertion of the *preretinal* tract. The particles do not migrate into the vitreous cortex. If particles are found behind the ora serrata in close proximity to the retina, they have either entered the vitreous at this point, or there is a retrovitreal space into which they have sedimented (Fig. 100). Preretinal hyphema-like or hypopyon-like deposits in the lower periphery are indicative of a posterior vitreous detachment.

In *children* there is a different pattern of sedimentation which corresponds, as demonstrated by biomicroscopic examinations, exactly to expectations based on the different pattern of vitreous framework [54]. With the lack of vitreal tracts, the sediments accumulate within fissures of the "radial fibres", forming oblong sacs that hang perpendicularly into the vitreous space (Fig. 87b). Mixed forms of sedimentation occur in *adolescents*, where there are vitreal tracts only in the anterior vitreous while the posterior vitreous retains its infantile radial pattern.

The nature of the particles and the degree of vitreous destruction determine the velocity of migration. *Inflammatory exudates* generally migrate rapidly, since they can alter the structure of the interceptive layers, and thus may accumulate in rather large clouds (Fig. 97). *Erythrocytes* usually move more slowly—at least if the vitreous is intact—often becoming decolorized before reaching the ora serrata. They closely follow the tractus vitreales in thin parallel layers. They are usually resorbed slowly and may be found years after the haemorrhagic infiltration as white clouds of a very characteristic arrangement. On the other hand, in a degenerated vitreous they migrate more rapidly and are resorbed more quickly.

Atypically arranged deposits, deviating from the pattern described, are indicative of changes in the vitreous structure, such as in *perforations of the vitreous*. The typical picture of the tractus vitreales disappears with the prolapse of vitreous substance through a hole (Fig. 34b) either into the retrovitreal space (through the prefoveal hole) as in the case of a posterior rhegmatogenous vitreous detachment, or through the coats of the eye, as in traumatic perforations. New vitreous strands become visible, converging to the point of perforation (Fig. 116). The clinically important sign of the "arrow head" indicating the hole in the vitreous is formed in this way. Responding to gravity, intravitreal particles become deposited in the plications of these newly formed perforation tracts illustrating by their very pattern of sedimentation the course of the tracts which otherwise for optical reasons may often be difficult to follow.

Similar "arrow heads" may be produced experimentally by piercing an unfixed vitreous specimen with a needle. Strands then appear converging to the point of the needle. Compression of the vitreous obviously causes a decrease of the distance between the submicroscopic vitreous fibrils in some directions. Not only does this change the optical density, but it also changes the size of the meshes and hence their permeability for particles.

Another atypical pattern of sedimentation is found in severe *vitreous destruction,* after which there are no vitreal tracts left. Instead, there are cavities containing liquefied vitreous at the bottom of which the particles accumulate.

Is this **movement of the particles** influenced by gravity alone, or must we assume a fluid current within the vitreous? While in rabbits a fluid current has indeed been demonstrated [102] (although in the opposite direction, i.e. from the periphery to the nerve head), in primates or in humans this has not so far been possible [12]. Clinical observation indicates that *gravity* evidently plays the main part in the migration. At any rate, in reclining patients the particles are deposited elsewhere, according to gravity. If a patient's head stays horizontal for a long period, as in a state of unconsciousness, the corpuscles are found in the posterior, not in the anterior, parts of the tractus vitreales. In patients with subdural haematoma of the optic nerve, for instance, the intravitreal haemorrhages are arranged in a funnel which is sharply delimited at the border of the papilla and fringed towards the periphery ("daisy"). The same happens in unconscious patients with septic dissemination, where the inflammatory exudates are also deposited at the posterior insertion of the tractus vitreales.

The fact that the space in the *lower periphery* of the fundus represents a **collecting basin** for all pathological sediments in the vitreous is of great clinical importance. If intravitreal infiltration is suspected, this is the area where the most striking signs are to be looked for, especially if only a few particles have penetrated. Moreover, the progression of a pathological process can best be evaluated here. There are cases where the morphological appearance of the causative lesion changes very little, so that signs of deterioration or healing are not perceptible; or else, the lesions themselves can scarcely be detected because of vitreal opacifications. In all such situations, the examination of the "collecting basin" in the lower periphery, which Goldmann [92] aptly compared to *Douglas' pouch* in the peritoneum, can yield valuable information. If the process deteriorates, the sediments increase; with the onset of healing, they decrease. This information is especially important when therapy with strong side-effects has to be used, which evidently ought to be discontinued as soon as possible. An increase of sediments in the collecting basin will quickly reveal whether the discontinuation of therapy has reactivated the pathological process, so that medication can be guided with precision.

2. Inflammations in the Peripheral Fundus

Inflammatory changes were already noticed by the first examiners of the peripheral fundus. In 1950, in one of his first reports on the methods of indentation ophthalmoscopy, Schepens [175] described patients with extensive inflammatory exudates. Subsequent examiners described the inflammation of the periphery as a new disease, calling it *peripheral uveitis, posterior cyclitis*, or *pars planitis*. Their descriptions, however, show that the disease is extraordinarily *polymorphic* with regard to morphological appearance, severity of the condition as well as its progression, and the nature and frequency of complications [14–17, 104–106, 121, 122, 137, 138, 189, 232].

Whereas only coarser changes are detectable ophthalmoscopically, slit-lamp examination reveals the microscopic minutiae. In addition, with the help of focal illumination in the optical section, it is possible to delineate opacifications precisely and to find their exact position within the different compartments.

Biomicroscopic examinations have led to the conclusion that exudates in the peripheral fundus are not a symptom complex and a disease in themselves [50], but a sign of *three different inflammatory processes* (Fig. 89):

(1) a concomitant sign of an *anterior* uveitis,
(2) a sign of inflammation in the *pars plana itself*, i.e. a true posterior cyclitis,
(3) a concomitant sign of a *posterior* inflammation.

A more exact description of these three basic forms of peripheral exudates and of the criteria for differentiation follows.

2.1. Concomitant Signs of Anterior Uveitis

Both the anterior and the posterior sections of the ciliary body are usually involved in iridocyclitis. This is well known from examinations of autopsy eyes, but it is difficult to detect in the living eye as the posterior ciliary body is usually not visible, owing to synechiae and exudation into the anterior chamber. In *mild cases*, however, the pars plana can be examined. The inflammatory changes present are similar to those in the anterior sections.

The anatomic structures of the pars plana become indistinct (Fig. 91). Precipitates are detected which are similar in type to those found between the zonula fibres and in the anterior chamber. They are scattered about the entire circumference of the pars plana, collecting in a denser belt at the white midline or at the ora serrata (Fig. 90). These inflammatory manifestations of anterior uveitis are situated *outside* the vitreous proper, i.e. anteriorly to the anterior hyaloid membrane, *within the previtreal space*. The latter may expand in the course of the inflammation owing to the ascension of the anterior hyaloid membrane in the lower periphery, together with the general ascension of the tractus vitreales.

A "restitutio ad integrum", at least biomicroscopically, may follow healing of iridocyclitis. The pars plana then resumes its normal granular and striated structure, the precipitates disappear, and the anterior hyaloid membrane returns to its normal position. In some cases, stronger reflecting areas, producing a "pseudo-white with pressure" phenomenon (see p. 36), may remain as the only residues of inflammation.

2.2. Inflammations of the Ciliary Body Localized in the Pars Plana

One of the most important issues involving "peripheral uveitis" has been: Is there a special type of inflammation that could be called "pars planitis"? Do the inflammatory phenomena of the pars plana really reveal special characteristics? There are, in fact, many anatomical peculiarities which might support such a hypothesis. There being no chorio-capillaris, typical choroiditis cannot occur. There being no retinal vessels, direct penetration of substances into the vitreous is impossible. On the other hand, as the uvea is covered by only two single-layered epithelia, indirect penetration of inflammatory cells from the uvea might be facilitated. The most significant feature however, is probably the presence of interlaminar connective tissue, containing vessels cut off from the surroundings by the two laminae of Bruch's membrane. This might, indeed, promote chronic, latent inflammation.

In practice, however, it is impossible to establish any specific syndrome precisely related to the special anatomical features. Too many concomitant signs make evaluation difficult. For lack of better criteria there are only two kinds of inflammation distinguishable in the pars plana area as in the other uveal sections: the *diffuse* and the *focal*.

2.2.1. Diffuse Inflammations

In diffuse cyclitis, there are only slight morphological signs, as would be expected. There is a moderate haze in the peripheral vitreous and the pars plana appears blurred (owing to the vitreous haze or swelling of tissues). Since there are no distinct morphological signs, the diagnosis is based on pathological permeability after intravenous *injection of fluorescein* [40]. The posterior ciliary body does not stain, being covered entirely by pigment epithelium, but there is a belt-shaped fluorescent zone above the pars plana in the late phase, situated in either the *vitreous* or the *previtreal space*. The staining of the *ciliary body* becomes visible only at the ciliary body band in the chamber angle, owing to the lack of a pigmented cover there.

While in slight, diffuse inflammation morphological signs are insufficient for the diagnosis of a pars plana involvement, in *chronic*, smouldering cases intensive *scarring* may occur. In some cases, however, the pars plicata of the ciliary body may remain free of scarring (Fig. 93), which seems paradoxical in a diffuse process; yet this may be explained by the fact that in the pars plicata exudates enter the previtreal space, from where they can be removed by the fluid current of the aqueous. In the posterior pars plana, however, they may be trapped within the dense framework of the vitreous base.

Diffuse inflammation, naturally, is in most cases not limited to the posterior ciliary body alone. Anterior chamber activity, nearly always present, is a proof of the involvement of the *anterior* segment. Concomitant cystoid macular oedema, slight oedema of the nerve head and splintered retinal reflexes suggest involvement of the *posterior* part of the eye. Cells, Tyndall's phenomenon, and frequently the ascension phenomenon of the tractus vitreales are observed in the *vitreous*.

2.2.2. Focal Inflammations

Circumscribed foci of the pars plana—despite their different anatomical substratum—do not differ morphologically from chorioretinitic foci.

Nevertheless, differences were observed following intravenous injection of fluorescein, as the exudative foci stained already in the early phase. However, there have been too few such observations to date to permit a definite interpretation.

Granulomatous foci on the pars plana may appear in the *entire circumference* and do *not* prefer any particular meridian. Initially, they are a dull grey, not clearly outlined, and slightly prominent (Figs. 92, 94). Atrophic pigmented scars remain after healing is complete and are occasionally covered over in the course of time by a normal-looking pigment epithelium. They may be very hard to detect later on, and can usually be seen only when their localization was previously known.

In the case of very abundant exudation, infiltration of the vitreous base as well as of the previtreal space may obscure the view of the pars plana foci so that differentiation from other forms of peripheral exudation may become difficult (Fig. 95). A first approach to *differential diagnosis* between true *pars planitis* and *sedimentation of intravitreal exudates* is based on the location of the exudates, sediments occurring exclusively in the lower periphery. Later on during the healing stage, differentiation is easier, as the position of the scars indicates the origin of the exudates: scars from *peripheral chorioretinitis* are posterior, those from a "*pars planitis*" anterior to the ora serrata.

In case of very pronounced inflammation a *cyclitic membrane* may result, which leads to a total amotio retinae and to phthisis. *Vessels from the ciliary body* may penetrate this cyclitic membrane.

In fact, it is only the *focal inflammations within the pars plana* that can be taken as an independent clinical picture. Terms like "peripheral uveitis", "posterior cyclitis", "pars planitis", etc. should be reserved for *this* type of inflammation only.

2.3. Peripheral Exudates Connected with an Inflammation of the Posterior Sections of the Fundus

Exudates penetrating the vitreous descend along the vitreal tracts, as described in chapter V/1. They then accumulate and form exudative sediments in the lower vitreous base, covering the region of the ora serrata (Fig. 87). In contrast to the two groups discussed previously, such sediments are always *within* the vitreous body, i.e. *behind* the anterior hyaloid membrane. The ciliary body and the previtreal space, as may easily be ascertained by an examination through the iridolenticular space, remain free of any inflammatory signs (Fig. 97). Localization in the *lower circumference* is characteristic of exudative sediments.

In case of **acute inflammations,** usually a morphological restitutio ad integrum follows, at least within slit-lamp microscopic dimensions. There remain no sequelae of the former infiltration of the lower vitreous base.

In case of **chronic inflammations**, which may persist for a long time, *secondary reactive processes* may surround the exudative sediments. Thus, scarred residues remain after healing. They affect primarily the cortical vitreous and the inner retinal layer, leading to *fibrous condensation of the vitreous base* and to diffuse thickening of the marginal retina (Fig. 98). Cicatrization may be widespread, with the formation of *cysts* or even large intraretinal cavities, sometimes filled with a yellowish material of unknown origin. *Newly formed vessels* may cover the surface, forming a "rete mirabile", or may even penetrate the vitreoretinal scar (Fig. 99). They originate from retinal vessels, in contrast to the vessels of cyclitic membranes which derive from the ciliary body. *Holes* may develop in the altered retina, leading eventually to retinal detachment [17]. The latter, usually caused by vitreous shrinkage, spreads slowly, with the result that pigmented demarcation lines are formed at its borders.

All this cicatrization initially affects only the *inner* retinal layers and the *vitreous*. Reaction in the external layers is not usually seen until later and is probably not the result of the initial inflammation but of the secondary cicatricial processes. This type of cicatrization characteristically respects anatomical borders for beneath the vitreous condensations the pars plana appears free (Fig. 102).

If the *vitreous* is *detached*, the picture changes: the exudates can now collect in the retrovitreal space. If there is only *slight* exudation, accumulation occurs at the posterior border of the vitreous base, forming a clearly defined, *preretinal hypopyon* (Fig. 100). In case of *abundant* exudation, the *entire retrovitreal space* is filled with opaque material obscuring the fundus (Fig. 101). Only the periphery of the retina within the vitreous base and the ciliary body remain visible.

In *chronic and recurrent inflammations* both types of sedimentation occur. At the beginning, while the vitreous is still attached, exudates penetrate it, collecting in its lower periphery, as described above. When, in the course of the inflammation, the vitreous becomes detached, the exudates now enter the retrovitreal space forming a hypopyon. Vitreal scarring and shrinkage may further complicate the picture (Fig. 102). Details can then only be correctly interpreted if the course of the inflammation has been followed from the onset.

There are *other views* [193] about the *connection between peripheral exudates* and *inflammations of the posterior parts* of the eye. The peripheral exudates are considered to originate in the ciliary body as a reaction to the inflammation of the posterior segment and to migrate through the vitreous from the periphery towards the focus of inflammation. Such a reaction, in fact, is well known in the case of *endophthalmitis* with a vitreous abscess, where massive infiltration into the vitreous from the adjacent structures (especially from the ciliary body) occurs. In the living eye such endophthalmitic reactions can seldom be followed, as observation is impeded by the violence of the widespread inflammatory exudation. Occasionally, however, cases do occur where the course takes a milder form under antibiotic treatment. The picture of endophthalmitis then differs clearly from that of the exudative sediments described above. In the case of a vitreous abscess, the *ciliary processes* are affected and are strongly vascularized, oedematous and adherent to the anterior hyaloid membrane. Clouds of cells penetrate into the vitreous from the ciliary processes. They form lines of exudates converging upon the causative intravitreal focus. In the healing stage, the ciliary processes remain for a long time covered by mutton-fat exudates which are in contact with the vitreous. When healing is complete, fibrous synechiae between the ciliary processes and the anterior hyaloid membrane remain. *Cyclitic reactions* therefore involve the ciliary body, not only in the pars plana, but also in the pars plicata. Consequently, this form of inflammation must be classified with the second group, which comprises the inflammations of the ciliary body itself. Conversely, in cases with *exudative sediments*, the ciliary body is unaffected, even with most violent inflammatory processes. This fact—as may be remembered—is easily confirmed by examination through the iridolenticular space (via contact glass or microzonuloscopy) (Fig. 97), which is possible as long as the anterior parts of the uvea are not inflamed.

The **source of such peripheral sediments** within the vitreous space are *all inflammations which have penetrated through the vitreous cortex*. Deposits may develop rapidly in focal chorioretinitis, especially if the foci are adjacent to holes in the vitreous cortex. In case of a *central chorioretinitis* with a focus near the macula, single cells arranged in layers along the inferior preretinal tract can be seen as early as a few days after, frequently even on the very day of entry into the vitreous (Fig. 96). Large sediments may form rapidly in more violent exudations. The exudates in the periphery disappear during healing, usually *prior* to those directly overlying the causative focus. The first signs of healing may be observed, therefore, in the inferior ora serrata region.

In *peripheral chorioretinitis* the exudates at first remain near the foci for a long time, since there the vitreous cortex is dense and rather broad. In disseminated peripheral chorioretinitis the exudates may cover the entire periphery of the retina, giving an initial impression of "posterior cyclitis" (though thorough examination will then show the pars plana to be free). It is only after a certain lapse of time that the exudates will reach the central vitreous layers and then sink downwards. Exudates are therefore more or less evenly distributed in the peripheral fundus at the *onset*, whereas later on they are concentrated mainly in the lower half of the globe.

The *relation between focus and sedimented exudates* is easily recognizable in **acute focal inflammations**. In **diffuse, chronic processes** this is much more difficult, since the peripheral accumulations of exudates may be the only striking sign. Despite the usually slight exudation in such chronic processes, these deposits may be quite extensive as a result of the long duration. It is usually only after careful searching that the *sources of these deposits* are found. There is often only very slight vascular inflammation, recognizable by a fine, greyish, ill-defined sheathing around the peripheral vessels [198]. In other cases, however, the vascular signs are completely lacking, and only diffuse retinal oedema (recognizable by splintered reflexes, cystic macular oedema, and slight oedema of the papilla) may suggest a diffuse inflammatory process. Vascular involvement may then only be demonstrable by fluorescein angiography. The appearance of the causative inflammation may change little in the subsequent course of the disease. *Improvement or deterioration of the condition can be evaluated only by the increase or decrease of the peripheral sediments.*

Finally, there is a **particularly mild form of inflammation** where the source of the peripheral deposits may *not be detected at all*. Sediments in the lower periphery are the *only* pathological finding. There is no external ocular irritation in such very mild cases. Symptoms are hardly noticed, since the larger vitreous opacities are situated outside the patient's visual field. Therefore changes in the inferior vitreous periphery are usually discovered accidentally during routine examination (Fig. 98). Subsequently, a smouldering inflammation with recurrent exacerbations may be observed, the content of cells and the form of the larger exudates changing constantly. However, no other inflammatory signs are to be found which might reveal the origin of this chronic basal "vitreitis".

Understandably enough, this picture has frequently been described as true "pars planitis" [137] and, since no inflammatory foci were detectable as their source, there was no reason to consider such peripheral exudates as sediments. Yet there are three definite criteria which prove that the exudates are not independent foci within the pars plana: the fact that (1) they are found exclusively in the lower periphery, (2) that they are purely intravitreal, and (3) that the pars plana is free of any inflammatory signs.

Some histological cases reported as "pars planitis" [138], when evaluated under these three criteria, have to be interpreted as exudative sediments of this type of mild peripheral inflammation.

That such a clinical picture may actually be caused by exudative sediments deriving from inflammation in the posterior fundus can be proved clinically only in the rare cases where the process has been observed from the onset. This was described in two pediatric cases [50]; one child (aged 10) initially had periphlebitis, the other (aged 8) had a broad, flat and only slightly infiltrative chorioiditic focus (Fig. 102). The inflammatory foci later disappeared completely in both children without leaving any visible scars. However, the exudative sediments, which had steadily increased during the first phase of inflammation, did not disappear. Instead, a permanent peripheral inflammatory process persisted for years, causing occasional, rather severe recurrences.

From these observations it may be concluded that such chronic mild "peripheral" inflammations are caused initially by a chorioiditis or angiitis in the posterior parts of the fundus. The initiating process may heal completely leaving no trace, whereas the exudates may persist and induce permanent inflammation, sui generis.

According to Goldmann (personal communication) such exudates may possibly contain displaced antigenic material which, separated from the general blood circulation, may independently produce a chronic inflammation.

Frequently, this form of inflammation occurs in children [106, 117, 233]. *Therapy* has little effect, but such mild inflammations may heal spontaneously after a lapse of many years [106]. The scars left in the inferior periphery are often found fortuitously during a routine eye examination in patients unaware of any previous eye disease. However, the scars may be a source of future complications, since vitreous traction and retinal holes in this area can lead to detachment of the retina [17].

2.4. Mixed Forms

The three clinical pictures described above, viz. the involvement of the pars plana in inflammations of the anterior and posterior sections, and diseases of the pars plana itself, are not always distinct from one another. The inflammatory process is often not confined to one circumscribed and restricted area only (Fig. 99), but usually involves many internal parts of the eye. The inflammatory signs may, however, be more pronounced in one particular section of the eye. This is specifically so in cases of *inflammation of the pars plana ("pars planitis")* where signs of involvement of the anterior and posterior uvea are nearly always observed [223].

Excessive and violent exudation may mask the clinical picture, since it does not respect the limits of the vitreous base. The causative process can then only be determined by the *localization of the scars* after healing is complete.

A routine histological examination of diseased eyes seldom yields information about the clinical pictures described here. In most of the usual (i.e. horizontal) sections, the connections in question have been destroyed. In addition, exudative sediments remain in their original position only if great care is taken during the fixation process to maintain the normal position of the eye.

In conclusion, peripheral exudates are not representative of any *one* particular disease classified under the term of peripheral uveitis, pars planitis, etc. Rather, there are three different types of exudates each of which is caused by an inflammation of a specific section of the eye. The interrelation of cause and effect therefore may be precisely inverse to the concept of "peripheral uveitis" generally established to date. Most of the peripheral exudates *do not induce* inflammations in other parts of the eye but on the contrary are the *result* of such inflammations.

Knowledge of the various causes of peripheral exudates is not only of theoretical, but also of practical importance, as it permits one to judge the state of inflammatory processes and to direct therapy accordingly.

3. Amotio Retinae

3.1. The Expansion of Retinal Detachment to the Ciliary Body

Retinal detachment usually arises in the region of the equator and spreads posteriorly and anteriorly. The separation of the retinal lamina from the pigment epithelium is usually halted at the ora serrata, where retroretinal adhesion begins. On occasion, especially in chronic conditions, retinal detachment may spread further anteriorly, leading to *detachment of the ciliary epithelium* [36].

This spreading beyond the ora is not difficult to diagnose *at the onset*, since all structures of the ora serrata area (cystoid spaces, marginal cysts, the transition of the retina into the ciliary epithelium, and the granular and striated structures of the latter, as well as the serrations) are clearly recognizable in the detached lamina. *In the late stages*, however, the gradual transition of retinal detachment into the ciliary body becomes more difficult to evaluate, since the inner layer has become atrophic and indistinct in its structure. The ora serrata is then barely recognizable in this hyaline membrane and may appear merely as an abrupt change in the thickness of the lamina. *Differentiation* between this condition and a *prebasal ora serrata tear* may be difficult, especially if in the latter case the anterior hyaloid membrane is densified (Fig. 104). Differential diagnosis is based on an examination of the *external layer* which, in cases of expanding retinal detachment, is the single-layered pigment epithelium; there is therefore no change in its thickness at the ora serrata, although the colour changes from red to brown. On the other hand, differentiation from a *schisis retinae* presents no difficulty, as a schisis cannot possibly extend beyond the ora serrata.

The diagnosis of an expanding retinal detachment may be made even without scleral indentation thanks to the displacement of the retina and of the ciliary epithelium towards the optical axis. Indentation is indispensable, however, for examination of the outer layer in the differential diagnosis of a prebasal ora tear (Fig. 104).

3.2. Changes in the Peripheral Fundus as a Cause of Retinal Detachment

In our present state of knowledge two varieties of retinal detachment are distinguished, arrhegmatogenous and rhegmatogenous.

In the **arrhegmatogenous form** the retinal lamina is intact. There are no holes to cause its onset (though they may arise secondarily through atrophy). Therefore, fluid cannot pass directly through a retinal defect from the vitreous into the retroretinal space. At present, it is not known how the retroretinal fluid is produced. Causes of arrhegmatogenous retinal detachments are, for example, traction caused by shrinkage of the inner surface of the retina (e. g. proliferative diabetic retinopathy) or exudation of fluid into the retroretinal interstice (e. g. in the case of inflammation or a tumour). An arrhegmatogenous retinal detachment may begin *anywhere* in the fundus. The problems connected with this form of detachment are not confined to the periphery of the fundus only and will therefore not be discussed here any further.

On the other hand, in the **rhegmatogenous form** of retinal detachment, changes in the peripheral fundus play an important part. At present, two factors are charged with the genesis of detachment: (1) a retinal defect which allows the free passage of fluid from the vitreous into the retroretinal space, (2) traction upon the retina.

Both factors depend on the condition of the vitreous base, since its traction may cause the formation of holes as well as the ensuing detachment [23, 69, 27].

For a **prognosis** as to whether a peripheral lesion will lead to retinal detachment, three criteria should be considered:

(1) the *quality of the retinal* tissue, from which one may determine whether a tear will arise or spread ("*cohesion*");

(2) the *strength of the retroretinal adhesion*, which might possibly prevent detachment of the retina;

(3) the force and the direction of the *traction*.

Which of these criteria can be evaluated *biomicroscopically?* As it is most difficult to deduce a dynamic process from purely morphologic signs, biomicroscopic observations must be interpreted with caution. However, on the basis of clinical experience and the results of experimental research, a prognosis is nevertheless possible in many cases.

Under *normal conditions*, topographical landmarks may provide information concerning "*adhesion*" and "*cohesion*", since these qualities change on either side of the ora serrata border. The inner "retinal" lamina (i.e. the ciliary epithelium) is less resistant anterior to the ora serrata, so that tears in the single-layered ciliary epithelium may spread more readily than in the multi-layered retina with its manifold intercellular connections. On the other hand, adhesion becomes stronger anterior to the ora serrata, since the retroretinal interstice ends at this point. From clinical observations it is well known, however, that this adhesion may halt an amotio but cannot always prevent its spreading beyond the ora serrata.

In *pathologic conditions* adhesion and cohesion change with regard to degree and topographical distribution. The *cohesion* of pathological retinal tissue is difficult to evaluate biomicroscopically; however, it can be anticipated, for instance, that a white necrotic retina will tear easily. The presence of an *adhesion* may be suspected from morphological signs, as it is well known that adhesion is stronger at pigmented scars. However, there is no direct correlation between pigmentation and the strength of adhesion, and it is well documented that even heavily pigmented foci, e.g. so-called demarcation lines, do not always prevent the spreading of an amotio. Tears are likely to occur even at well established chorioretinal adhesions, viz. at their marginal zones, where fixed layers are adjacent to those which are displaceable above the retroretinal interstice.

Since it is very difficult in practice to evaluate adhesion and cohesion of the tissues, prognosis has to be based principally on analysis of the *vitreal traction*, especially since adhesion and cohesion are of practical interest only in relation to the tractional forces present. Is it possible to evaluate vitreous traction biomicroscopically? Clinical and experimental research have in fact revealed that vitreous tracts of greater *mechanical* density (therefore mainly responsible for the traction) also have a greater *optical* density and can thus be made visible. It must be borne in mind, however, that, for optical reasons, only those tracts are clearly recognized which run at a *large angle* to the retinal surface. Tracts *parallel* to the surface are scarcely visible and their presence is recognizable only when the retinal surface is deformed by their traction.

Of all the denser vitreous membranelles, the most important are the *limiting membranes*. The "whipping" movements of the vitreous are transferred to the retina mainly by the anterior and posterior hyaloid membranes. Other dense tracts may develop as a result of pathologic processes, e.g. through inflammatory foci or through perforations of the eye (see p. 79). These newlyformed *atypical* tracts do not follow the direction of the normal vitreal tracts (Fig. 116). They are pathognomic of so-called "vitreous shrinkage". Their rate of traction is slow but continuous, gradually tearing even strong retroretinal adhesions.

In *summarizing* the various factors which determine the prognosis with regard to the genesis of a retinal detachment, it may be stated that, as a general rule, vitreous traction *posterior* to the ora serrata is always more dangerous than traction *anterior* to it. On the other hand, tears anterior to the ora serrata will more easily develop into giant tears than those situated in the multi-layered retina. This discussion is the basis of the following scheme of prognosis for the various locations of tears (Fig. 103).

Posterior to the ora serrata in the normal eye there is no insertion of vitreous membranules. Only after a posterior vitreous detachment is a membrane formed (the *posterior hyaloid membrane*) which is inserted here (Fig. 103c). If this membrane produces traction, this is effective above the retro-retinal interstice. Tears posterior to the ora serrata, which are connected to the posterior hyaloid membrane, are therefore the *most frequent cause of a retinal detachment*. This danger is diminished only through retroretinal adhesions, e.g. chorioretinitic scars. The shape of tears depends on the shape of the vitreoretinal adhesions, which in the region posterior to the vitreous base are usually quite small. Thus, either *round holes* are produced here with an operculum corresponding to the adhesion, or *horseshoe tears* with a raised flap. The flap is formed as the retina on either side of the vitreo-retinal adhesion is torn further in the direction of the traction, i.e. anteriorly. The original adhesion is consequently at the apex of the horseshoe, the sides ending at the posterior boundary of the vitreous base.

Anterior to the ora serrata the tears are subject to the traction of the *anterior hyaloid membrane* [213, 41]. This is usually fixed to the ciliary body (at the ligamentum medianum or at the ligamentum coronarium), with the result that the direction of the traction is tangential to the surface of the eye and does not, at least initially, detach the edges of the tears (Fig. 103b, 108). Even if the anterior hyaloid membrane were to float, only a slight displacement would occur. The tears anterior to the ora serrata are further protected by the retroretinal adhesion, so that the slight vitreous traction is seldom able to detach the ciliary epithelium. In fact, if the retina becomes detached at all, it is through vitreous shrinkage, which, however, may occur only after a long period of latency, sometimes lasting several years. Corresponding to the shape of the vitreo-ciliary attachments at the anterior vitreous base, the tears are long and run parallel to the ora serrata. Because of the thinness of the ciliary epithelium, tears can easily spread (Fig. 110).

Tears directly at the ora serrata are more complex (Fig. 103 d–f). The anterior and posterior edges of such a tear are subject to *various degrees of adhesion, cohesion*, and *traction*, which results in numerous possible combinations.

In addition, it must be borne in mind that, among apparently similar conditions of traction, certain individual variations may occur, owing to the fact that the boundaries within the three different layers at the ora serrata do not always coincide precisely, e.g. the transition of the retina into the ciliary epithelium may not coincide exactly with the beginning of the retroretinal adhesion. Thus, if the first row of cells of the ciliary epithelium lies above the retroretinal interstice, there may be a predisposition to a giant tear; if, however, the retroretinal adhesion extends under the retina, this suggests a greater degree of safety.

The mode of *traction* is decisive for prognosis. Both the posterior and the anterior hyaloid membranes can produce traction at the ora serrata, since their insertion lines almost coincide at this point. According to the different conditions of traction, three varieties of tears can be distinguished:

(1) *prebasal ora serrata tears*: anterior to the vitreous base (Fig. 103 d);

(2) *retrobasal ora tears*: posterior to the vitreous base (Fig. 103 e);

(3) *intrabasal ora tears*: within the vitreous base (Fig. 103 f).

In a **prebasal tear**, the rupture is anterior to the vitreous base, i. e. the entire *traction* will be *behind* the tear. The anterior hyaloid membrane is inserted at the posterior edge of the tear, whereas the anterior edge is free of traction.

The *traction* produced by the anterior hyaloid membrane is much the same as in a tear of the ciliary epithelium above the pars plana. Nevertheless, the prognosis for the prebasal ora tear is less favourable, since the posterior edge of the tear, which is under traction, is not protected by retroretinal adhesion (Fig. 106a and b). Thus, even slight traction of the anterior hyaloid membrane is capable of detaching the retina. The detachment usually spreads slowly because initially the direction of traction is parallel to the surface. If there is a *giant* tear prebasally, the prognosis may be better than for other forms of giant tears, because the anterior hyaloid membrane prevents the inversion of the edges and the penetration of vitreous substance into the retroretinal space.

In the *biomicroscopic picture* prebasal ora tears may easily be confused with an old retinal detachment which has gone beyond the ora serrata and detached the ciliary epithelium (Fig. 104). The detached ciliary epithelium and a shrinking hyaloid membrane may present a similar appearance: on the one hand, the detached ciliary epithelium may become hyalinized, losing its characteristic structure; on the other hand, the anterior hyaloid membrane may become densified. The two membranes are the more easily confused because pars plana texture may also be seen on a detached anterior hyaloid membrane as a cast-like relief of unknown origin. Thus, a retinal detachment caused by a prebasal ora tear may be misinterpreted as an arrhegmatogenous retinal detachment that has expanded beyond the ora serrata.

What are the criteria for the *differential diagnosis?* Examination of the detached lamina is, as explained above, of little value. The necessary proof is provided by an examination of the still-attached pigment epithelium. In the case of a *spreading arrhegmatogenous retinal detachment*, the pigment epithelium merges from the retina to the pars plana without a step. In the case of a *prebasal ora tear*, however, the pigment epithelium anterior to the ora is covered by the still-attached ciliary epithelium. Thus a step is formed at the ora serrata, where the ciliary epithelium begins. The region of the pars plana then still has its granular and striated surface and, even if intact ora processes are visible upon it, the diagnosis of a prebasal ora tear is established. This differential diagnosis is very important in practice, since a prebasal ora tear should be closed surgically, whereas an arrhegmatogenous retinal detachment is usually a nonsurgical condition.

In a **retrobasal tear,** where the lesion is posterior to the vitreous base, the *traction* will occur *anterior* to the tear. The posterior hyaloid membrane is inserted at the anterior edge of the tear, the posterior edge of the tear thus being free of traction (Fig. 106e and f). The full force of vitreous traction will be exerted on the *ciliary epithelium*, which consequently becomes detached. The tears may readily expand in the thin epithelial layer, going on to become giant tears of nearly the whole circumference (Fig. 105). If no residual adhesions to the posterior edge remain, retinal detachment *need not* necessarily follow. If it does occur, it is caused by traction at the lateral edges of the tears, which is the more effective the shorter the tear, being concentrated within a small area (Fig. 113). Conversely, *giant* retrobasal tears may have a good prognosis after all.

This is illustrated by the case of a 54-year-old man who, as a result of a contusio bulbi, developed a retrobasal ora tear involving almost the entire circumference. The ora serrata was intact in only a very narrow area (2–4 o'clock). In an observation period covering 44 years no retinal detachment has developed.

Residual adhesions to the retina posterior to the tear are, however, very dangerous since the resulting traction is not neutralized by any retroretinal adhesion. Even weak vitreous strands may then cause a rapidly expanding retinal detachment. Giant retrobasal ora tears differ from other giant tears in that the vitreous is still protected by a membrane, viz. the posterior hyaloid membrane. If this is intact, no unformed vitreous will pass behind the retina.

The *biomicroscopic appearance* of retrobasal ora tears is quite characteristic. The detached ciliary epithelium is drawn anteriorly towards the centre of the eye by vitreous and zonula traction, thus forming a crest upon the pars plana (Fig. 105). The characteristic granular and striated structure, the cristae ciliares, and sometimes even residual ora teeth may be recognized in the semi-opaque, greyish lamina. The detached epithelial leaf may appear directly behind the lens border; in retro-illumination it has a fine black filigree pattern against the glowing red of the fundus.

Differential diagnosis between this membrane and other membranes above the ciliary body is usually not difficult: the posterior hyaloid membrane is inserted at the edge of the detached lamina. The pigment epithelium lies exposed beneath it. A very abundant dissemination of pigment, presumably a result of pigment epithelium cells being injured by the tearing of the retroretinal adhesion, is a highly characteristic sign of retrobasal ora tears.

In **intrabasal tears,** i. e. those lying within the vitreous base, the edges are not in direct contact with the hyaloid membranes. The vitreous probably becomes split above the tear (Fig. 106a and d). This split, however, does not offer enough contrast to be visible and becomes recognizable biomicroscopically only when outlined by pigment or blood cells.

No *traction* occurs directly at the edges of the tear, so that the likelihood of a retinal detachment depends principally on the degree of vitreal destruction. If the vitreous is *intact*, retinal detachment either never develops at all, or does so very slowly (Figs. 109, 112). This is well known from, for instance, ora tears in adolescents, which are observed predominantly in the lower periphery.

With the vitreous *liquefied*, the situation is more precarious. The posterior hyaloid membrane then usually detaches. Although it is inserted at quite a distance from the ora serrata, its "whipping" movements are transmitted to the posterior edge of the tear. The retina then not only detaches, but the tear itself frequently becomes enlarged, with its edges inverting [99, 110, 127, 183]. The liquefied vitreous, which is then not restrained by any membrane, flows into the retroretinal space.

This fact is most important for therapy, for attempts to re-attach the retina through injections into the vitreous body will only force more vitreous fluid into the retroretinal space. Therefore, methods of re-attaching the retina in such cases by injection of air into the vitreous are likely to be more successful if vitreous substance has previously been evacuated [134].

The *prognosis* of intrabasal giant tears is far less favourable than that of prebasal and retrobasal giant tears.

The *criteria for the prognosis* of lesions in the peripheral fundus discussed here may appear to be dealt with too schematically. However, they are based on well known mechanical and anatomical facts. Even though not supported by extensive statistics, a careful analysis of individual cases has shown them to be reliable. Cases deviating from this schema must be examined all the more thoroughly, for new insights into the genesis of retinal detachments may be obtained in this manner. To illustrate this, we may refer to detachments in aphakia or in acute traumatic retinal necrosis (see p. 78).

4. Traumatic Lesions in the Extreme Periphery of the Fundus

There are so many possibilities of mechanical damage to the eye that the number of clinical syndromes anticipated may be legion. All traumatic lesions, however, may be explained by just two different mechanisms:

    (a) the straining of textural elasticity in blunt trauma (contusions),

    (b) displacement of tissues (perforations).

4.1. Contusions

Contusions naturally deform the ocular globe. Tissue damage relates to the degree of deformation, i.e. to the force involved as well as to the velocity. Maximum deformation occurs at the point of application, i.e. generally in the anterior segment of the eye. Other zones of strong deformation result wherever the displacement of the eyeball is impeded. But it is the quality of the tissues that determines what kind of lesion will be caused by any given deformation. A rupture may be expected wherever tissues with differing distensibility are connected: during ocular deformation, the distensible tissues will exert traction on the less distensible—more inert—structures. Clinical observations and recent experiments [35, 230, 231] confirm these theoretical speculations.

In the region of the ciliary body, *contusion damage* will be anticipated at the insertion of the ciliary body (at the scleral spur) [3, 73, 234], at the suspension of the lens, at the "insertion" of the retina at the ora serrata, and at the insertion of the anterior and the posterior hyaloid membranes. Lesions following a blunt trauma, despite the manifold causative agents, have thus a striking uniformity and a characteristic appearance. They occur at the site of the greatest deformation, so that nearly all of them are found *along the same meridian*. Barely visible lesions of the peripheral fundus are therefore to be sought in that meridian which has the most marked traumatic alterations in the chamber angle.

Lesions in the area of the ciliary body are important in practice, since they are the source of two of the most serious late complications following ocular contusion: *secondary glaucoma* and *retinal detachment* [28, 38, 130]. As the latter always begins in a region visible only by means of scleral indentation, this examination is indispensable for early diagnosis and prognosis (for contra-indications see p. 11). In the following paragraphs contusional lesions of the peripheral fundus will be discussed in detail.

4.1.1. Post-Traumatic Vitreous Detachment

There is no doubt that *small* vitreous detachments quite frequently occur after blunt trauma, as shown by the preretinal hemorrhages observed. These small detachments are usually not progressive and seem to be of little clinical importance. On the other hand, it is still controversial whether a large rhegmatogenous vitreous detachment can be caused by ocular contusion. Since such an event would induce a chain reaction culminating in retinal detachment, this problem is of interest, especially forensically. At present, however, no morphological signs are known to distinguish a post-traumatic from a degenerative, i.e. senile or myopic, rhegmatogenous vitreous detachment. A *traumatic etiology* can thus be postulated only upon the basis of a *temporal correlation*.

This coincidence cannot be established unless the patient has been examined immediately before and after the injury. Otherwise one must rely upon the patient's statement that "muscae volantes" appeared suddenly after the contusion. It is obvious that such subjective statements are often unreliable: accidents so frequently create the occasion for patients to check the function of their eyes and to notice unilateral symptoms for the first time. Even objective signs, such as recent haemorrhages, do not exclude the possibility that there may have been a posterior vitreous detachment prior to the trauma.

There are other unanswered questions: Does ocular contusion worsen the condition of a pre-existing vitreous detachment, i.e. will new tears occur, or will so-called silent tears become detached? Whatever hypotheses may be brought forward definite proof is difficult to establish.

4.1.2. Partial-Thickness Tears of the Retina

From a theoretical point of view, one might assume that the *inner layers of the retina* could be torn off by vitreous traction during ocular contusion. This phenomenon, however, is exceptional and has been observed only in cases of schisis retinae. In the normal retina the cellular connections are presumably so much interwoven that they are not torn by the traction produced by blunt trauma. In a cystoid degeneration minute fragments from the inner layer between supporting pillars might indeed be avulsed, but since such small particles cannot be distinguished from micro-adhesions, it would be difficult to establish their traumatic nature.

4.1.3. Full-Thickness Tears of the Retina

The attachment of the retina to the pigment epithelium is weak and full-thickness tears can easily occur. Tearing is anticipated at the edges of retroretinal adhesions, at the ora serrata or at chorioretinal scars. Tears can also occur at *vitreoretinal adhesions*, i.e. at the anterior and posterior borders of the vitreous base and at pathological vitreo-retinal adhesions [49]. As a result of the retinal laceration there is now a free passage between the pigment epithelium and the vitreous space so that pigment may reach the vitreous. Tearing of the retina must be suspected if, after trauma, *brown pigment granules* are observed in the vitreous cavity. It is important to trace carefully the *origin of this pigment*.

(a) When "**cysts**" at the edge of the retina are ruptured, brown pigment granules may penetrate into either the vitreous or the previtreal space, depending on the location of the rupture. Only the emerging clouds of pigment (Fig. 107) may call attention to the lesion, for the defects themselves are so minute that they are barely recognizable in the irregular cystoid structure of the retinal edge. The pigment granules gradually disappear, after which the ruptured cysts are scarcely to be made out. They are of no clinical significance; no complications have been reported.

(b) Tears in the region of the **posterior vitreous base** are usually horseshoe-shaped and cannot be distinguished in appearance or in location from those arising in an idiopathic posterior vitreous detachment. Only if there is a temporal correlation may a connection with trauma be postulated. Oblong and ora-parallel tears at the posterior edge of the vitreous base are exceptional and usually appear only in connection with avulsion of the whole vitreous base (see p. 77).

(c) **At the ora serrata,** prebasal, retrobasal and intrabasal tears can appear. They are not always exactly at the edge of the retina, but sometimes slightly anterior or posterior (Fig. 109). The reason for these individual variations is probably the dissimilar position of the ora serrata border in each of the layers (see p. 51). Biomicroscopic appearance and prognosis of **prebasal** and **retrobasal** ora tears are described on pp. 72ff. In an **intrabasal** ora tear the edges are initially only slightly detached and tend to withdraw from one another, so that the pigment epithelium lies exposed. As explained on p. 74, a retinal detachment need not necessarily develop; the edges of the tear may re-attach in the course of time and be held in place by scar tissue, making the rupture difficult to recognize. Only the partly exposed pigment epithelium, which often must be traced through kinetic indentation, will indicate an intrabasal tear. If a retinal detachment does follow, it cannot be distinguished in appearance from intrabasal ora tears of unrelated etiology.

(d) **Tears of the ciliary epithelium** are usually situated at the anterior border of the vitreous base, at the white midline (Fig. 108). Further posteriorly, tears occur only if the anterior vitreociliary connections have been torn. At first, the edges of the tear are slightly detached, the thin ciliary epithelium then appearing greyish (Figs. 110, 111). A distinct contrast in colour is offered by the dark brown base of the tear where the velvety, gleaming pigment epithelium is exposed. If the edges of the tear later re-attach [41, 59], the ciliary epithelium may remain slightly opaque as a result of fine vesiculation; mostly, though, it regains its normal appearance. Such tears are frequently overlooked (Fig. 108). Only very careful kinetic indentation will expose them. Clouds of pigment issuing from the bottom of the tear help in diagnosis.

Theoretically, the onset of tears in the ciliary epithelium might be anticipated to result, not only from traction of the anterior hyaloid membrane, but also from zonular traction. Such a rupture would be at the linea serrata and would have to be serrated, not straight. Ruptures of this type can indeed be produced in *autopsy* eyes by traction on the lens, but it has to be borne in mind that in this case the lacerated tissue is necrotic. In the *living* eye no ruptures have been observed at this site. This might be due to unsatisfactory viewing conditions. Probably, however, the zonula fibres are more likely to tear than the ciliary epithelium, as suggested by the frequency of traumatic subluxation of the lens.

(e) **Avulsion of the whole vitreous base.** If tears arise at the anterior as well as at the posterior border of the base, the entire vitreous base is avulsed, i.e. the vitreous along with an *adherent strip* of tissue from the ciliary epithelium and the retina (Fig. 103g). The anterior hyaloid membrane is then inserted at the anterior edge of the strip, and the posterior hyaloid membrane at its posterior edge. In many cases the limiting membranes, having torn, are hard to follow.

In short avulsions the edges of the tears may re-attach and scar spontaneously (Fig. 114). In long avulsions however, the strip of tissue is drawn towards the centre of the eye, floating freely. In the early stages, it presents the typical pattern of retinal and pars plana tissue, with pigment granules upon its external surface. Later, the strip shrinks (Fig. 115), becomes twisted and hyalinized, appearing finally as a greyish, fibrous and sharply delimited vitreous opacification. To prove its origin the points of insertion at the retinal border must be sought. Between these two points of insertion, there is a retinal defect which corresponds to the floating strip. The anterior and posterior edges of this defect, not being under traction, become slightly detached initially but may later re-attach spontaneously. The traction of the vitreous base is effective only where the detached strip is inserted at the lateral ends of the defect. This traction is usually not very strong, so that a retinal detachment seldom follows. When it does occur, it starts from the lateral ends so that these points must be closely watched and if necessary coagulated.

(f) **Traumatic tears of the uvea.** Tears affecting not only the retina but also the underlying tissue form oblong, ora-parallel defects in the pigment epithelium and the inner uveal layers. The white sclera, as well as large uveal vessels with their characteristic parallel and meridional direction, will then be seen at the bottom of the defect (Figs. 112, 113). The edges of the tear are sharply outlined, showing a more or less pronounced proliferation of pigment. While most of these scars are found at the ora serrata, some occur in the middle of the pars plana. Abundant haemorrhage into the vitreous is usually produced by these uveal ruptures (in contrast to tears in the avascular retinal border or the ciliary epithelium). On account of the haemorrhage such ruptures may be suspected early but become visible only in the late stages. They look like chorioiditic scars, differing from them in their form and location, and the absence of other inflammatory signs. Yet other traumatic lesions may be present.

What is the mechanism involved in uveal tears? Specific anatomical weakness of the uvea in the periphery of the fundus cannot be the explanation, since the uvea continues without any definite borderline from the choroid into the ciliary body. The location of the ruptures points to a connection with traction of the vitreous base. Traction in this area will also affect the deeper layers owing to the strong connections of the retroretinal adhesion. Such uveal ruptures can be replicated experimentally: if vitreous traction is induced before fixation of autopsy eyes, uveal tears will appear at exactly the same site as after a contusion.

4.1.4. Traumatic Retinal Necrosis

As becomes apparent in the chapter on the prognosis of peripheral lesions following trauma, usually a retinal detachment will develop only after a long *period of latency*. There is, however, a special form of "amotio retinae" which may appear *within hours* of the contusion. The picture differs in many respects from that of a rhegmatogenous retinal detachment, even though holes may be present in the retina. On the one hand, the difference lies in the fact that the vitreous has usually remained *intact* so that no strong traction is expected at the onset, especially not a tractional force sufficient to bring about detachment so precipitously. On the other hand, there is also a difference in the shape of the tears, which fail to develop the typical horseshoe picture but are usually of dendritic or round shape, or are ora tears of considerable length. *This atypical shape of tears* (if present), and even more the unexpected fact that, despite their considerable extent, these retinal detachments may *re-attach spontaneously* within a few days, exonerate vitreous traction as the culprit.

There is little doubt that this form of traumatic detachment depends on *other mechanisms* than the rhegmatogenous variety produced by traction. The etiology, however, becomes evident only in the late stages: After the detachment has subsided, there is no retina left in the previously detached area. Only the most careful examination will reveal an extremely thin membrane infiltrated by pigment proliferations. No vessels, only some white fibrotic strands are visible here and there. In the visual field there is an absolute scotoma corresponding to the entire previously detached area.

This is the typical picture of *retinal necrosis*. The pathogenesis of the retinal detachment in these cases is, at present, unknown. It may be of some interest here that Gloor *et al.* [84] produced segmental retinal detachments in cats by simultaneous occlusion of the supplying retinal artery and vein.

The *diagnosis* of retinal necrosis presents no problem in the late stages, whereas in the early phase it is rather difficult. Early differential diagnosis could be made by examination of the visual field or by fluorescein angiography; the latter, however, is usually impossible immediately following trauma. A suspicion of retinal necrosis will therefore be based mainly on the *rapid onset* of detachment.

Usually the necrosis is part of severe overall damage to the eye. However, there are cases where it occurs without any other signs, especially without any lesions of the anterior sections of eye. This at first seems surprising considering the severity of the retinal damage. How can it be explained? Heavy damage confined to a restricted area will result from the action of forces with high velocity. The affected small area may be situated as far posteriorly as the equator if the patient's eyes in this attempt to close them were rotated upwards (Bell's phenomenon). This type of isolated retinal necrosis posteriorly is to be suspected whenever a large (i.e. visible) object hits the globe at high speed as for example a shoe trown from nearby. In such a case the only significant finding may well be a lesion of the eyelid yet one always has to keep in mind the possibility of a retinal necrosis.

4.2. Perforations of the Eye

In perforations, in addition to more or less severe damage from contusion, there is a loss of tissue. Loss of vitreous affects mainly the most peripheral parts of the fundus. If part of the vitreous has herniated through the wound, the prolapse is amputated by the surgeon. If, however, some vitreous substance has remained trapped in the wound (Fig. 117), new zones of discontinuity (Fig. 116) are formed in atypical directions, converging arrow-like onto the site of perforation.

No complications arise in the periphery of the fundus in the early stages, since the volume lost in the vitreous space is replaced by fluid. But later on the vitreous usually shrinks. The ensuing complications differ from those of vitreous shrinkage of non-traumatic etiology. In the intact eyeball, the vitreous generally shrinks between the two physiological adhesions, the anterior vitreous base and the posterior pole. The tractional force then works, at least at the beginning, in a direction parallel to the surface of the retina. Following perforation, a new and particularly strong adhesion is created at the globe wall by the trapped vitreous. Owing to the atypical position of this adhesion traction upon the retina is now exerted in atypical directions, which in most cases are perpendicular to the retinal surface. This leads to complications characteristic of perforations.

After partial vitrectomy the remaining vitreous develops a typical configuration [87]. There is incarceration of either the *anterior hyaloid membrane* alone (Fig. 117a) or of *both* hyaloid membranes (anterior and posterior) (Fig. 117b). With the first form, vitreous shrinkage will produce an arrhegmatogenous posterior vitreous detachment which is similar to an arrhegmatogenous detachment of non-traumatic etiology. But where the posterior hyaloid membrane is also incarcerated, shrinkage will pull the vitreous base from the *opposite side* towards the wound

(Fig. 119). Thus, a retinal detachment may result when the vitreous remains attached to the retina. In other cases the vitreous becomes detached from its base. Whereas the vitreoretinal connections are hardly ever torn there, after perforation the force and abnormal direction of traction may be able to detach the vitreous even from its *absolute base*, the ora serrata.

If the vitreous is detached from its *anterior base* only, the connecting fibres at the white midline and accessory lines are torn. The anterior hyaloid membrane is now inserted directly at the ora serrata. At the edge of the anterior vitreous detachment residual adhesions may remain in the region of the ligamentum medianum, forming equidistant fibrous fascicles (Fig. 120). In contrast to the constitutionally floating hyaloid membrane, the circular fibres of the ligamentum medianum can still be seen within the traumatically detached anterior hyaloid membrane.

In the case of a *complete basal detachment*, the vitreous is detached also from the ora serrata (Fig. 121) so that a direct passage between the previtreal and retro-vitreal spaces is formed—a very unusual situation. The diagnosis is often difficult as the structures of the ora serrata, pars plana and adjacent retina are reproduced—as in a prebasal ora tear—on the external side of the detached hyaloid membranes. The picture is, therefore, easily confused with a detachment of the retina and ciliary epithelium. It is only by careful examination that a second retinal and pars plana structure (that of the still attached, actual inner retinal layer) can be recognized under the detached hyaloid membrane. As a late complication retinal detachment may follow. Naturally, the vitreous will not exert any traction on the retina where it is detached but it can pull at the lateral edges of the basal detachment, where it again comes into contact with the retina.

4.3. Indications for Indentation after Trauma

The importance of examining the peripheral fundus after trauma is evident on account of the significant part played by the vitreous base in post-traumatic complications. But, as explained on p. 11, in order to avoid additional damage *indentation should not be attempted immediately after trauma*. Large lesions likely to cause early complications are usually readily visible even without indentation. For detection of small peripheral lesions, one has to rely initially on indirect signs.

Suspicion will arise, of course, in all lesions involving the ciliary region, such as detachment of the ciliary body from the scleral spur, subluxation of the lens, or a partial, circumscribed detachment of the anterior hyaloid membrane.

Signs produced by the lesion itself are:

– *Brown granules* within the vitreous space indicate a lesion of the retinal layer or of the ciliary epithelium. If no corresponding lesions are detected in the posterior fundus, the origin of the pigment must be suspected in the periphery.

– The very pattern of a *vitreous hemorrhage* may indicate its origin. Blood deriving from retinal vessels initially remains trapped in the adjacent vitreous cortex, descending only later into the lower vitreous base. A hemorrhage into the pre-retinal tract in the early phase is indicative of a lesion at the ora serrata and—since the retina is avascular there—of uveal involvement.

But even if signs indicative of peripheral injury have been detected, there need not necessarily be rapid onset of grave complications. In most lesions of the ora serrata or in those anterior to it, complications will not arise until later, owing to the retro-retinal adhesion. It is only in changes *posterior* to the ora serrata, i.e. at the posterior boundary of the vitreous base, that early complications must be expected. These are visible without indentation.

In conclusion, early indentation is not generally necessary. It is sufficient for protection and prophylaxis to examine the ora serrata and pars plana in greater detail some weeks after the trauma. This rule may be disregarded only if it is feared that a rapidly progressing cataract will later prevent proper examination and prophylactic procedures.

5. Tumours

5.1. Ciliary Body Tumours

The great usefulness of indentation biomicroscopy in cases of ciliary body tumours is obvious, as it can serve to evaluate their posterior extent. Quite often, however, the latter may be difficult to distinguish from the protuberance produced by the indenter itself. Reliable conclusions are arrived at only by painstaking comparison with adjacent indented areas. Indentation diaphanoscopy is useful but must be interpreted with special caution, as melanomata may have unpigmented flat extensions which do not stand out in diaphanoscopy.

5.2. Retinal Tumours

Retinoblastomata may extend to the very edge of the retina, or be present there as isolated small foci. These peripheral tumours should be investigated carefully if conservative treatment is planned. Howard and Ellsworth [109] have shown in a series of seventy children that the most obvious tumours are found mainly in the posterior segments, but in two thirds of the cases foci were also found anterior to the equator; in one tenth of the cases, they were only visible by means of indenta-tion. As such peripheral tumours may nowadays be treated by coagulation or by X-rays, all children with suspected retinoblastoma should be examined with in-dentation.

Small tumours, particularly intravitreal seeds, are easily confused with harmless developmental variations (ectopic ciliary epithelium, see p. 52) if the examination does not include biomicroscopy. With the biomicroscope the random agglomerations of tumour cells become distinguishable from the cystoid, sharply outlined tissue ectopies. If a cystic formation is nevertheless suspect as a tumorous focus, particular attention must be paid to its relation to the structures of the vitreous base (holes in the preretinal tract, see p. 56). If the findings are inconclusive, follow-up will demonstrate a progression in the suspected tumour.

Conclusion

A survey of the pathology of the peripheral fundus explains the clinical significance of the vitreous base. Its anatomical structures determine many of the clinical syndromes. The interest in a morphological examination is based on the fact that the optically denser vitreous structures have special mechanical qualities: on the one hand they can exert traction on the retina and, on the other hand, they can act as a filter to prevent the passage of certain substances. An exact knowledge of the peripheral vitreous structures provides important information concerning the behaviour of pathological processes and is consequently essential to prognostication.

The structures of the vitreous are visible in the living eye only with the aid of the slit lamp. Biomicroscopy of the vitreous base provides so much valuable information that the additional effort is richly rewarded.

Illustrations

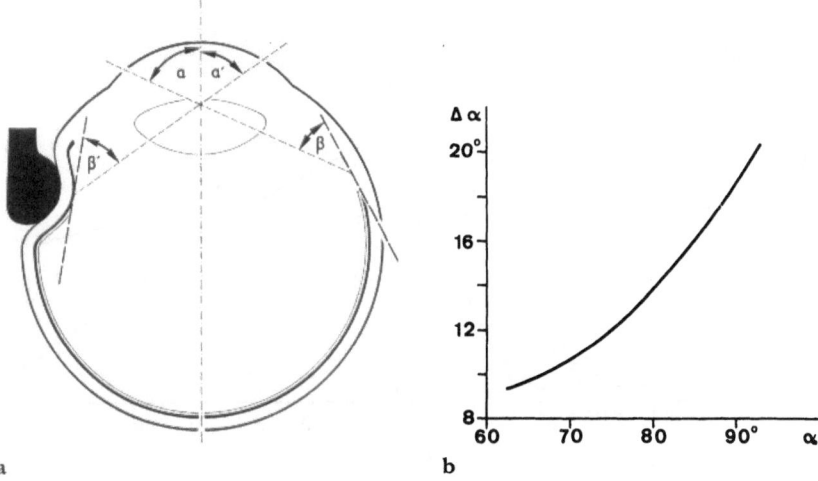

a

b

Fig. 1a and b. *The principle of indentation.*

a The angle of eccentricity α is decreased by indentation (α′), the area to be examined being displaced towards the optical axis.

The angle of acceptance β (i.e. the angle between the observation beam and the tangent to the eye wall at the point examined) is changed (β′). In principle this angle may assume, at any point, values between 0° and 90°, according to the position of the indenter.

b Decrease of the angle of eccentricity by Δα when locations that in the non-indented eye are observed under the angle α are indented by 2.5 mm (after Fankhauser and Lotmar, 1970 [58])

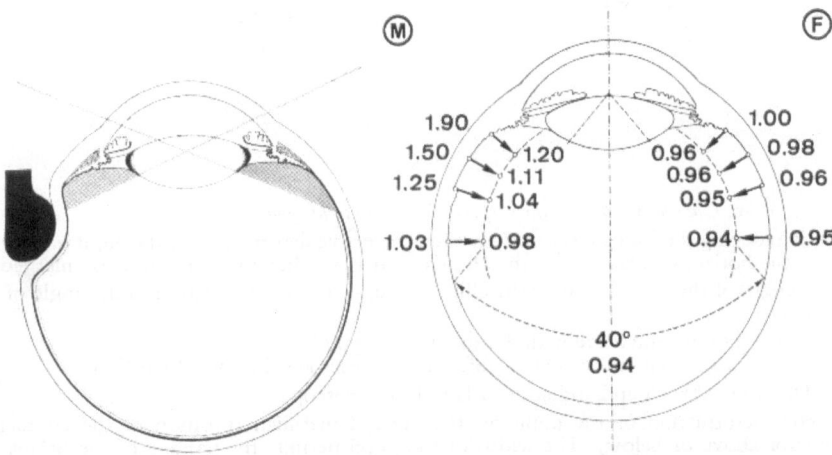

Fig. 2. *Static examination.*

With indentation, normally invisible areas of the eye may be seen. Reducing the angle of eccentricity will bring the region of the ora serrata out of the "shadow" of the lens border (right) so that it becomes visible (left)

Fig. 3. *Change of magnification by indentation.*

With the use of the contact glass the magnification depends on the angle of eccentricity. The latter changes with indentation and so does, therefore, the magnification. The figure shows the change of magnification with an indentation 2.5 mm deep. Left, magnification on the meridional plane (*M*); right, magnification on the frontal plane (*F*) (after Lotmar [132])

85

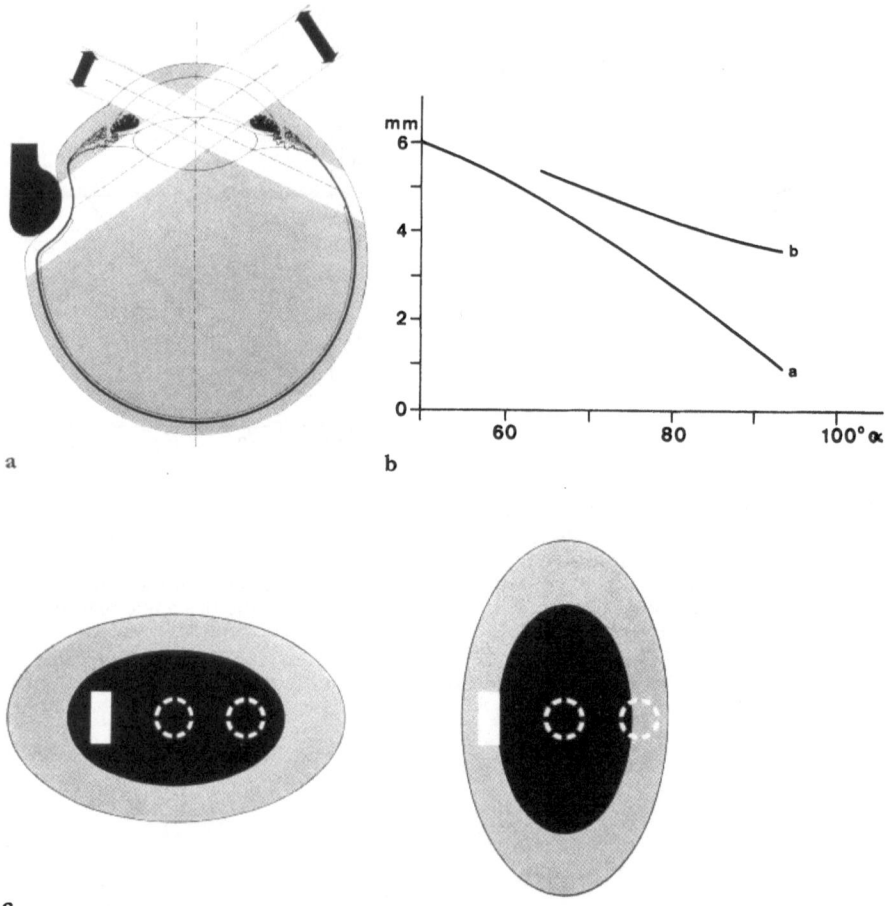

a   b

c

Fig. 4a–c. *Changes in the pupillary aperture due to indentation.*

a By reducing the angle of eccentricity the perspective deformation of the pupil is diminished, i.e. the horizontal diameter of the ellipsis increases. Thus the visual field is enlarged.

b Length of the shorter axis of the elliptical pupil (in mm) in relation to the angle of eccentricity.

Curve *a*: non-indented eye with 8 mm width of pupil.

Curve *b*: with 2.5 mm indentation (after Fankhauser and Lotmar, 1970 [58]).

c Diameter of the pupil and stereopsis in biomicroscopy.

Left: Deformation of the pupil on the vertical meridian (position of the contact glass mirror above or below). The width of the pupil permits the passage of the beams of the two objectives as well as of the slit lamp.

Right: Deformation on the horizontal meridian (contact glass mirror lateral). The pupillary aperture is not wide enough for the passage of all three beams. Stereopsis is therefore lost. Circles: beams of microscope. Rectangle: Slit beam

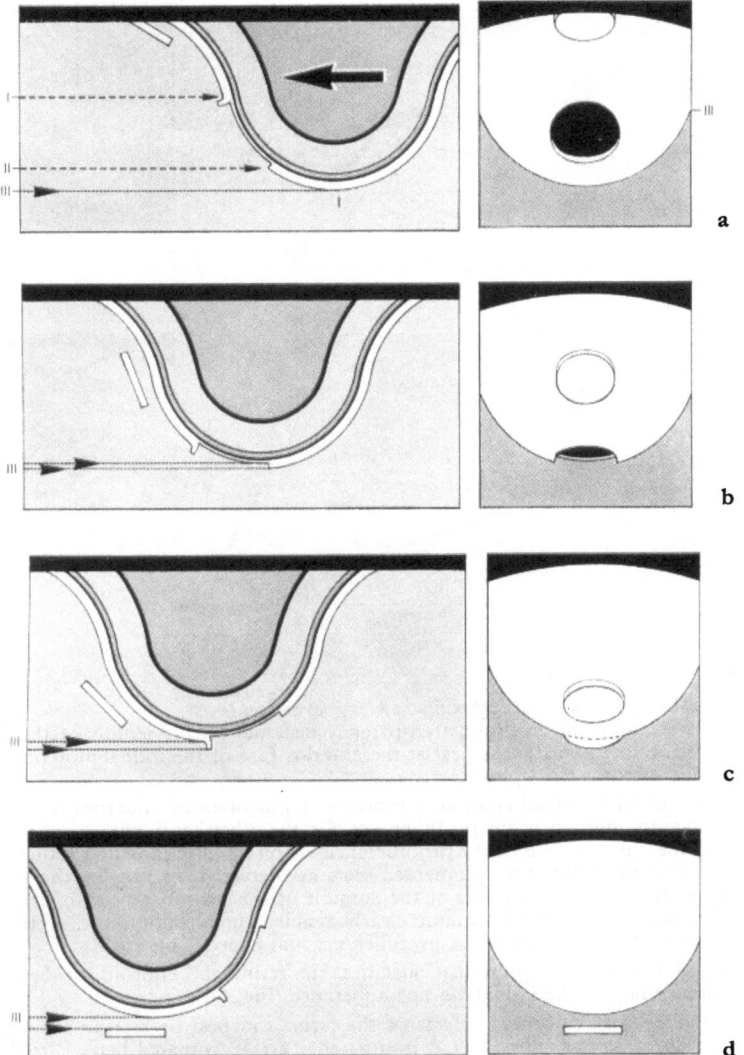

Fig. 5a–d. *Kinetic examination: Parallaxis.*
I. Examination on the anterior face of the indentation protuberance.
II. Examination on the summit of the protuberance.
III. Examination in silhouette.
Perspective changes are demonstrated in the example of a retinal tear with raised anterior border and with an operculum floating in the vitreous. The figures left show the movement of the indenter in a postero-anterior direction (from right to left). The figures right show the effect produced in the contact glass mirror.

By examination in silhouette the anatomical structures are observed in profile, i.e. without perspective distortion.

a The retinal tear is on the anterior face of the protuberance.

b With the indenter shifted, the tear now appears in silhouette: its actual depth may be seen.

c The anterior border is now in silhouette: its prominence becomes evident.

d When the floating operculum is in silhouette, both its thickness and distance from the retina may be estimated

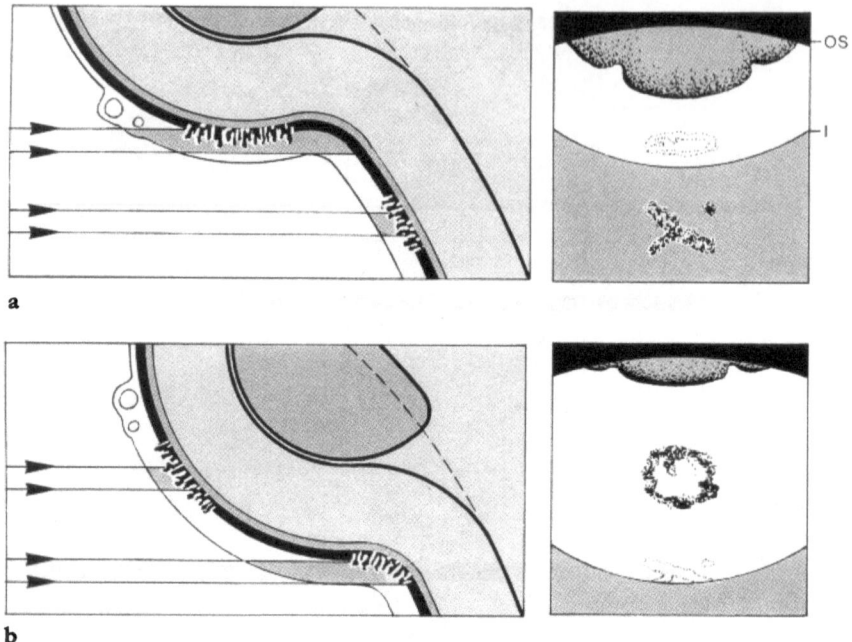

a

b

Fig. 6a–f. *Change of transparency in kinetic examination.*
In a semi-opaque medium, transparency depends on the length of the path of the transgressing rays. This is shortest at the anterior face of the indentation protuberance, longest at its summit. Examples:

a and b With a small angle of acceptance, pigmentations underneath the retina are scarcely seen at the summit of the protuberance. On the other hand, with a large angle of acceptance (on the anterior face of the protuberance, or on the non-indented retina, respectively) they are seen distinctly. Two pigmented scars are depicted. In Fig. 6a, the anterior scar cannot be seen very well, as it lies at the summit of the protuberance; in Fig. 6b, it appears on the anterior face, thus becoming clearly visible. The posterior scar, on the other hand, now appears at the summit of the protuberance and hence is invisible

c and d In case of preretinal opacities, the retina and choroid are best examined on the anterior face of the indentation protuberance (Fig. 6d).

e and f Partial-thickness defects of the retina can best be seen at the summit of the protuberance, as the differences in transparency are accentuated here. Partial-thickness defects or epiretinal appositions are therefore examined at that position (Fig. 6e)

I   Indentation protuberance
OS   Ora serrata

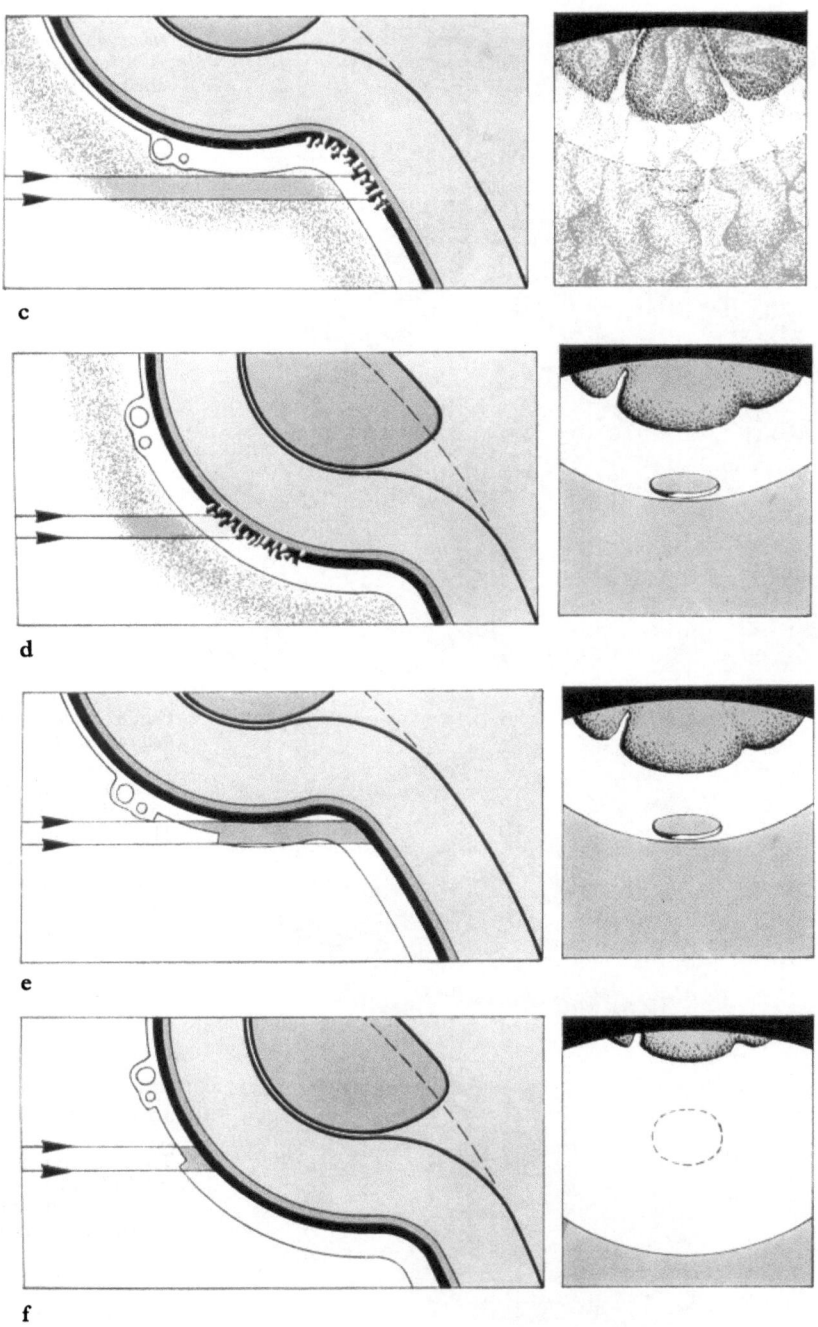

c

d

e

f

Fig. 6 c–f. Legend see opposite page

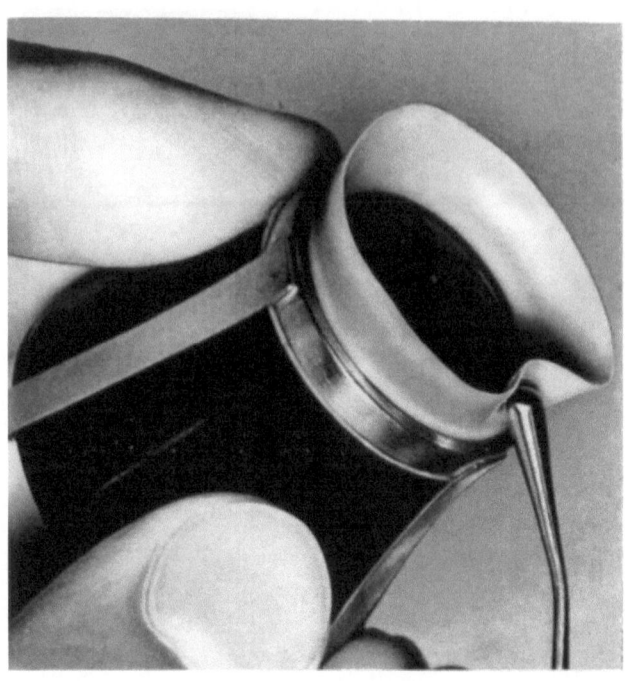

Fig. 7. *Liesenhoff's indentation cuff.*
A soft plastic cuff is attached to the lower (corneal) part of a three-mirror contact glass with the aid of spring clips. A blunt instrument, held in the other hand, serves as an indenter

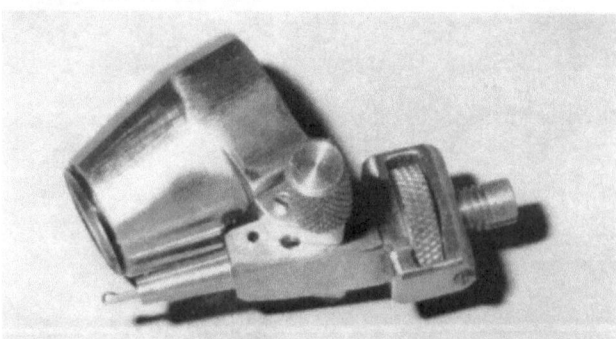

Fig. 8. *Fankhauser's indentation contact glass.*
A special contact glass is fixed in a metal case in such a way that it may be rotated. The indenter may be brought into various positions by means of several screws

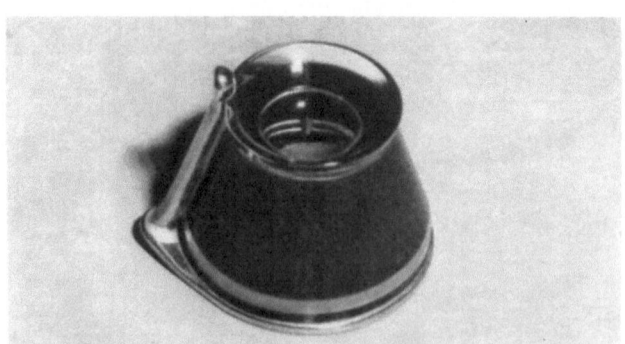

Fig. 9. *Goldmann's and Schmidt's indentation contact glass.*
The indenter is locked on the front plate of a contact glass specially constructed for the ora serrata region

Fig. 10. *Goldmann's three-mirror contact glass.*
Specific sections of the fundus may be examined with each of the three mirrors. Each section overlaps the next even when the contact glass is not moved. However, if the latter is shifted on the surface of the globe, the various sections may be extended (arrows). The ora serrata region may be examined both with the middle mirror (*3*) and with the gonioscopy mirror (*4*)

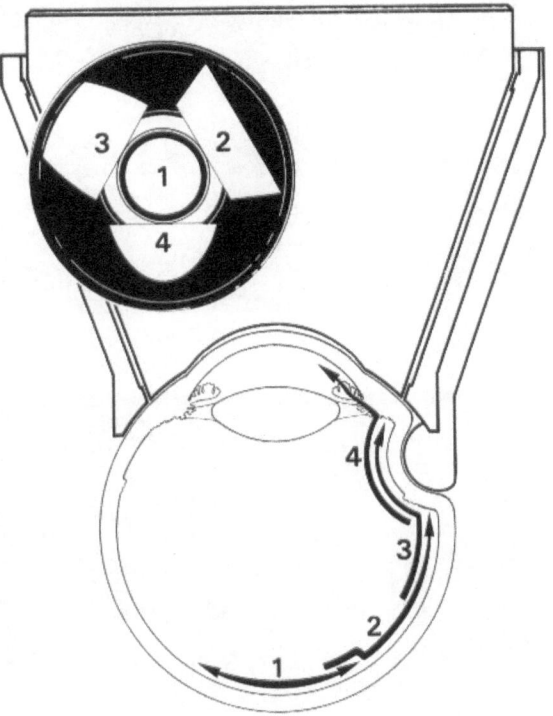

Fig. 11. *Position of the indenter in examination of different sections of the fundus.*
The nearer to the equator indentation is applied, the greater must be the distance of the indenter from the axis of the eye

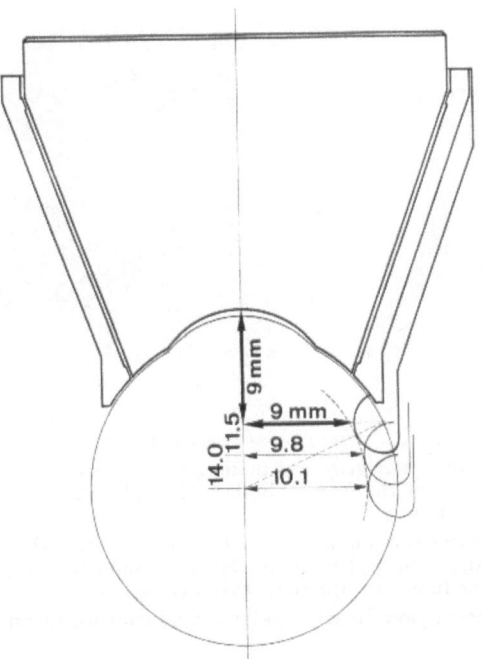

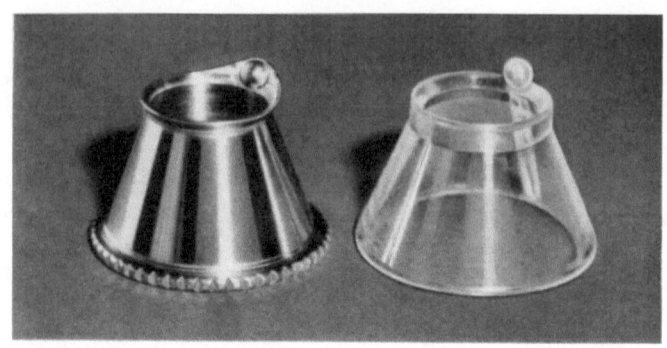

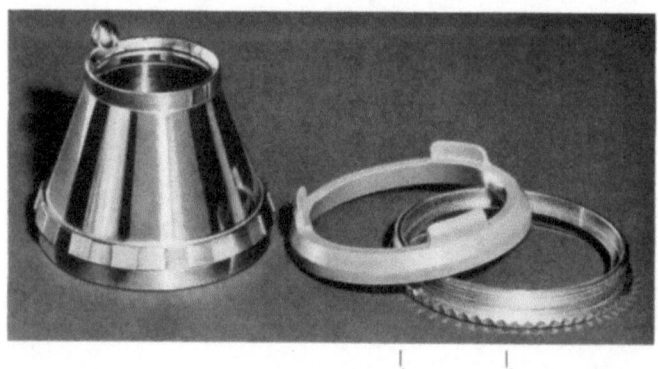

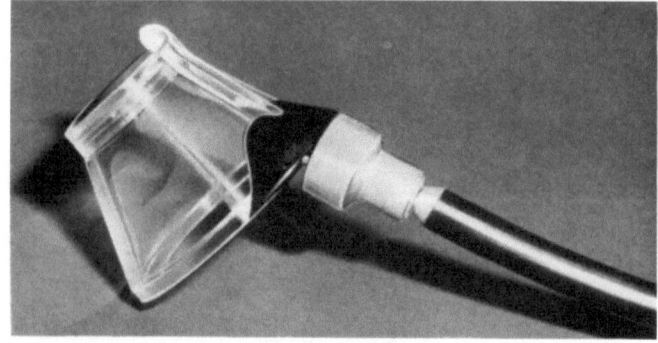

Fig. 12a–c. *Various types of indentation funnel with immovable indenters.*

a Simple plexiglass indentation funnel (original model) with which, depending on the position of the fingers, both static and kinetic examinations can be made (right). Similar model in steel (left).

b Indentation funnel (model by Haag-Streit) with two additional rings: (*1*) additional ring on the contact glass for the kinetic examination, (*2*) screw ring for fixing the contact glass in the funnel for the static examination.

c Indentation funnel with light conductor for diaphanoscopic examination

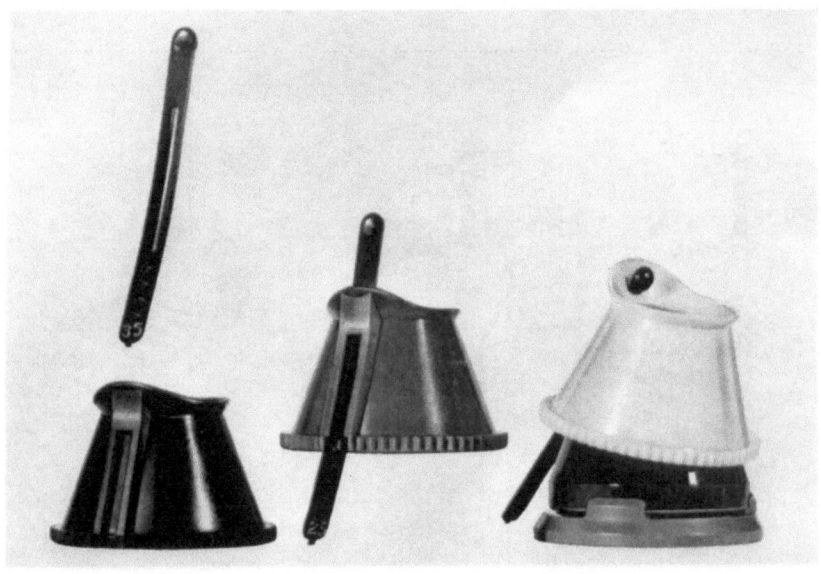

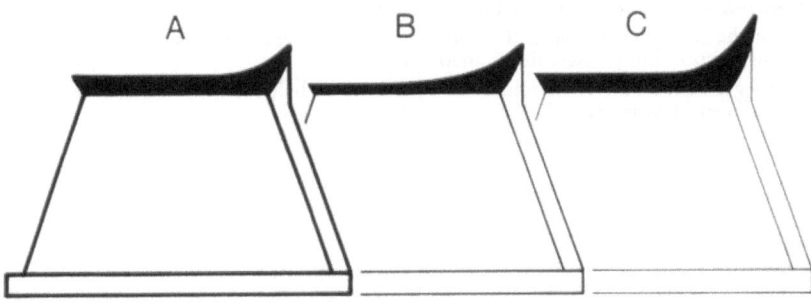

Fig. 13. *Indentation funnel with movable indenter* (Model by Huber-Stöckli).
The indenter is fixed on a flat spring. The latter is inserted along a guiding track on the indentation funnel and can be moved forward and backward. There are three types of funnel: *A* for normal eyes, *B* for narrow palpebral fissures, *C* for long myopic eyes

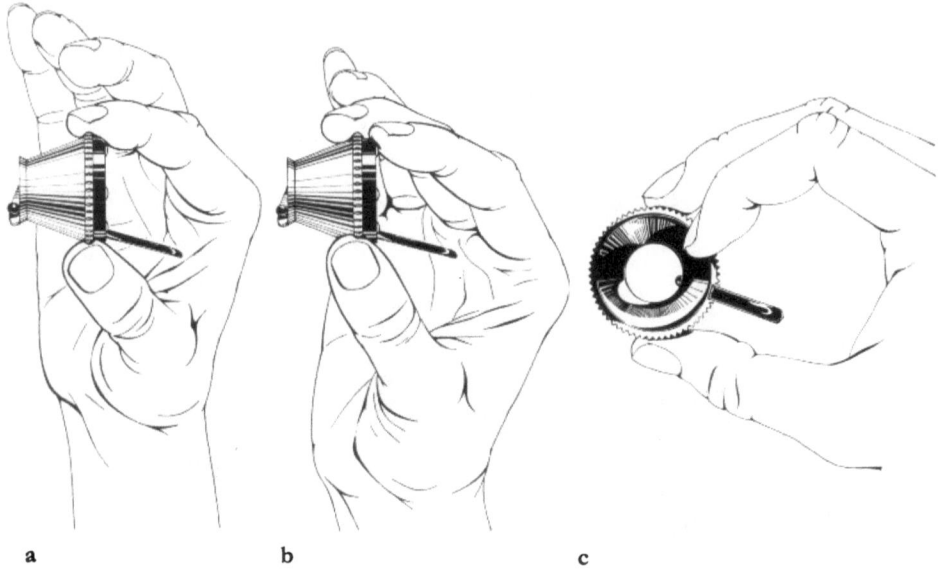

a   b   c

Fig. 14a–c. *Technique of manipulating the indentation funnel.*

a For the static examination, the contact glass and the funnel are held firmly together with the finger tips and rotated simultaneously.

b and c For the kinetic examination, the funnel is held with thumb and middle finger and the contact glass is rotated with the index finger

---

Fig. 15a–f. *Technique of inserting the indentation funnel into the palpebral fissure.*

a Application of a cotton tip to the upper eyelid with slight pressure against the bony orbital rim. The patient looks downwards.

b The cotton tip is rotated, thus raising the upper lid.

c Insertion of the empty funnel into the palpebral fissure. The indenter lies laterally towards the temporal angle of the eyelids.

d Now the funnel is situated correctly in the upper palpebral fissure.

e Application of the cotton tip to the lower eyelid with slight pressure against the inferior bony orbital rim.

f By rotating the cotton tip, the lower lid is pulled down. The patient looks straight ahead. The funnel now lies free in the palpebral fissure. Care must be taken that neither lid tissue nor cilia are trapped in its opening. Then the three-mirror contact glass is inserted

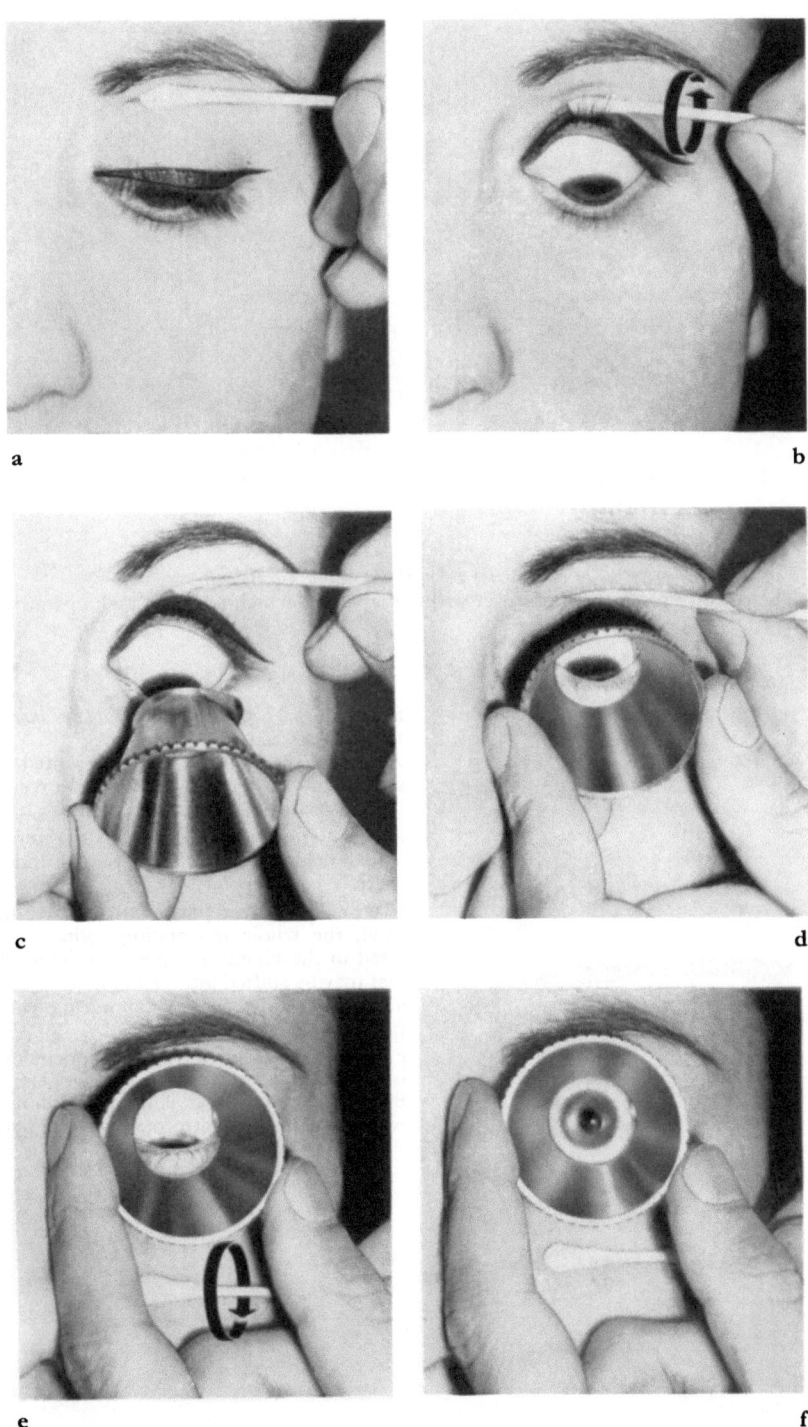

Fig. 15a–f. Legend see opposite page

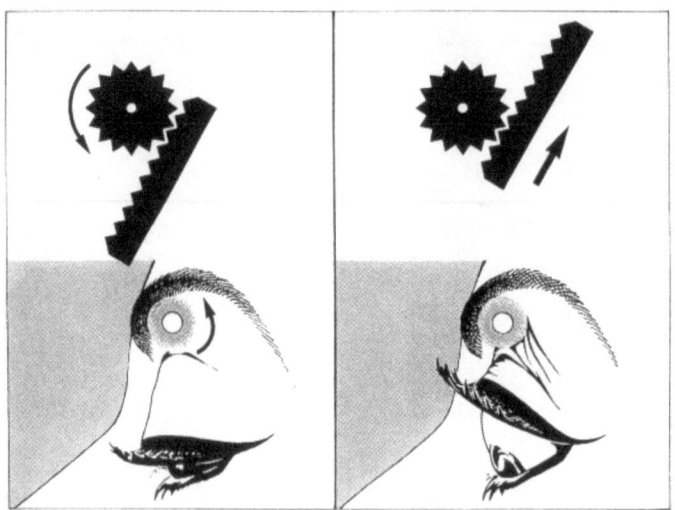

Fig. 16. *The principle of opening the lid with the aid of a cotton tip.*
The cotton tip may be compared with a cogwheel, which pushes a rack upwards by means of friction

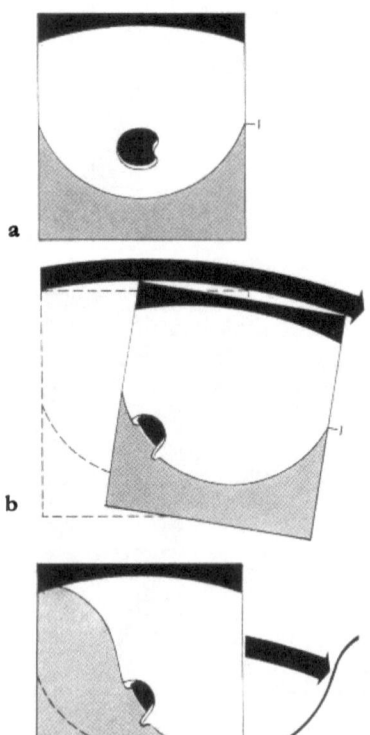

Fig. 17a–c. *Lateral movement of the indentation protuberance for kinetic examination.*
A tear in the retina may be presented in various states of indentation by a lateral movement alone (in a direction parallel to the limbus).

a Indentation protuberance in the centre of the visual field. In the middle of the indented area there is a retinal tear.

b When a contact glass with a fixed indenter is used, the whole indentation contact glass is rotated in the kinetic examination. Thus the retinal tear may be shifted into "silhouette", with the disadvantage, however, of appearing only on the periphery of the visual field.

c In kinetic examination with an indentation funnel, only the latter is shifted, the contact glass remaining fixed: the retinal tear is seen in silhouette while remaining in the centre of the visual field

I Indentation protuberance

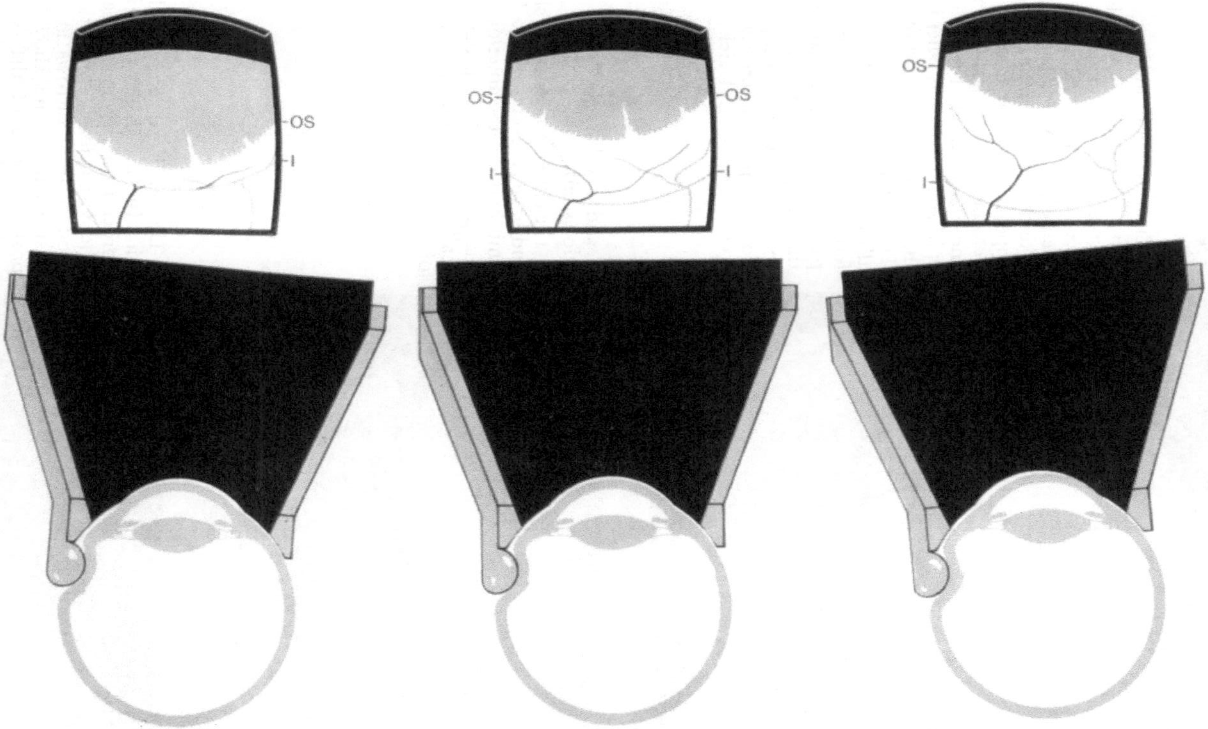

Fig. 18. *Displacement of the indentation protuberance in a meridional direction (i.e. anteriorly and posteriorly) with a fixed indenter.*
If the examination is performed with a fixed indenter, the position of the whole indentation contact glass must be changed with respect to the globe. For this purpose, either the contact glass is shifted on the surface of the bulbus, or the patient is asked to move his eye. The top row of drawings shows the effect obtained in the mirror by displacing the contact glass along the surface of the eye (lower row)

I Summit of indented area
OS Ora serrata

97

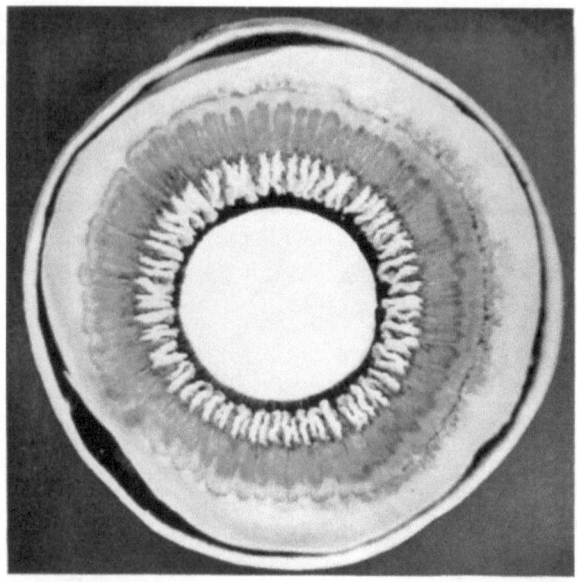

a

a Ciliary body in old age.
The ciliary processes are depigmented and corrugated with accessory processes between them. The anterior pars plana is dark, the posterior pars plana appears bright as a result of post-mortem changes (oedema and opacification of the ciliary epithelium, which is taller here than in the anterior pars plana). The anterior pars plana is equally broad in the whole circumference, while the posterior pars plana is nasally narrower than temporally. Striae ciliares (bright) extend from the posterior pars plana anteriorly. (By courtesy of Dr. B. Daicker.)

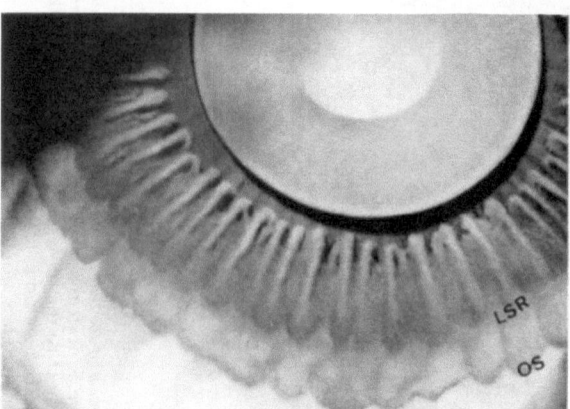

b

b and c Ciliary body of an adolescent.

b The ciliary processes are slim and have an even surface. The limit between the anterior and the posterior pars plana is a scalloped line, the linea serrata of the pars plana.

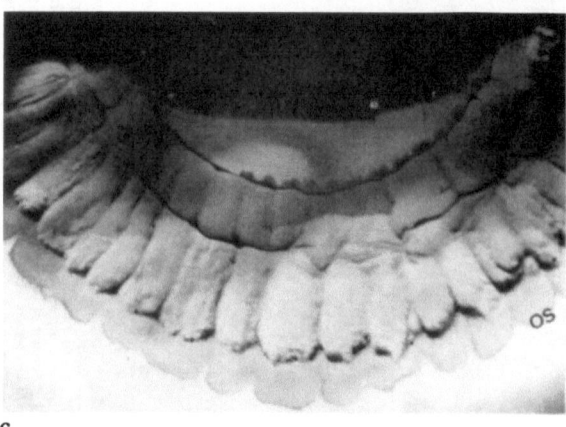

c

c The previtreal space is filled with Indian ink. Its posterior border is at the linea serrata. The vitreociliary connections produce deep furrows at the cristae ciliares and above the posterior third of the ciliary processes (ligamentum coronarium)

LSR Linea serrata
OS   Ora serrata

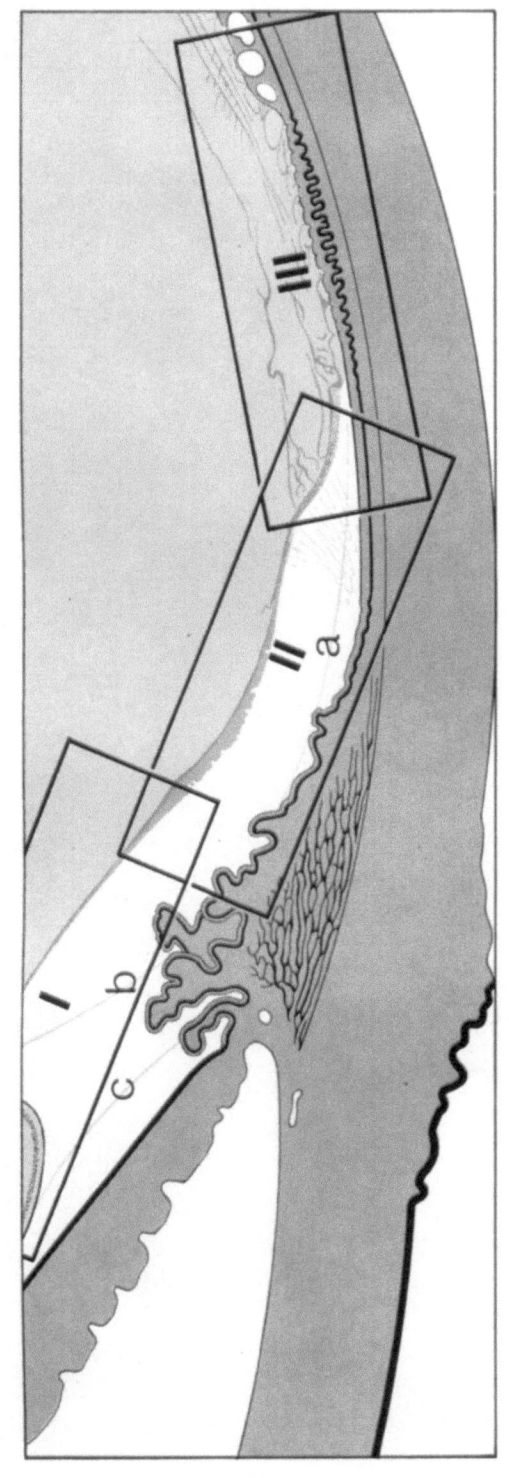

Fig. 20. *Histological section through the periphery of the fundus* (43-year-old woman, enucleation because of melanoma of the uvea). Phase-contrast microscope. Schematic drawing of the entire section, in which the position of the detail sections is marked *I, II, III* (see following pages).

a epiciliary zonular leaf; *b* posterior zonular leaf; *c* anterior zonular leaf

99

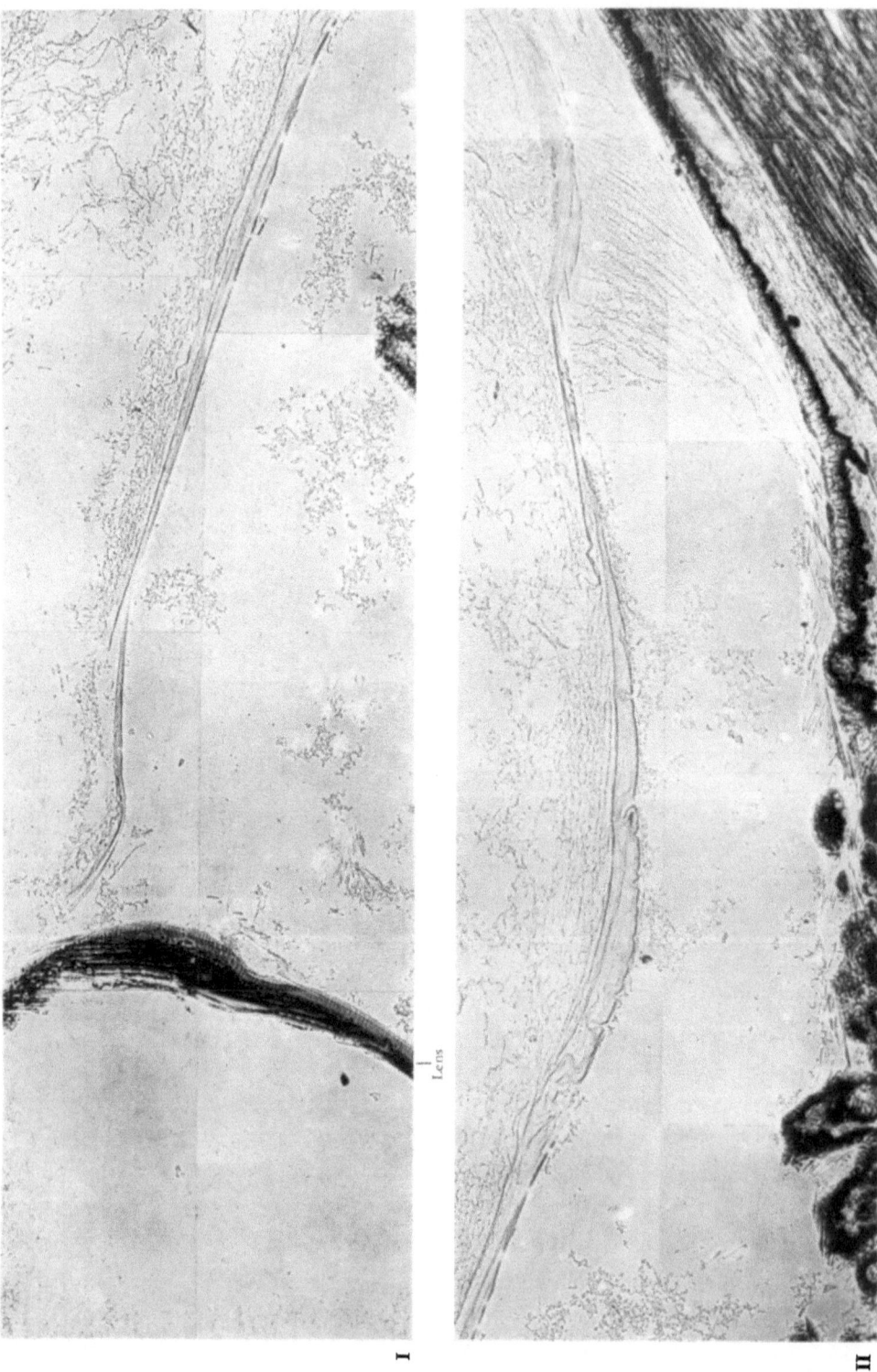

Lens

I

II

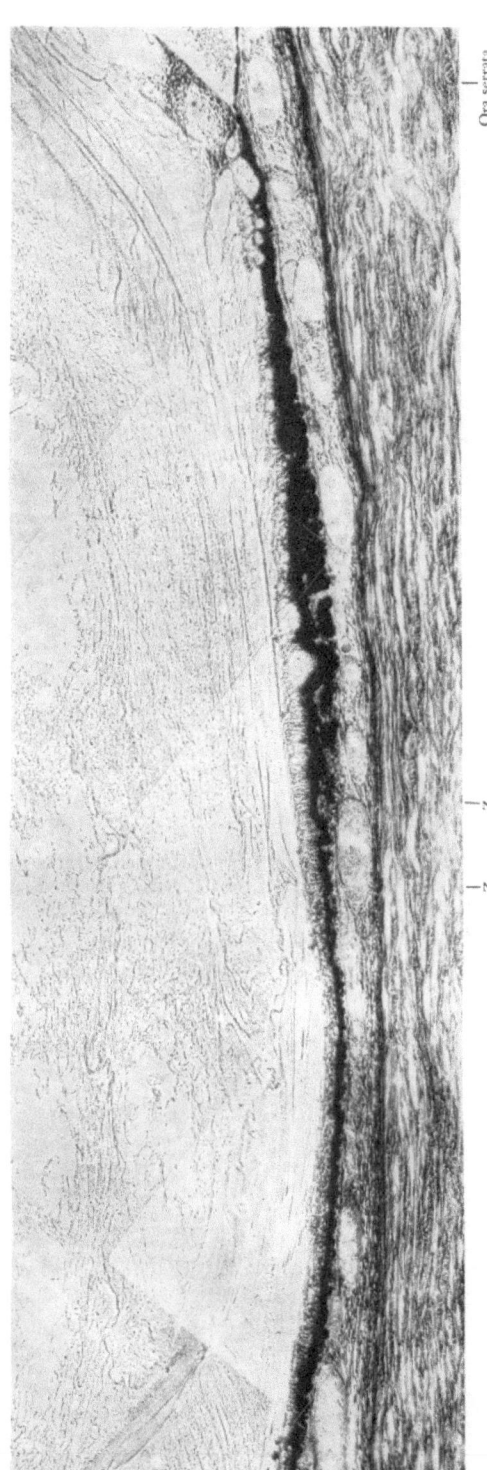

III

Ora serrata

Z_1 Z_2

Fig. 20. Section I—III

I *Perilenticular space.* The zonular fibres have been sectioned obliquely and are therefore visible only for short distances. The anterior vitreous cortex consists of parallel lamellae densely apposed to each other. Anteriorly and posteriorly it is clearly defined ("anterior hyaloid membrane"). Further lamellae coming from the central vitreous are apposed at the posterior surface. Towards the periphery the anterior vitreous cortex therefore continuously increases in thickness

II *Pars plicata and anterior parts of the pars plana of the ciliary body.* The single-layered ciliary epithelium overlies the dark pigment epithelium. In the *posterior part of the pars plicata*, flat cells are apposed on it ("covering cells" = Deckzellen, after Rohen [158]). Above them there are zonule fibres crossing each other ("tensing fibres" = Spannfasern, after Rohen [157]). The pars plana is covered by the zonule fibres of the epiciliary leaf. The anterior vitreous cortex forms a fairly broad layer here which is clearly defined towards the previtreal space; towards the vitreous cavity, however, there is no sharp borderline. In the region of the *ligamentum coronarium*, the anterior surface of the cortex is finely plicated. The circular zonule fibres of the ligamentum coronarium cannot be seen in this reproduction because of the low magnification

III *Pars plana of the ciliary body and ora serrata.* In the posterior pars plana the cells of the ciliary epithelium are taller and denser. The pigment epithelium follows the meshwork of Müller's reticulum, so that in the section it seems to proliferate into the choroid. Between the two epithelial layers there are several "cystic" cavities ("microcysts" of the pars plana). The vitreous cortex is now broad with the framework disintegrated, and no sharp borderline is to be seen either towards the outside or towards the inside. In the region of the *ligamentum medianum* zonular fibres form peaked extensions towards the pars plana. One of these extensions obviously originates from a marginal area (Z_1), a second one (lying somewhat further to the right and at the top of the picture) branches off from layers of the cortex further inwards (Z_2). In the same region the membranelles of the *tractus medianus* join the vitreous cortex. At the *ora serrata* the inner border of the retina is extended anteriorly (spiculae of the ora) [32]. The retina is detached and contains rather large cystoid cavities. Posterior to the ora serrata the retina is covered by the posterior vitreous cortex. The vitreous membranelles are parallel to the retina here; they are crossed by fibres which are inserted on the retinal surface at right angles

101

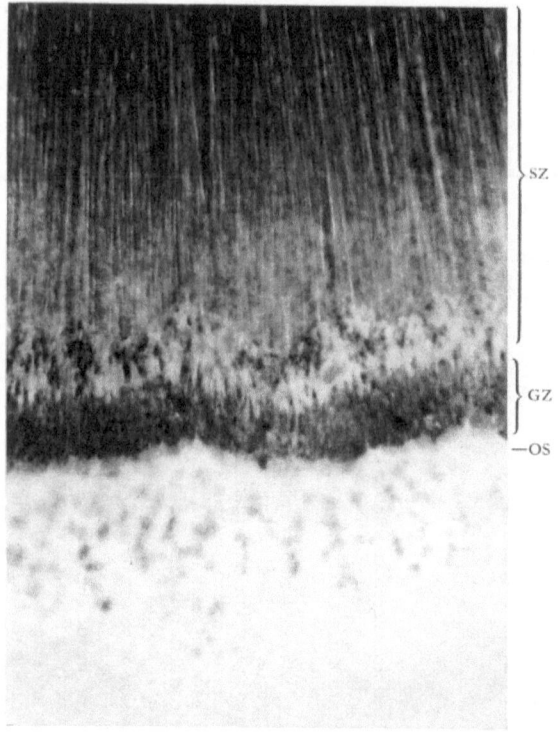

SZ

GZ

—OS

Fig. 21. *Epiciliary zonule.* Anterior to the linea serrata there are fine fibres arranged parallel to each other, forming a dense layer above the pars plana. The surface of the posterior pars plana lying behind it is irregularly granular. In the peripheral retina there are coarse cystoid cavities. (By courtesy of Dr. B. Daicker)

Fig. 22a and b. *Ligamentum medianum.* In the midst of the pars plana, a strand of circular fibres passes across the fibres of the epiciliary leaf. a Low magnification, b higher magnification
(By courtesy of Dr. B. Daicker)

CP   Ciliary processes
GZ   Granular zone
OS   Ora serrata
SZ   Striate zone

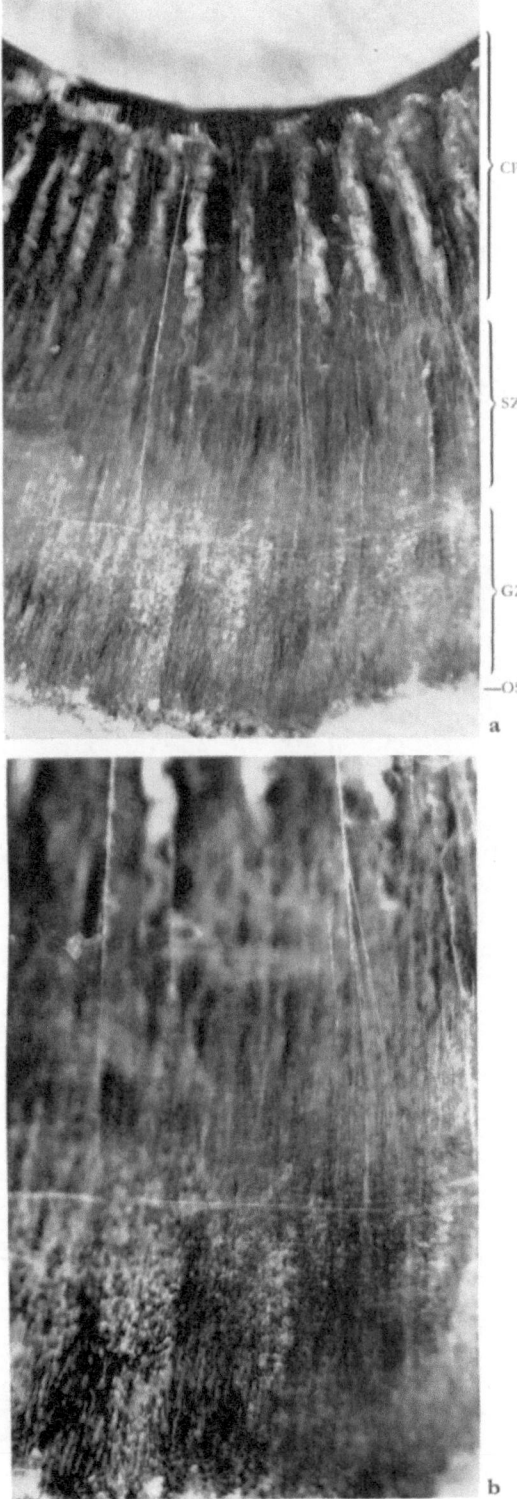

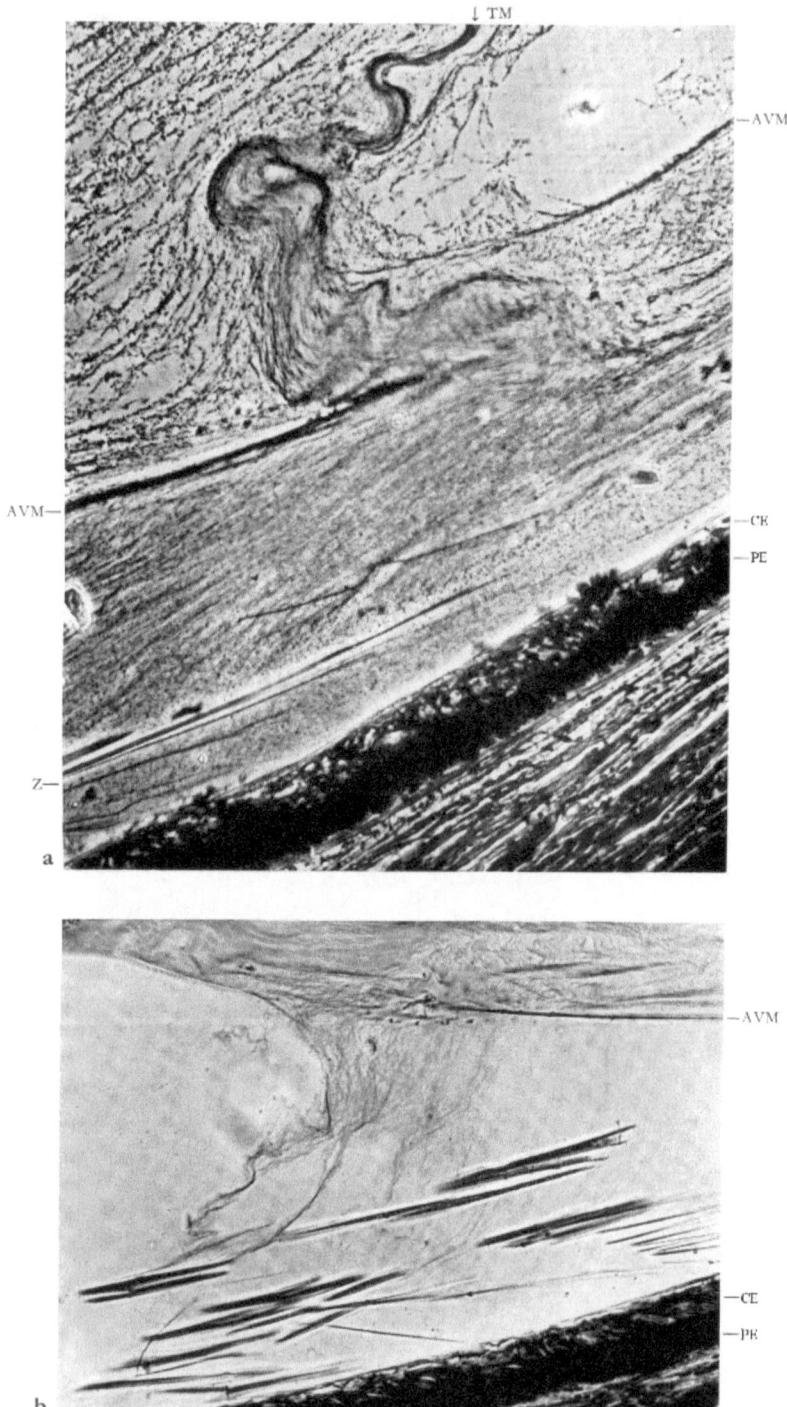

Fig. 23a and b. Legend see opposite page

Fig. 23 a and b. *Ligamentum medianum, histological section.* The picture of histological sections through the ligamentum medianum varies according to the plane of section.

a Insertion of the tractus medianus in the region of the ligamentum medianum (same specimen as in Fig. 20).

b Vitreous processes from the ligamentum medianum to the ciliary body. The fibres of the circular zonule band that are sectioned at a right angle appear as black dots. From here loose vitreous fibres extend between the zonule fibres of the epiciliary leaf on their way to the ciliary epithelium. (By courtesy of Dr. B. Daicker)

Fig. 24. *Vitreous body. Schematic drawing of the division into zones:*
a Posterior vitreous cortex, ending at the ora serrata.
b Central vitreous.
c Central canal limited anteriorly by the posterior surface of the lens

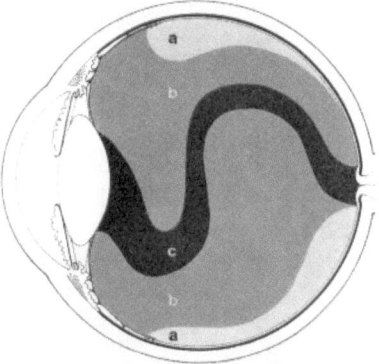

Fig. 25 a and b. *Schematic drawing of the variations of the tractus vitreales.*

a *S-shaped course.* The individual "fibres" of the tractus vitreales are curved in an S-shaped course, first sinking downwards behind the lens, then rising slightly upward in the centre of the vitreous body, then reaching the papilla. The individual fibres appear to be twisted spirally round the axis of the S-shaped tractus hyaloideus.

b *Retrolental folding.* In the anterior sections the tractus vitreales are folded in the form of a Z

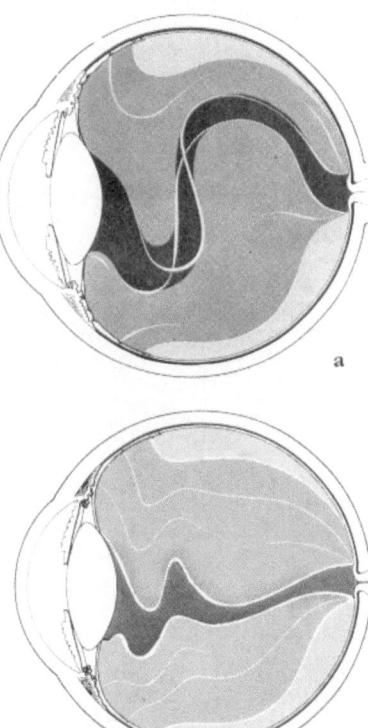

AVM	Anterior hyaloid membrane
CE	Ciliary epithelium
PE	Pigment epithelium
TM	Tractus medianus
Z	Zonule

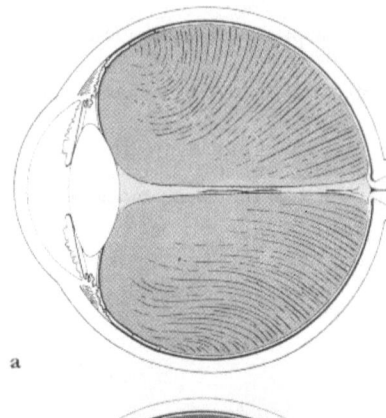

a

Fig. 26a–c. *Development of vitreous structure.*

a Newborn. There is a relatively homogeneous pattern of radial "fibres". Cloquet's canal is still present.

b Adolescent. In the anterior sections the vitreal tracts are already formed, and there is a subdivision into cortex and semifluid central vitreous. The posterior sections have retained the infantile radial pattern.

c Adult. Tractus vitreales traverse the vitreous space

TC	Tractus coronarius
TH	Tractus hyaloideus
TM	Tractus medianus
TP	Tractus praeretinalis

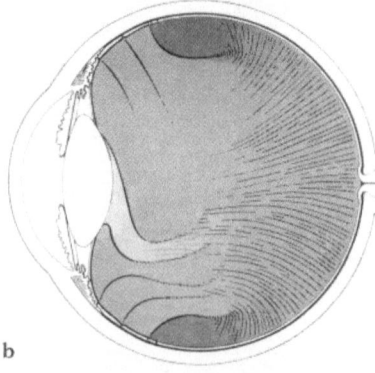

b

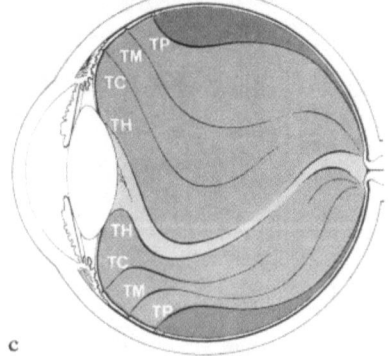

c

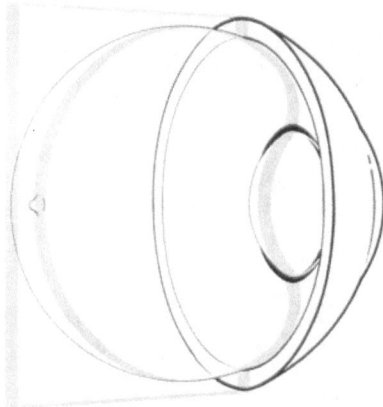

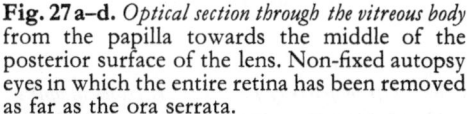

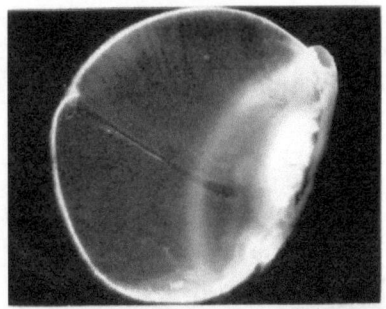

a

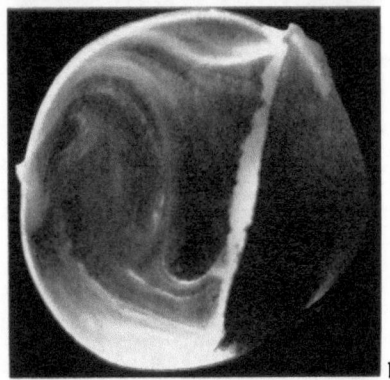

b

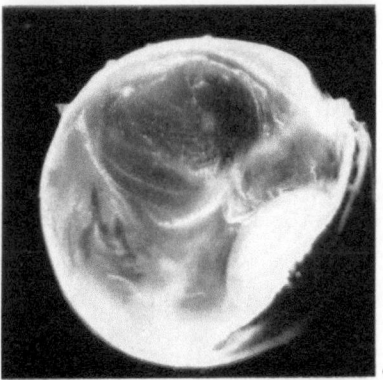

c

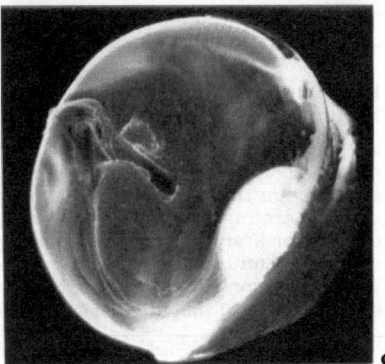

d

Fig. 27 a–d. *Optical section through the vitreous body* from the papilla towards the middle of the posterior surface of the lens. Non-fixed autopsy eyes in which the entire retina has been removed as far as the ora serrata.

a 7-month-old child. The vitreous body appears almost homogeneous. The tractus vitreales are not developed and there is no division into the typical zones. There is a pattern of a fine parallel striation, the "fibres" running perpendicularly from the retina towards the centre of the globe. Cloquet's canal is a narrow, optically empty tube in which there is still a filiform residuum of the hyaloid artery.

b 40-year-old man. Tractus vitreales with S-shaped course (see Fig. 26a). The vitreous cortex is delimited from the central vitreous by the preretinal tract. The tractus medianus is scarcely visible in the upper half of the globe; in the lower half it appears as an opacified strip above the tractus praeretinalis. The tractus hyaloideus contains in its anterior parts brightly reflecting "fibres".

c 35-year-old man. Retrolental folding of the tractus vitreales (see Fig. 26b). The framework of the central vitreous is destroyed in the upper half of the globe. The tractus medianus is not a membranella there but forms a rather coarse meshwork. In the lower half, however, it is still a typical membranule overlying the tractus praeretinalis. The tractus hyaloideus runs in an almost straight path, except for the Z-like folding behind the lens.

d 60-year-old man. Pronounced fibrous destruction of the vitreous framework. The inner tractus vitreales form a rather coarse fibrous network which traverses the vitreous space in the typical S-shaped curve. The tractus praeretinalis and the vitreous cortex are still intact

107

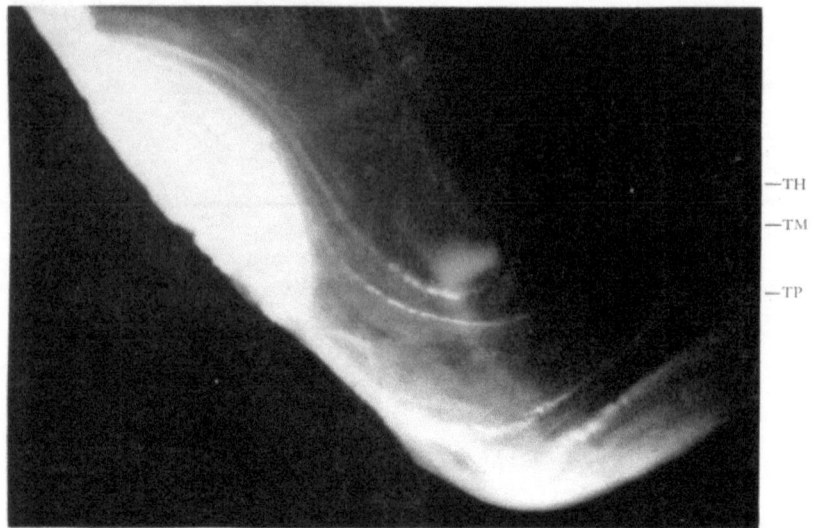

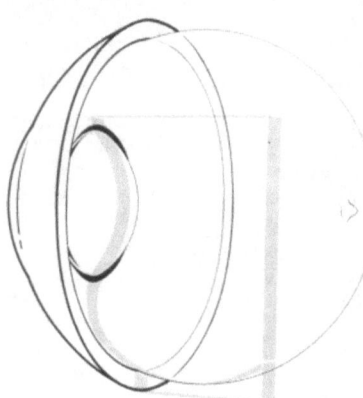

—TH

—TM

—TP

Fig. 28. *Anterior parts of the tractus vitreales in optical section* (same specimen as in Fig. 27 b). Sagittal section (see diagram). The lens with a Mittendorf's dot is on the left of the picture. The pars plicata of the ciliary body is hidden from view. The slit beam above the ciliary epithelium is seen only in the region of the pars plana, which bulges slightly interiorly. Just below the lens, the anterior hyaloid membrane arches posteriorly. From the posterior surface of the lens the tractus hyaloideus runs downwards. The tractus coronarius is only faintly visible. The tractus medianus runs towards the middle of the pars plana, the tractus praeretinalis to the ora serrata

Fig. 30 a and b. *Vitreous cortex and tractus praeretinalis.* ▶
Region of the equator, oblique light incidence from below (autopsy eye).

a Optical section. At right angles to the vitreous surface (*A*) there are parallel "fibres" running perpendicularly and at regular intervals towards the tractus praeretinalis (*TP*); at that point they are deflected, continuing in the form of loose, wavy bands towards the vitreous centre, thus creating the spiral-shaped structures of the central vitreous. When observation beam and slit beam are at right angles, dispersion phenomena produce maximum brightness and the vitreous cortex appears as a rather opaque substance. Under biomicroscopy conditions, however, there is a small angle between the observation beam and the slit beam, so that the vitreous cortex appears practically transparent.

b Wide slit beam: plicated reflexes on the exterior surface of the vitreous (*A*) and on the tractus praeretinalis

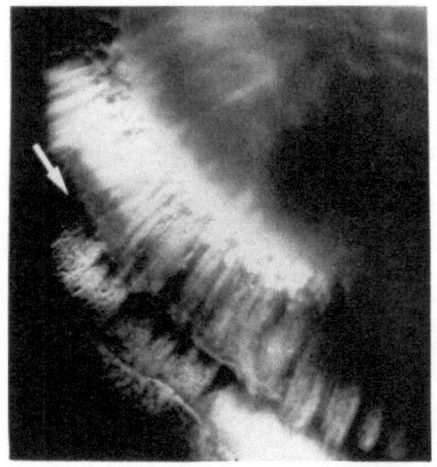
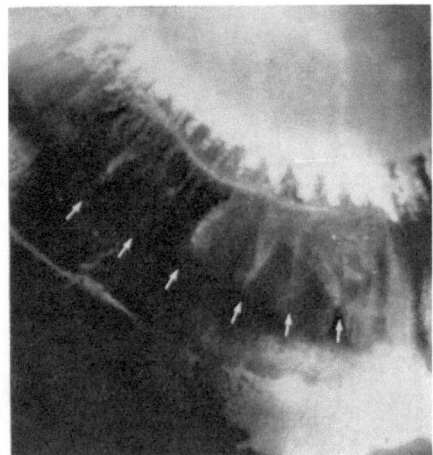

a   b

Fig. 29a and b. *Tractus medianus seen from above* (autopsy eye). Wide slit beam, incident from above right.

a The insertion line of the tractus medianus runs along the middle of the pars plana, crossing the teeth of the linea serrata (arrow). Since the tractus medianus, which arches anteriorly, is more opaque, the anterior sections of the ciliary body are veiled while the posterior pars plana appears more distinct in the picture.

b When the slit beam is moved slightly anteriorly, there appear in the tractus medianus strands which reflect more strongly (arrows). These silky, shining strands correspond to the meridional axis of the linea serrata bays

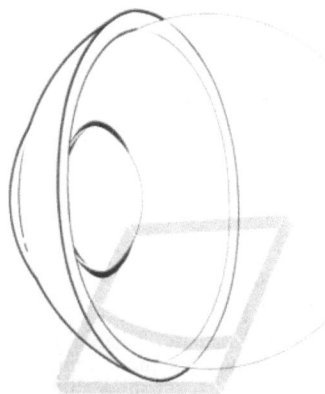

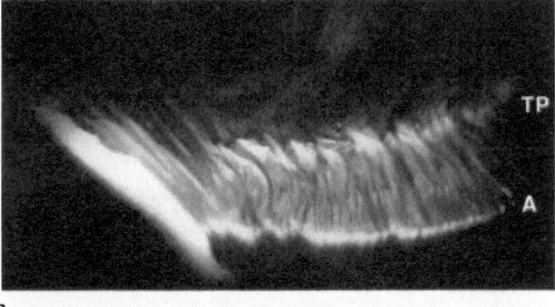

a

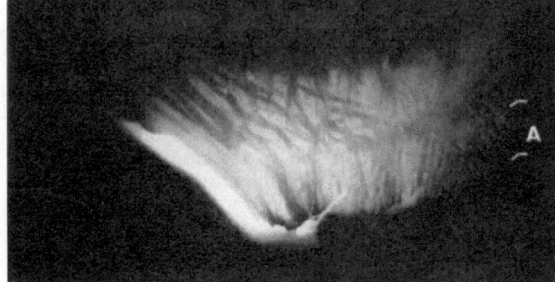

b

Fig. 30a and b. Legend see opposite page

A   surface of vitreous body
TH   Tractus hyaloideus
TM   Tractus medianus
TP   Tractus praeretinalis

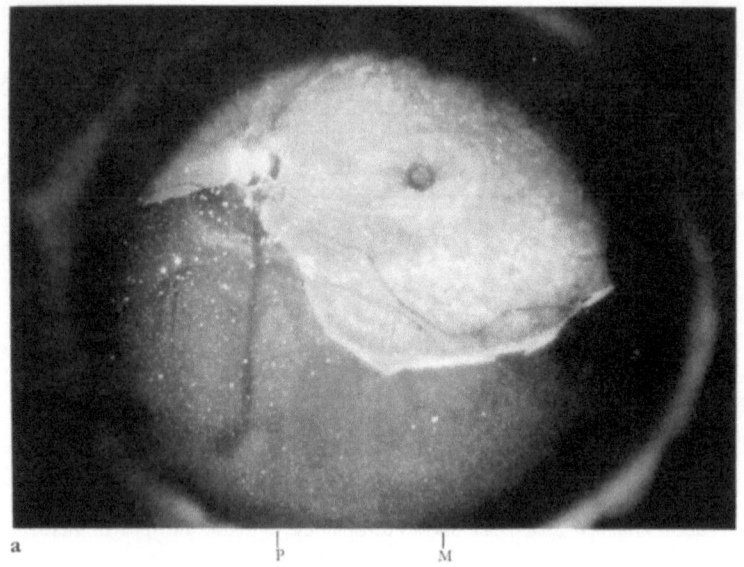

a ‎ P ‎ M

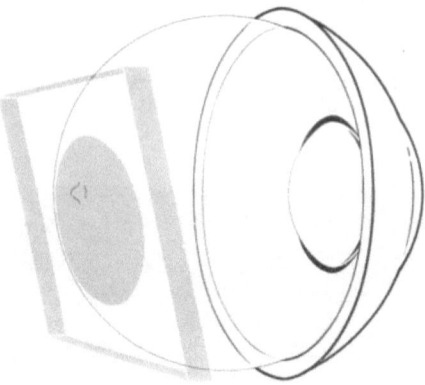

Fig. 31a and b. *Holes in the vitreous cortex at the posterior pole* (autopsy eye).

a Posterior pole of the vitreous in diffuse illumination. In the upper half the "membrana limitans interna" is still adherent to the vitreous body. It appears slightly opaque in diffuse illumination. Where it is thin, it is more transparent and the black background shines through. The macula region (*M*),the region of the papilla (*P*) and the vessels therefore appear dark. In the lower half the vitreous cortex is uncovered.

b By an inclination of the slit beam from posterior above towards anterior below (see diagram) the vitreous cortex is optically sectioned in the lower half of the picture; the cortex holes are transparent and appear as black spots. The prepapillary hole and the prefoveal hole appear behind the corresponding attenuations of the "inner limiting membrane". The other two holes (left in picture) are enlargements of prevascular fissures

110

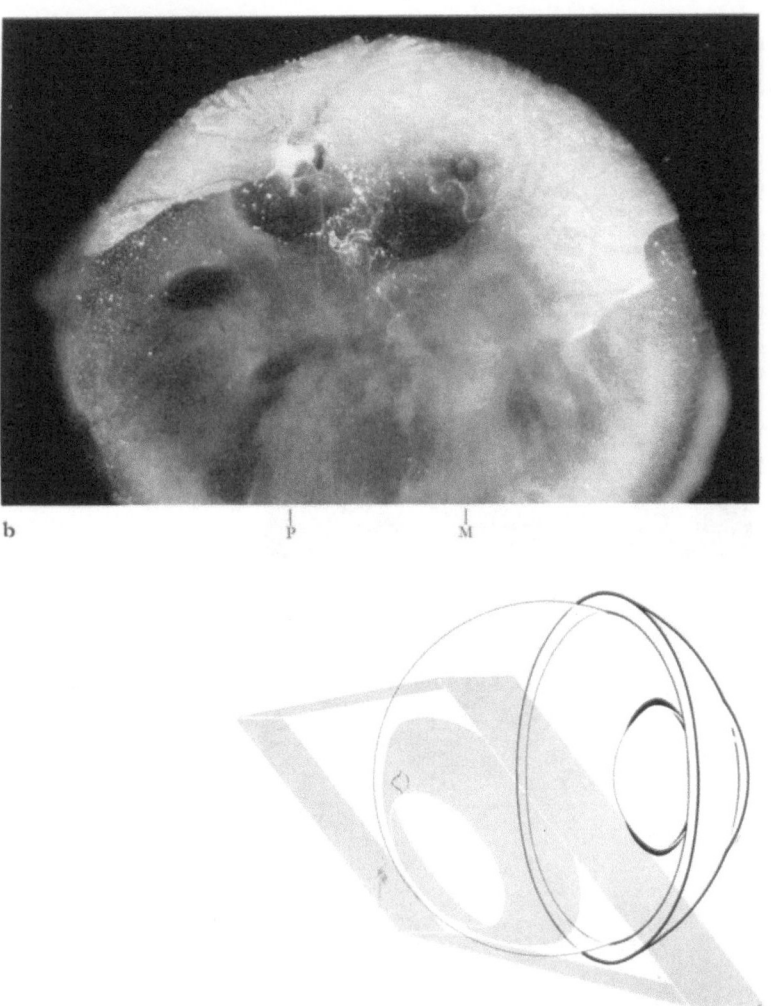

b   P   M

Fig. 31 b. Legend see opposite page

P   Papilla region
M   Macula region

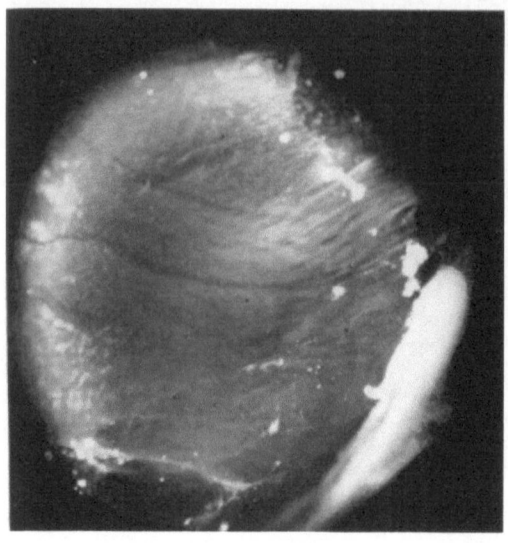

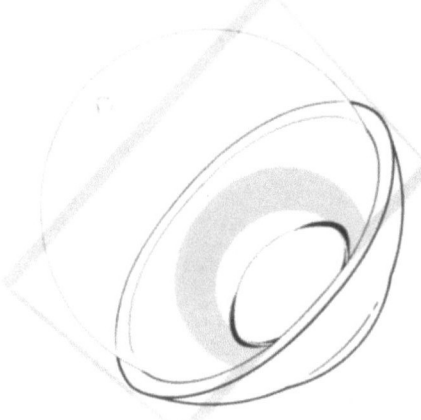

Fig. 32. *Prevascular fissure in the vitreous cortex* (autopsy eye).
Parasagittal wide slit beam through the nasal equatorial region (see diagram). Left in the picture the slit beam forms a bright crescent on the surface of the vitreous. Attenuated zones, caused by the retinal vessels, appear there as dark striae. In the centre of the picture, the entire thickness of the cortex is optically sectioned and hence the prevascular fissures can be seen penetrating into the deeper-lying parts of the cortex

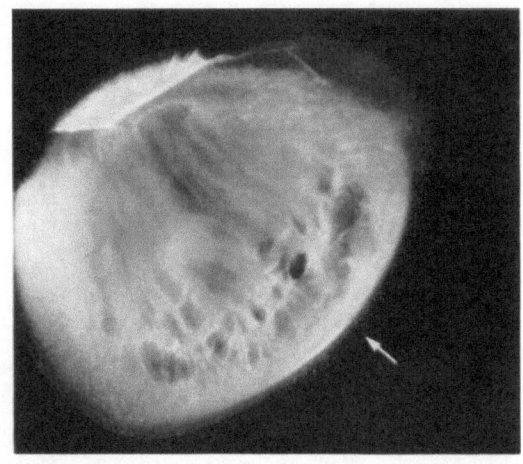

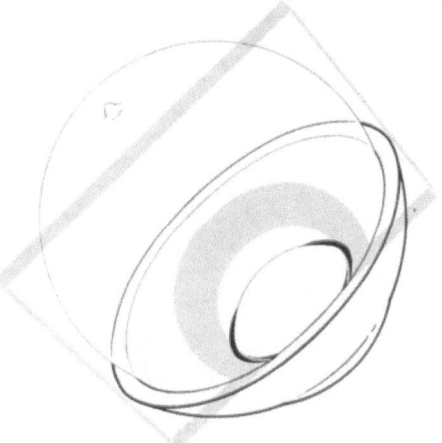

Fig. 33. *Cortex holes at developmental variations of the ora serrata* (autopsy eye). Parasagittal wide slit beam (see diagram).

Anomalies of the ora serrata are not visible here, since they were removed from the vitreous, together with the retina. The vitreous cortex here does not display its normal homogeneous pattern, but is pierced by several circular holes corresponding to ora bays and meridional ridges. The most apparent hole (arrow) corresponds to an enclosed ora bay

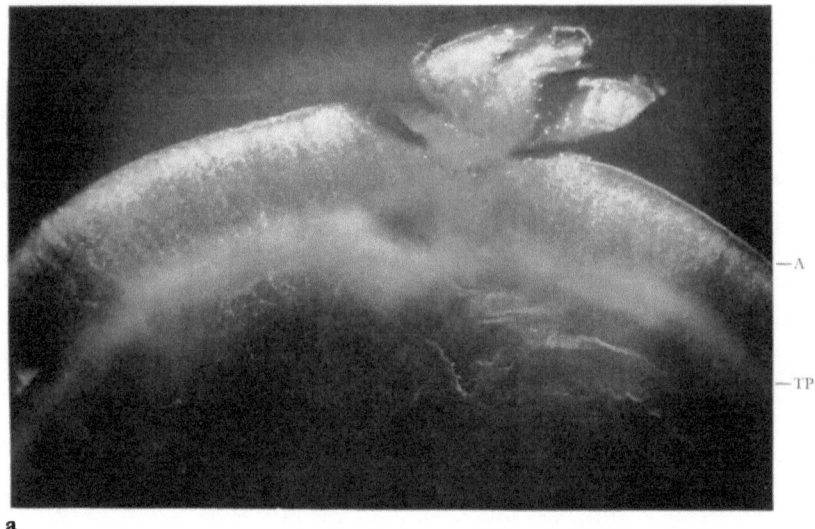

—A

—TP

a

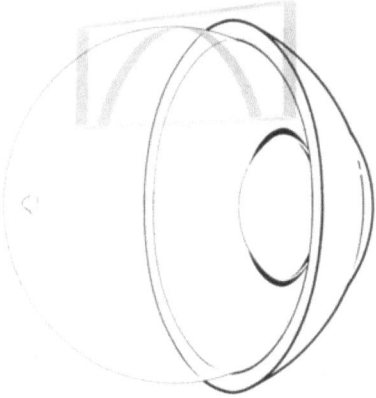

Fig. 34a and b. *Injuries of the vitreous cortex* (autopsy eye).

a With scissors a piece was cut out of the broad equatorial vitreous cortex. It has kept its shape and can be re-inserted in the defect. As long as the cortex is not cut right through its entire thickness, there is no prolapse of semi-fluid vitreous, and the pattern of the tractus vitreales is not changed.

b In the region of the prefoveal hole, a gentle touch with a pointed object is sufficient to cause a large defect. The central vitreous prolapses immediately, and consequently the vitreous globe collapses. The formerly S-shaped tractus vitreales now run straight to the site of the perforation

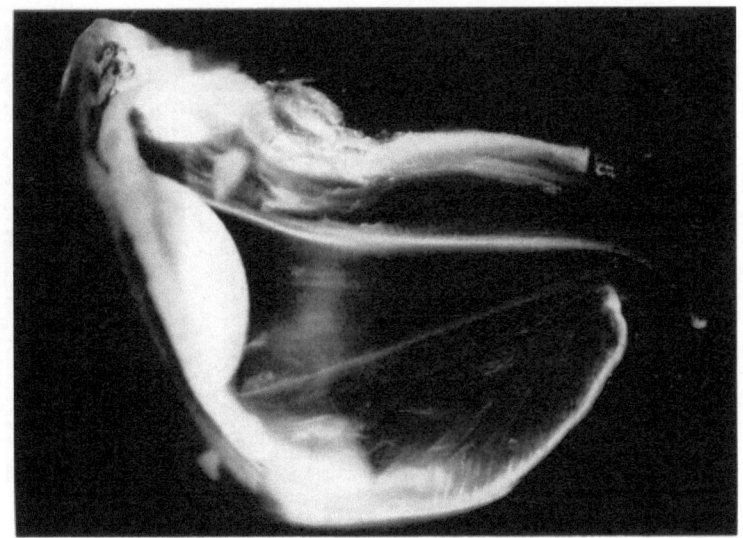

b

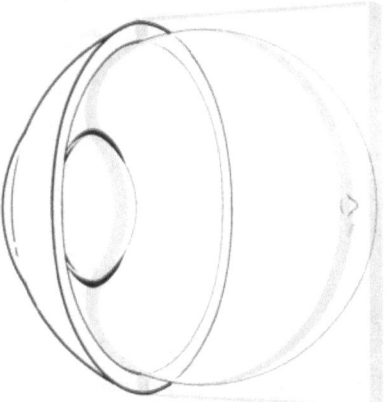

Fig. 34 b. Legend see opposite page

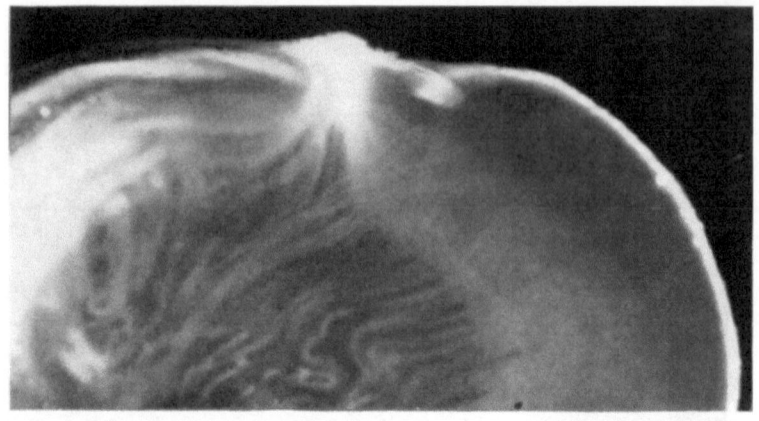

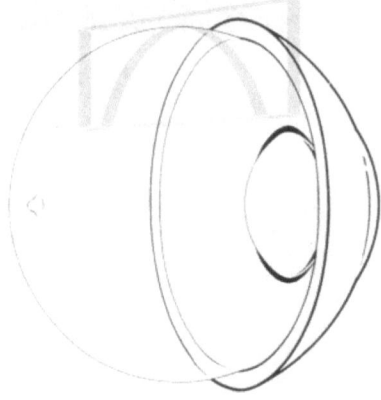

Fig. 35. *Cortex holes at chorioretinal scars* (autopsy eye).

In contrast to the constitutional holes, which appear to be cut out of an intact cortex, the surrounding cortex is condensed around the "secondary" hole shown here. The lamellae, normally parallel to the surface of the vitreous cortex, converge towards the edges of the scar, forming an adhering "fibrosis" there

Presentation of drawings of the peripheral fundus in the following figures

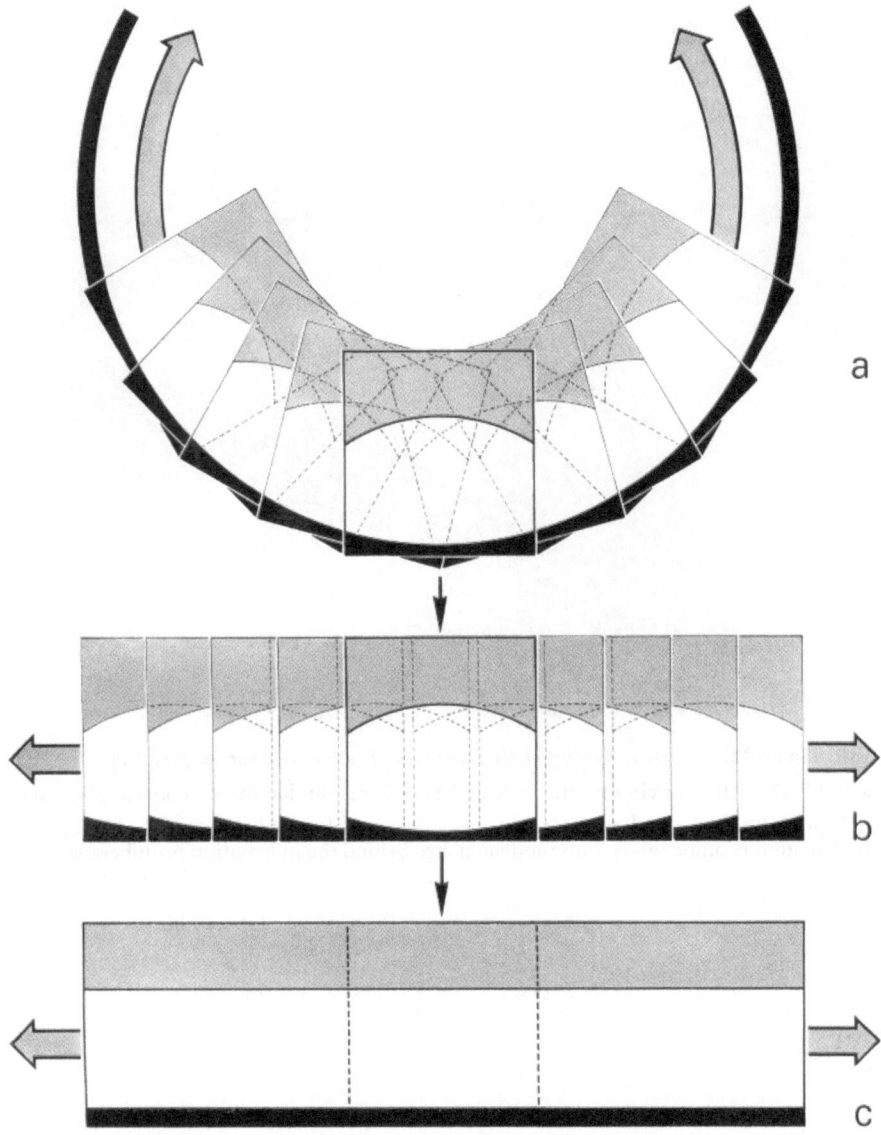

In the pictures, the position of the indentation protuberance is, with a few exceptions, always at the bottom. The actual position of the area depicted is mentioned in the text.

The incidence of the slit-beam is indicated by an arrow

Composite drawings are presented either in a semicircle (a), or in a linear extension (b), the summits of the protuberances then forming a straight line (c)

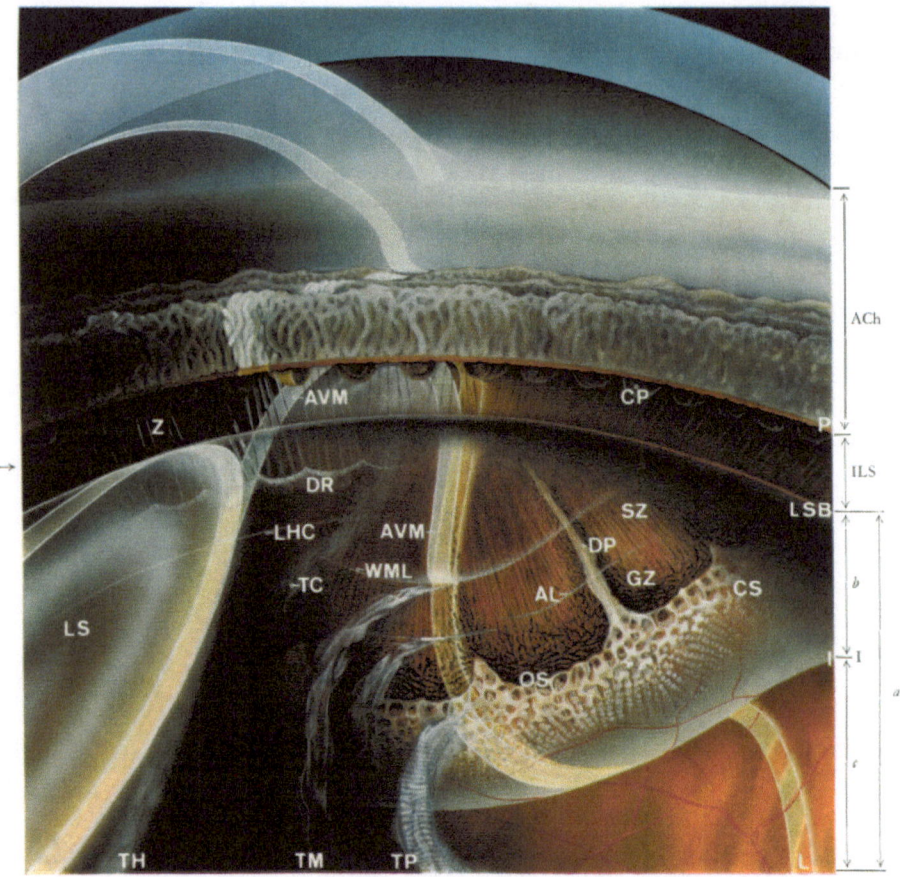

Fig. 36a and b. *Schematic drawing of the biomicroscopic aspect of a normal periphery.*

a Semi-schematic drawing of the indented peripheral fundus in the contact glass mirror.

b Sagittal section through the indented area. *a* Section observed translentally, *b* indented area (indentation protuberance), *c* non-indented area behind the indentation protuberance

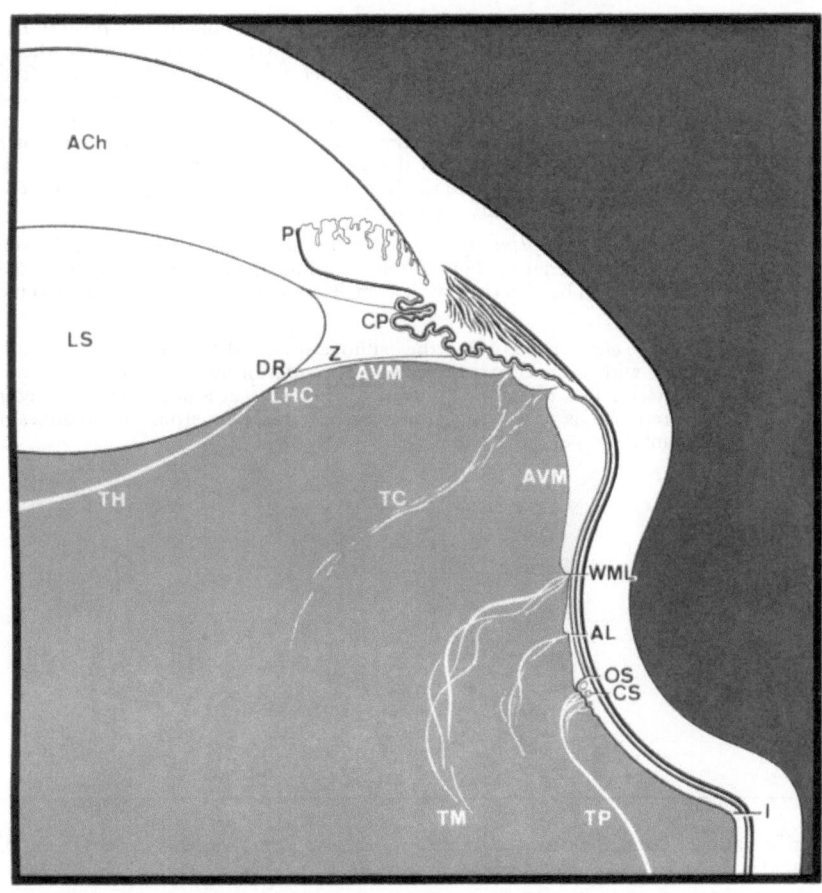

Fig. 36b. Legend see opposite page

ACh	Anterior chamber	LS	Lens
AL	Accessory line	LSB	Lens border
AVM	Anterior vitreous (hyaloid) membrane	OS	Ora serrata
CP	Ciliary processes	P	Pupillary border
CS	Cystoid spaces	SZ	Striate zone
DP	Dentate processes of the ora serrata	TC	Tractus coronarius
DR	Dentate reflex	TH	Tractus hyaloideus
GZ	Granular zone	TM	Tractus medianus
I	Summit or border of indented area	TP	Tractus praeretinalis
ILS	Iridolenticular space	WML	White midline
L	Light of wide slit beam	Z	Zonule
LHC	Ligamentum hyalocapsulare		

Fig. 37 a–c. *Normal fundus periphery. Various positions of the indenter* (R. K., 30 years of age).

a *Indentation of the posterior pars plicata of the ciliary body.* The middle and posterior parts of the ciliary processes appear in the picture. They are pressed deeply against the anterior hyaloid membrane. The latter is stretched out over them and folded. These folds exist only during indentation. At the summit of the protuberance there is the anterior pars plana, which is covered by the fibres of the epiciliary zonule leaf (best visible at left edge of picture). The white midline is posterior to the indented area. Up to this point, the anterior hyaloid membrane is clearly visible. Posterior to the white midline it appears only as an extremely fine line. In the vitreous body there are the bright membranelles of the tractus praeretinalis, the tractus medianus and the tractus coronarius.

b *Indentation of the middle pars plana region.* The white midline now appears on the silhouette of the indentation protuberance. The anterior hyaloid membrane is visible also further posteriorly, as far as it can be observed with a small angle of acceptance (tangential incidence of light).

c *Indentation of the ora serrata.* On the silhouette of the indentation protuberance the retinal border with cystoid spaces appears. The anterior hyaloid membrane is no longer visible on the anterior face of the protuberance when seen at a large angle of acceptance. the tractus praeretinalis is inserted at the ora serrata. Numerous micro-adhesions are visible in the granular zone

---

Fig. 38 a and b. *Normal fundus in a female Caucasian with slight skin pigmentation* (D. G., 35 years of age).

a Nasally: Deep indentation: The pars plana appears on the anterior face of the indentation protuberance. From the ora serrata two long teeth extend anteriorly. The border of the retina is edged with cystoid spaces. The pars plana is altogether darker than the region of the retina lying behind it. The very dark posterior pars plana is narrow and has a granular surface structure. In the striate zone the blurred outlines of large uveal vessels can be discerned. The white midline is clearly visible only on the sides of the indentation protuberance. Of the tractus medianus only isolated striate opacities can be seen. The tractus praeretinalis is well developed, separating into several lamellae.

b Temporally: The indentation is not as deep as in Fig. a. There are no ora teeth, and the retinal border is only slightly scalloped. The granular zone extends to the summit of the protuberance and is seen with a small angle of acceptance. It is broad and its surface has an irregular structure. The white midline is clearly visible as a white fibrous band. At this band there are inserted several densified strands of the tractus medianus. The latter otherwise appears only as an extremely delicate membranelle. At an accessory line, immediately anterior to the ora serrata, there are further vitreous membranelles inserted. The tractus praeretinalis is inserted at the ora serrata

---

AL	Accessory line		TC	Tractus coronarius
AVM	Anterior vitreous (hyaloid) membrane		TM	Tractus medianus
I	Summit or border of indented area		TP	Tractus praeretinalis
L	Light of slit beam on retina and ciliary body		WML	White midline
OS	Ora serrata			

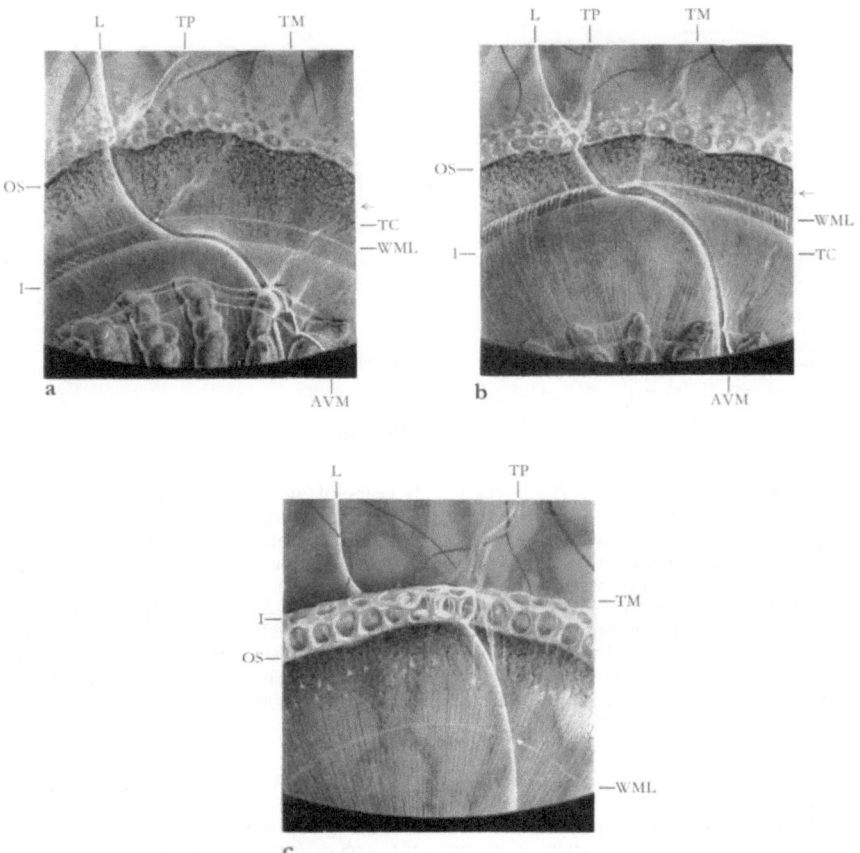

Fig. 37a–c. Legend see opposite page

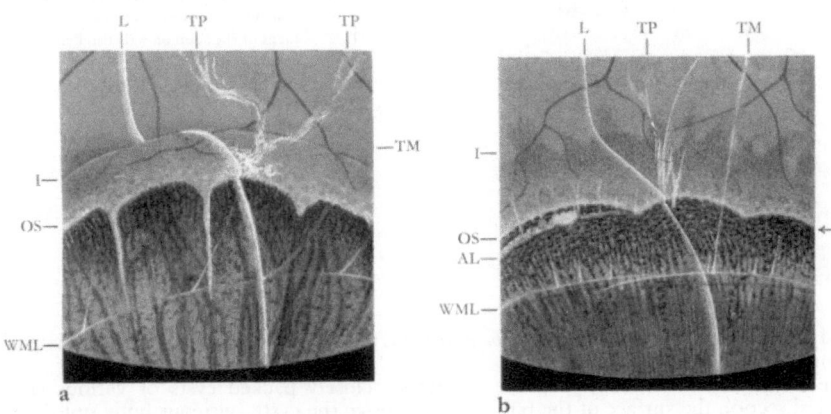

Fig. 38a and b. Legends see opposite page

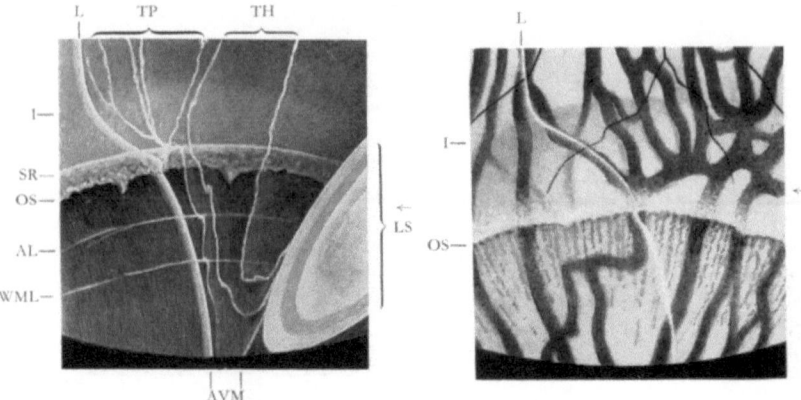

Fig. 39.   **Fig. 40.**

Fig. 39. *Normal fundus in a male Negro* (G.K., 27 years of age, upper fundus periphery).
Against the darkly pigmented background the zones of discontinuity of the vitreous body
form a particularly strong contrast. The anterior hyaloid membrane extends from its lens
attachment directly towards the ciliary processes (not visible here). It then re-appears
upon the indentation protuberance running over the pars plana to the ora serrata. At the
white midline and at an accessory line a fold is formed in it. Anterior to the ora serrata,
it bends in a sharp curve towards the retinal border, a silhouette reflex occurring at this bulge.
From the lens the tractus hyaloideus proceeds posteriorly in two fairly large membranelles.
The tractus medianus and the tractus coronarius cannot be seen. The tractus praeretinalis
separates into several lamellae. It is inserted together with the anterior hyaloid membrane
at the retinal border

Fig. 40. *Fundus periphery in a case of partial albinism* (A.C., 38 years of age, upper fundus
periphery).
The eye is not entirely free of pigment, since there is a slight pigmentation of the posterior
layer of the iris. In the fundus there is no pigment, except for a narrow band anterior to
the ora serrata. No retinal or vitreous structures can be discerned owing to the intense
reflected light

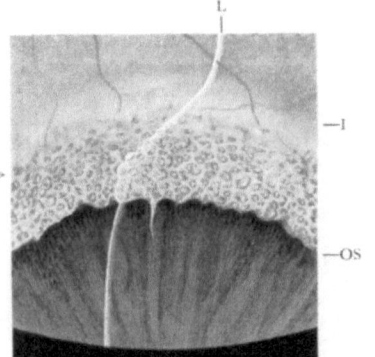

AL	Accessory line
AVM	Anterior vitreous (hyaloid) membrane
I	Summit or border of indented area
L	Light of slit beam on retina and ciliary body
LS	Lens
OS	Ora serrata
P	Pupillary border
SR	Silhouette reflex
TH	Tractus hyaloideus
TP	Tractus praeretinalis
WML	White midline

Fig. 41. *Broad belt of peripheral cysts in the retina* (G.R., 62 years of age, upper fundus periphery).
In the entire circumference there are numerous closely packed cysts of various sizes.
In optical section the surface of the retina bulges above the cysts (vitreous body not drawn
in the picture)

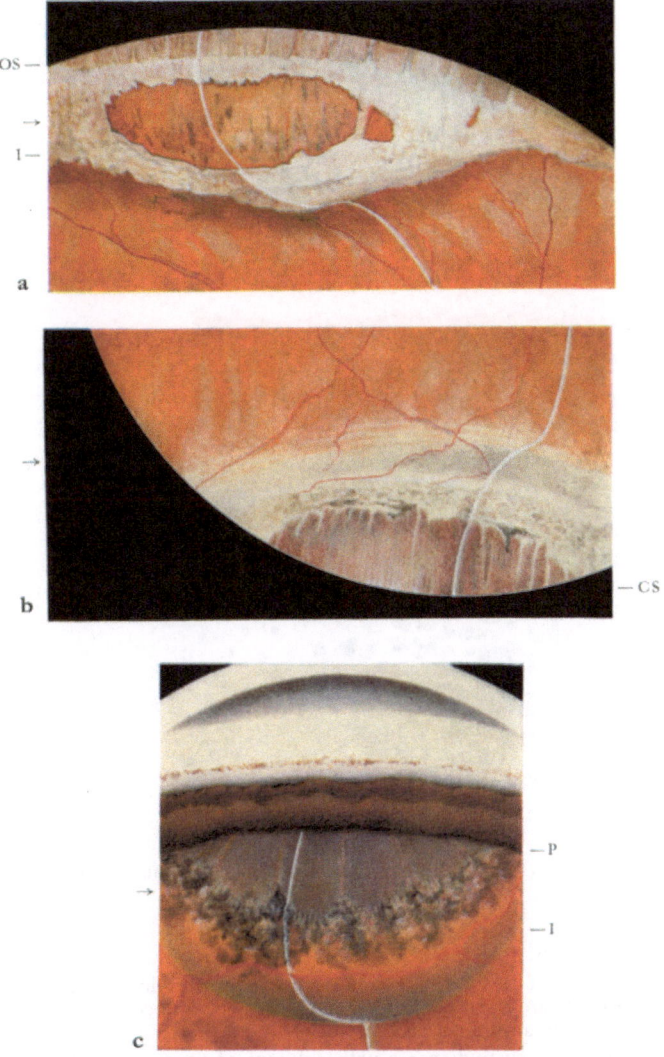

Fig. 42a–c. *Unilateral belt of retinal cysts with retinal defect* (R.S., 36 years of age). Brown corpuscles accidentally discovered in the vitreous led to further investigation. A large retinal defect posterior to the ora serrata was discovered as the source. The etiology is unknown.

a O.d., upper periphery at 12 h. Posterior to the ora serrata, the retina is thickened and opaque. Both on the anterior face and at the summit of the indentation protuberance it appears to have a whitish tinge. In it are interspersed numerous small cysts, closely juxtaposed. In the peripheral retina there is a large, elongated retinal defect with irregularly jagged edges. A second, small, slit-shaped defect, without operculum, is present on the right side. No vitreous traction is apparent at the edges of the holes.

b O.d., lower periphery at 6 h. Here, too, the retina is thickened and exhibits cystic changes.

c O.s., upper periphery at 12 h. Deep indentation; the ora serrata appears on the anterior face of the indentation protuberance. The contrast with the right eye is striking. The peripheral retina here is thin and transparent, containing only a few cysts. Owing to the thinness of their walls, they are visible only in the optical section. Examination on the anterior face of the indentation protuberance shows clearly the irregular pigmentation of the deep layers

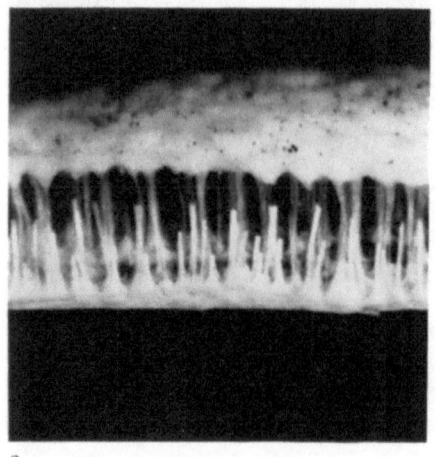

a

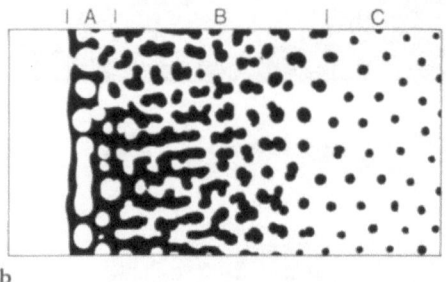

b

Fig. 43a. *Cystoid spaces in an autopsy eye.* (By courtesy of Dr. B. Daicker.) The intraretinal confluent cavities are crossed by pillars

Fig. 43b. *Schematic drawing of a flat section through cystoid cavities.*

A Belt of cysts at the extreme border of the retina. Some cysts are still delimited by walls. Others are open posteriorly, merging with the coarse cystoid spaces. Other cysts are confluent in an ora-parallel direction.

B Coarse cystoid spaces with columns of varying thickness and shape. They are placed at irregular intervals.

C Fine cystoid spaces with columns of equal size at regular intervals, circular in cross-section

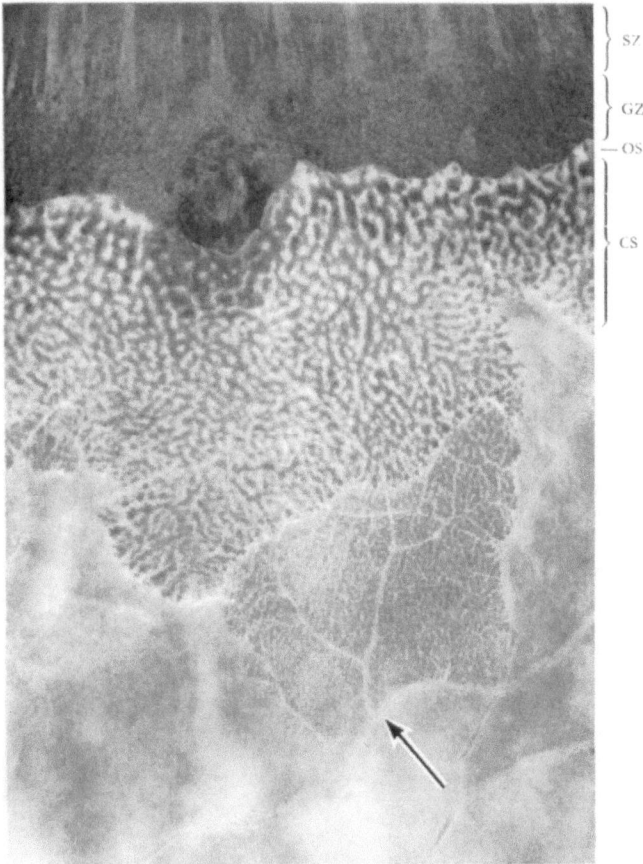

SZ

GZ

— OS

CS

CS   Cystoid spaces
GZ   Granular zone
OS   Ora serrata
SZ   Striate zone

Fig. 44. *Coarse cystoid spaces and reticular cystoid degeneration in an autopsy eye* (lower temporal quadrant). (By courtesy of Dr. R. Y. Foos.)

Owing to post-mortem tissue swelling the columns appear white. Posterior to the coarse cystoid spaces there follows an area of reticular (inner) cystoid degeneration. This is typically delimited by branched vessels (arrow). The individual columns are much finer there and arranged at regular intervals. The pattern of the fine vessels is retained in the areas of reticular cystoid degeneration.

At the border of the retina there is a deep, heavily pigmented ora bay, such as can occasionally be seen in the lower periphery as a developmental anomaly

125

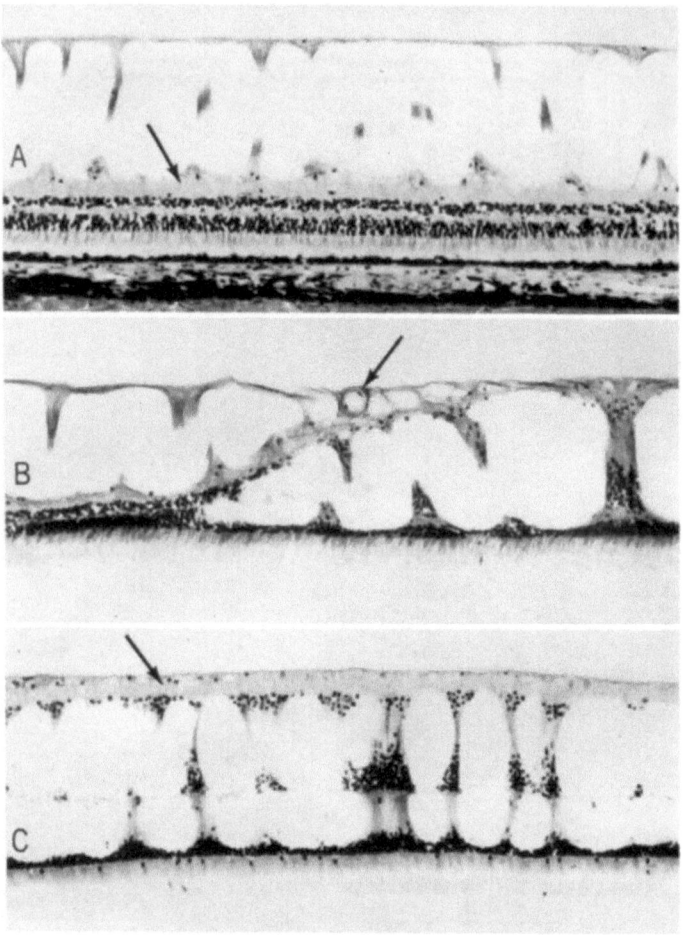

Fig. 45. *Histological section through an area of typical cystoid and reticular-cystoid degeneration.* (By courtesy of Dr. R. Y. Foos.)

A Reticular cystoid degeneration: The nerve-fibre layer is disintegrated, the ganglion cells have nearly all disappeared. The fibrous columns are partly sectioned obliquely. The inner plexiform layer (arrow) and the exterior layers of the retina are preserved.

B Transitional zone between reticular and typical cystoid degeneration. The two systems of cavities are separated by a membrane composed of the preserved inner plexiform layer. The reticular cystoid degeneration ends at an arteriole (arrow).

C Typical cystoid degeneration affecting predominantly the inner plexiform layer (arrow) and the outer parts of the retina. The cavities are traversed by a delicate membrane (membrana limitans media)

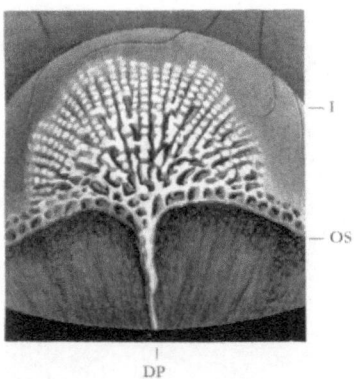

Fig. 46. *Coarse cystoid spaces at ora teeth* (nasally).
In an area almost symmetrical to the axis of an ora tooth, there are columns of varying thickness at irregular intervals

Fig. 47 *Broad belt of coarse cystoid spaces* (temporally). (A.N., 43 years of age).
The coarse cystoid spaces form a broad band posterior to the ora serrata. The columns are arranged in meridional rows extending anteriorly as far as the border of the retina. There the individual columns are clearly recognizable, since they are examined in silhouette. The surface of the retina is smooth and even in optical section

AVM	Anterior vitreous (hyaloid) membrane
DP	Dentate process of the ora serrata
I	Summit or border of indented area
L	Light of slit beam on retina and ciliary body
OS	Ora serrata
SC	Scar
TP	Tractus praeretinalis
WML	White midline

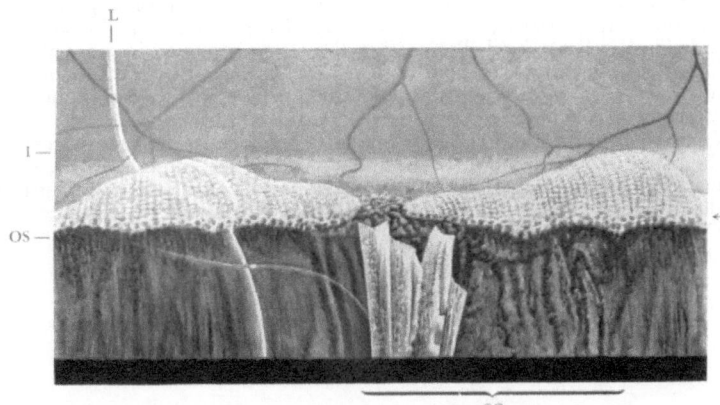

Fig. 48. *Coarse cystoid cavities adjacent to a foreign body* (K.S., 32 years of age).
Perforation by a splinter of aluminium. Initially the foreign body floated in the vitreous. A few weeks later it moved towards the site of perforation, where it remained fixed. The picture illustrates the appearance two years post trauma. Around the foreign body a scar has developed in the pars plana, with an irregular pigmentation and an atrophy of the ciliary epithelium. The scar extends beyond the ora serrata and into the retina. At either side of the scar there are coarse cystoid spaces, which had slowly developed during the two years. These are the only cystoid areas in this eye, since the remaining peripheral fundus shows only a narrow band of small cysts at the retinal border

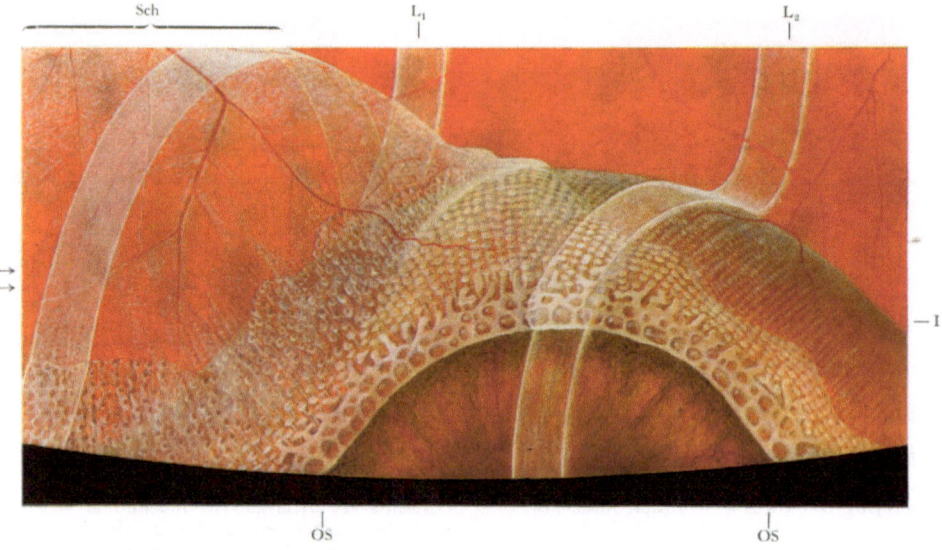

Fig. 49. *Coarse cystoid spaces, fine cystoid spaces, and schisis retinae* (B. Z., 70 years of age).

The indentation protuberance is situated at the bottom of the picture. The pars plana can be recognized as a dark half-moon, posteriorly is the retina. At the ora serrata there are one or two rows of cysts behind which a broad area of coarse cystoid spaces follows. The individual columns are thick and of irregular shape. With focal incidence of light the insertion points of the columns on the inner layer reflect brightly. Their surface pattern is best seen in reflected light. Towards the summit of the protuberance, owing to perspective distortion, the cystoid area seems to consist of "cysts".

Posterior to the coarse cystoid spaces there are fine cystoid spaces. They are delineated anteriorly by a clear-cut, wavy boundary. Their columns are fine and cannot be identified individually. With focal illumination the retina seems to be normal. Only with reflected light does the anomaly become apparent in the form of typical meridional striation. Here, too, a "cystic" picture is formed towards the summit of the protuberance. Posteriorly the transition to the intact retina is without a clear-cut boundary.

On the left in the picture, the margin of a high schisis cavity is represented. Near the edge the pattern of the cystoid spaces first continues, the columns of the coarse cystoid spaces being extended in length. There follows a zone where the same pattern is produced by naps on the inner layer. Then the wall of the schisis cavity becomes thin and completely transparent. Only in reflected light does a honeycomb structural pattern appear. The vessels on the schisis are sheathed

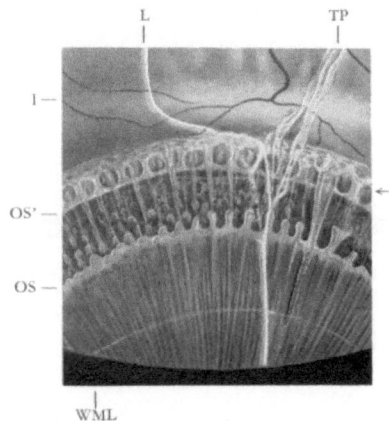

Fig. 50. *Marginal schisis* (M.W., 55 years of age).

This patient has a typical bilaterally symmetrical vesicular schisis. This is not visible in the picture, for the schisis cavities do not extend as far as the ora serrata. They are separated from it by a belt of normal coarse cystoid cavities. At the border of the retina itself, there is in the same sectors also an intraretinal splitting, but of a different pattern: The retina border is not easily identifiable here. At a superficial glance the ora serrata would be located where the typical coarse cystoid cavities end (*OS'*). Immediately anterior there is a broad band with a brown bottom, from which numerous "columns" protrude towards the vitreous body. This zone might be interpreted as the posterior pars plana with epithelial prolifera- tions; however, it is remarkable that these "proliferations" are all of equal size and at regular intervals—intervals that correspond to those of the columns in cystoid areas. More precise examination demonstrates the presence of the inner layer of the marginal schisis, which is delicate and completely transparent, forming a fine line in the optical section. In silhouette an extremely fine striation appears in it, connecting the columns at the posterior border of the marginal schisis (*OS'*) with those of the actual retinal border (*OS*)

I	Summit or border of indented area
L	Light of slit beam on retina or ciliary body
OS	Ora serrata
OS'	Posterior boundary of marginal schisis
Sch	Schisis retinae
TP	Tractus praeretinalis
WML	White midline

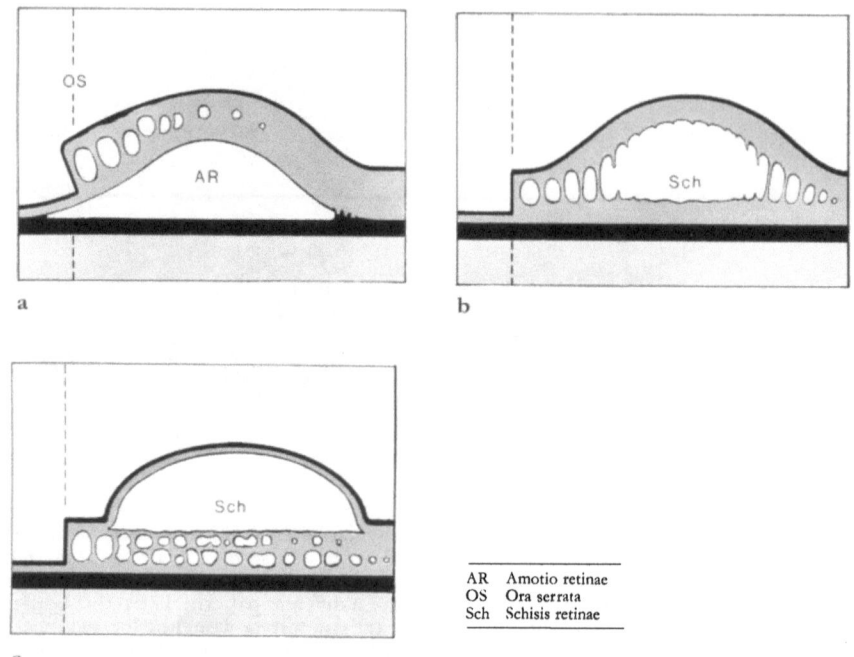

a

b

Sch

c

AR	Amotio retinae
OS	Ora serrata
Sch	Schisis retinae

Fig. 51a–c. *Schisis and retinal detachment (schematic drawing).*

a In a case of retinal detachment the fluid is in the retroretinal space, i.e. external to the cystoid degenerated retina.

b In the case of schisis the fluid is intraretinal. In the marginal areas of the schisis there are elongated columns of cystoid cavities.

c Schisis of the inner layer ("retinal cyst"). The cystoid spaces are still present underneath

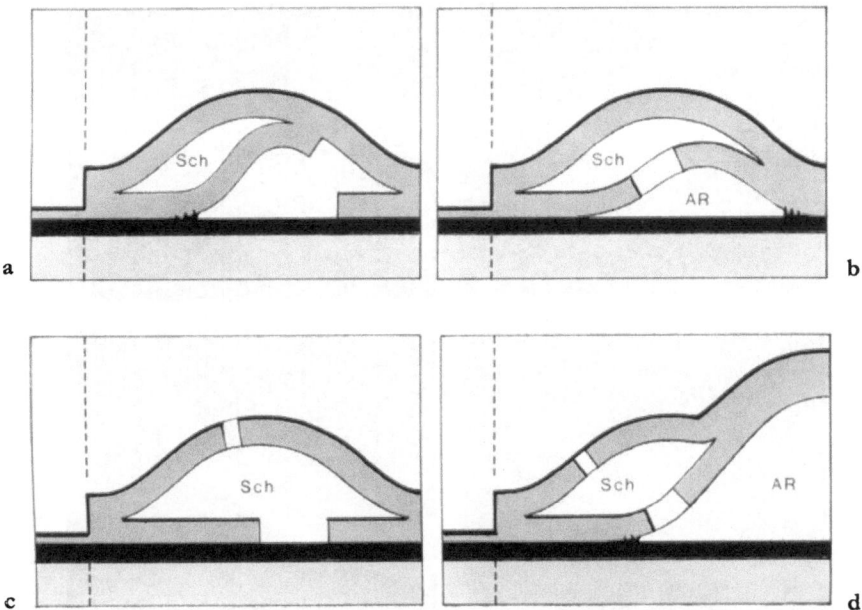

Fig. 52a–d. *Holes in the external layer of a schisis (schematic drawing).*

a The cavity is bridged by a strand of tissue extending from the edge of the hole to the inner layer, where it adheres.

b The external layer is detached. Through the hole there is a communication between the schisis cavity and the subretinal space.

c Holes in the outer and in the inner layer of the schisis.

d Through the holes free communication exists between the vitreous space and the subretinal space

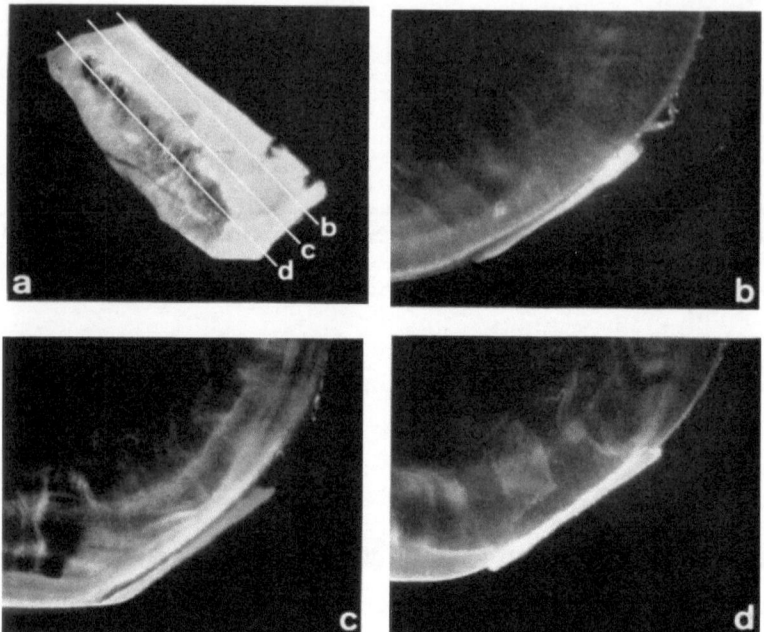

Fig. 53a–d. *Equatorial degeneration in an unfixed autopsy eye.*

a The retina is removed from the vitreous surface except for the equatorial degeneration and an adjacent strip of normal retina.
The planes of the optical sections b–d are marked.

b Optical section through the normal vitreous cortex.

c In the vicinity of the equatorial degeneration the cortex becomes narrower.

d Above the equatorial degeneration the regular cortex pattern is interrupted. There is a large fissure, giving free passage towards the central vitreous

---

Fig. 54a. *Paravascular attachments (autopsy eye).* ▶
Posterior to the ora serrata there are irregularly outlined areas of coarse cystoid spaces with a continuation into fine cystoid areas (left in the picture). The detached posterior hyaloid membrane is perceived as a delicate veil, which is sharply defined posteriorly. In the bifurcation of vessels there are areas with full- and partial-thickness defects of the retina, which are anteriorly delineated by the insertion line of the posterior hyaloid membrane. (By courtesy of Dr. R. Y. Foos)

Fig. 54b. *Paravascular attachments after a posterior vitreous detachment* (H.B., 61 years of age). ▶
At the summit of the indentation protuberance there appear circular retinal partial-thickness defects in groups near vessels. The posterior hyaloid membrane is detached and near its retinal insertion it is bent anteriorly. There are stripes of higher density on it, appearing like a cast of the retinal vessels. In their vicinity there are circular opacities corresponding to the paravascular partial-thickness defects ("opercula")

Fig. 54c. *Schematic drawing of the course of the posterior hyaloid membrane in sagittal section.* ▶
In Fig. b only that part of the posterior hyaloid membrane is visible which is bent, whereas the vertical part is not in focus. Arrows: Partial-thickness tears; corresponding "opercula" on PVM

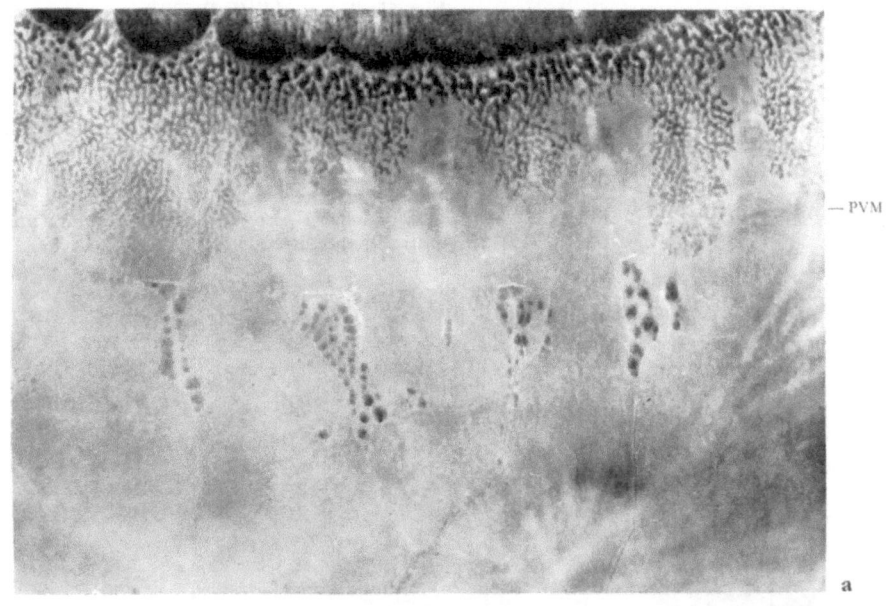

— PVM

a

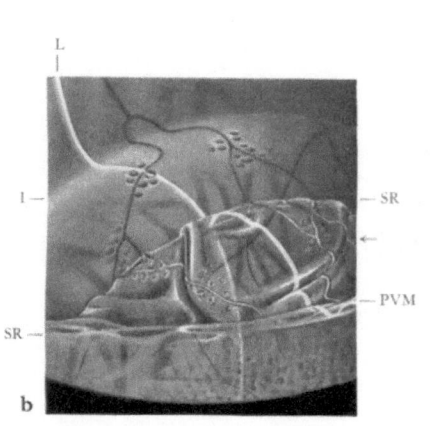

L

I —

SR —

b

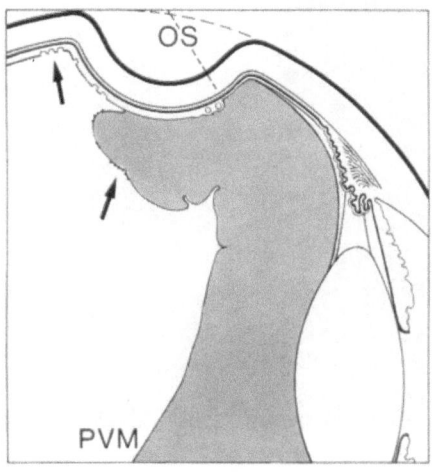

OS

PVM

— SR

— PVM

c

l	Border of indented area
L	Light of slit beam on retina and PVM
OS	Ora serrata
PVM	Posterior vitreous (hyaloid) membrane
SR	Silhouette on reflex PVM

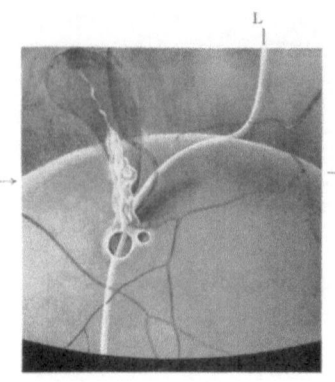

Fig. 55. *"Angioids"* (F.P., 37 years of age).
Upper temporal fundus periphery. Indentation of pre-equatorial region. The "angioid" originates from an irregularly formed retinal protrusion. At its base, there are two partial-thickness holes: abnormal vessels penetrate the protrusion and seem to anastomose there. The "angioid" is surrounded by a "hole" in the vitreous cortex. From the top of the retinal protrusion, the "angioid", a fibrous, very shiny, clearly defined vitreous strand, extends towards the centre of the vitreous cavity

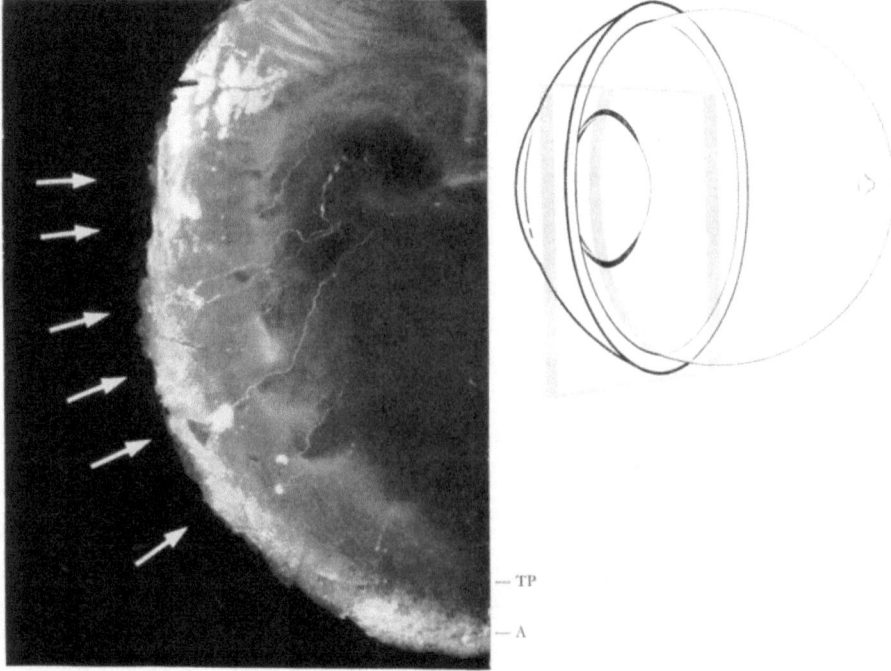

Fig. 56. *"Angioids"* in an autopsy eye.
The retina has been removed from the vitreous body, except for the retinal protrusions connected to the "angioids". The vitreous is illuminated with a wide slit beam (for direction of incidence see schematic drawing). The obliquely sectioned surface of the vitreous resembles a crescent, the cortex forms a grey half-moon, which is limited interiorly by the reflecting tractus praeretinalis. The "angioids" are fine whitish fibres that start from the retinal protrusions, traversing the cortex in a straight line. On entering the central vitreous they curve sharply, joining the twisting corkscrew course of adjacent "fibres". The angioids are surrounded by holes in the cortex, which do not stand out in this picture. But there are corresponding defects in the tractus praeretinalis, which appear as dark discs in the whitish reflecting surface of this tract. (The arrows indicate the retinal protrusions from which the angioids originate)

Fig. 57. *Microcysts on the pars plana* (autopsy eye).
Anterior to the ora serrata, in the granular zone, there are numerous small vesicles of various sizes. The striate zone is normal. In the retina there are coarse cystoid spaces. (By courtesy of Dr. B. Daicker)

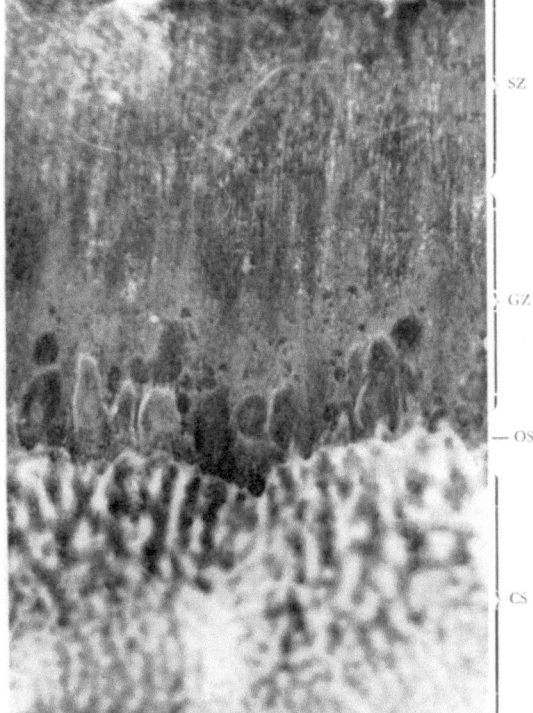

Fig. 58. *Macrocysts on the pars plana* (autopsy eye).
The large vesicles fill the space between two striae ciliares. In the striate zone they are oval. In the granular zone they are narrower, a constriction occurring at the linea serrata. Posterior to the ora serrata, coarse cystoid spaces. (By courtesy of Dr. B. Daicker)

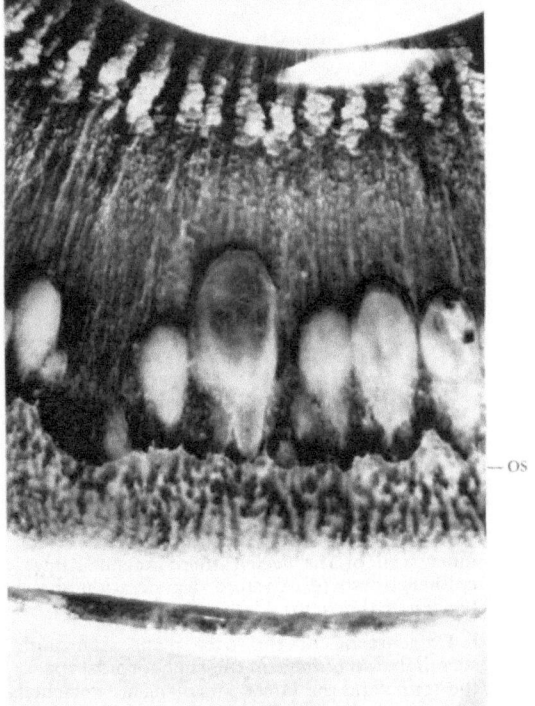

A	Surface of vitreous body
CS	Cystoid spaces
GZ	Granular zone
I	Summit of indented area
L	Light of slit beam on retina
OS	Ora serrata
SZ	Striate zone
TP	Tractus praeretinalis

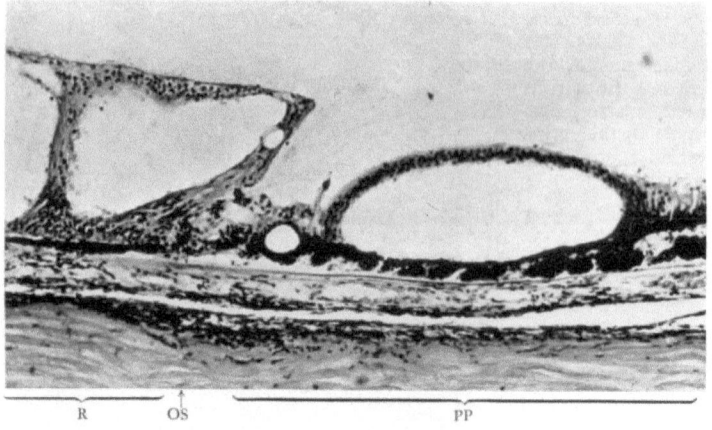

Fig. 59. *Pars plana cysts in histological section.*
In the posterior pars plana there is a small microcyst; in the anterior pars plana a macrocyst, both of which are formed by a separation between the ciliary epithelium and the pigment epithelium. The meshes of Müller's reticulum are clearly developed, and between them the pigment epithelium seems to proliferate into the deeper parts. Posterior to the ora serrata are cystoid spaces. (By courtesy of Dr. B. Daicker)

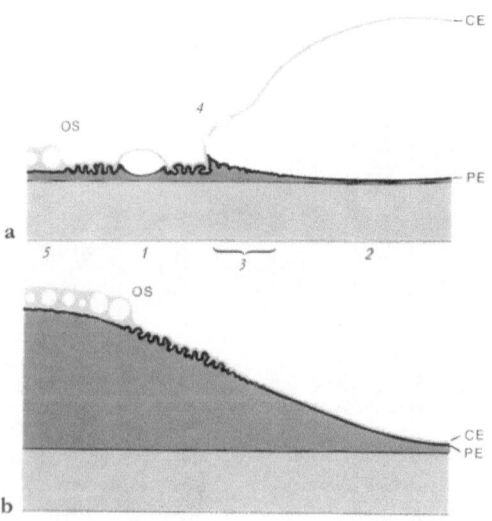

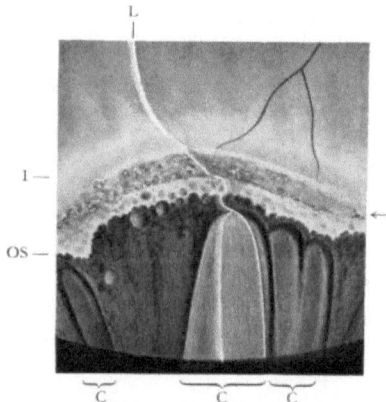

Fig. 60a and b. *Schematic drawing of "pars plana cysts" and "pars plana detachment".*

a Microcyst in the granular zone (*1*), macrocyst in the striate zone (*2*), with a constriction (*3*), where it encroaches on the granular zone. In the inner wall of the vesicle there are small intra-epithelial cysts (*4*). Cystoid degeneration at the border of the retina (*5*).

b Detachment of the pars plana. Through accumulation of fluid in the subchoroidal space, the retina and the intact pars plana are detached from the wall of the eye

Fig. 61. *Pars plana cysts* (biomicroscopic appearance, H.H., 69 years of age).
On the pars plana there are several macrocysts, whose walls are completely transparent and practically structureless. The cysts can therefore best be detected in optical section. In the granular zone there are small microcysts. At the ora serrata cystoid spaces; posterior to it an atrophic attenuation of the retina

Fig. 62. *Extent of the vitreous base* (schematic drawing).
a Anterior (variable) base.
b "Absolute" vitreous base (ora serrata).
c Posterior (variable) base

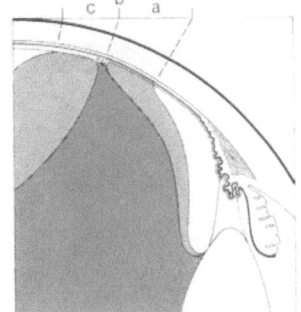

C	Cysts of the pars plana
CE	Ciliary epithelium
I	Border of indented area
L	Light of slit beam on retina and pars plana cyst
OS	Ora serrata
PE	Pigment epithelium
PP	Pars plana
R	Retina

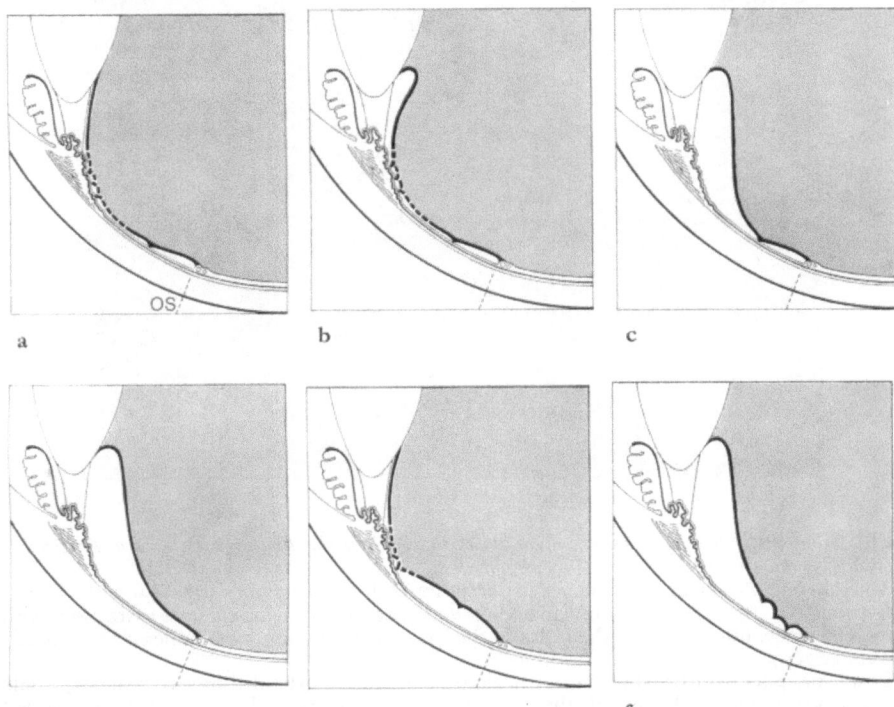

Fig. 63 a–f. *Variations of the course of the anterior hyaloid membrane* (schematic drawing).
Drawn in an interrupted line are those parts which are invisible in the normal eye even with indentation (their course is taken from observation of aphakic eyes).

a Normal course: the anterior hyaloid membrane is closely apposed against the zonule and the ciliary body.

b The most anterior part of the hyaloid membrane floats between the ligamentum hyaloideocapsulare and the ligamentum coronarium.

c The hyaloid membrane floats between the ligamentum hyaloideocapsulare and the white midline.

d The hyaloid membrane floats between the ligamentum hyaloideocapsulare and an accessory line.

e The hyaloid membrane floats between the ligamentum coronarium and the ora serrata.

f The hyaloid membrane floats between the ligamentum hyaloideocapsulare and the ora serrata

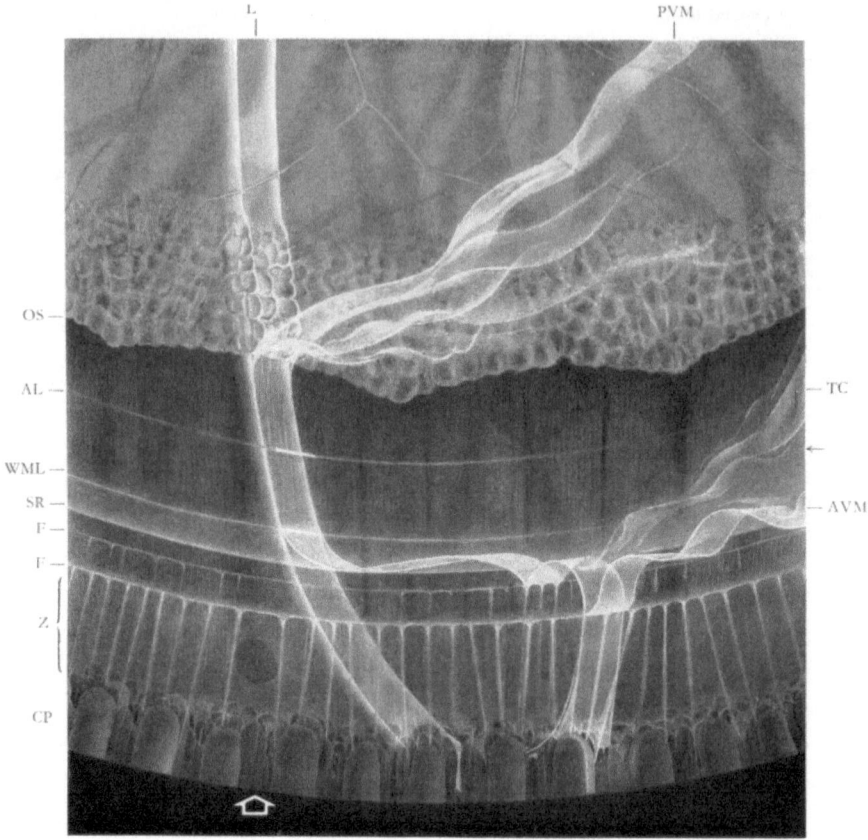

Fig. 64. *Anterior hyaloid membrane in an aphakic eye. "Posterior limiting membrane of the zonule"* (R.S., 62 years of age).

The drawing was made three months after an intracapsular cataract extraction with chymotrypsine. (On the other eye a similar finding was observed after the cataract extraction, with the difference, however, that the holes in the "posterior limiting membrane of the zonule" were larger.)

Lower periphery at 6h: The anterior hyaloid membrane is extended by two belts of zonule fibres into circular folds towards the ciliary processes. These zonule fibres are not connected into fascicles, but stand singly at regular intervals. Stretched between the zonule fibres there is a delicate membrane. Here we find a hole (arrow). The connection of this membrane with the ciliary processes is hidden by fibrous meshwork. Posterior to the belt of zonule fibres the hyaloid membrane takes on an S-shaped course towards the white midline. A silhouette reflex appears at the point of sharpest angulation. Posterior to the white midline the anterior hyaloid membrane is no longer seen. The lamellae of the tractus praeretinalis and the posterior hyaloid membrane are inserted at the ora serrata

AL	Accessory line	LSR	Linea serrata
AVM	Anterior vitreous (hyaloid) membrane	OS	Ora serrata
CP	Ciliary processes	PVM	Posterior vitreous (hyaloid) membrane
DR	Dentate reflex	SR	Silhouette reflex
F	Folds on AVM	TC	Tractus coronarius
I	Border of indented area	TM	Tractus medianus
LHC	Ligamentum hyalocapsulare	TP	Tractus praeretinalis
L	Light of slit beam on retina and ciliary body	WML	White midline
LSB	Lens border	Z	Zonule

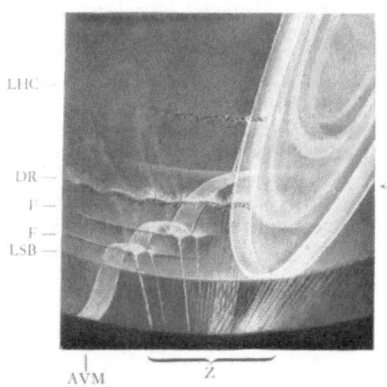

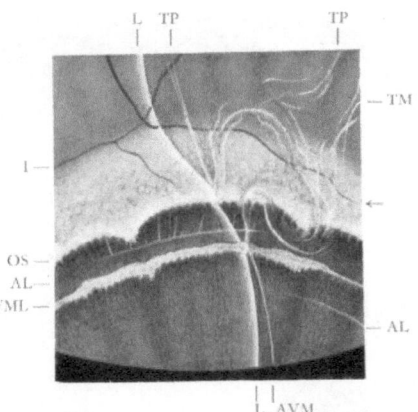

Fig. 65. *Floating anterior hyaloid membrane. Connections with the ciliary body* (E.N., 25 years of age).

Large previtreal space. Marked pigmentation on the posterior surface of the cornea (Krukenberg's spindle), on the trabeculum, zonule fibres, hyaloid membrane and in the hyalocapsular sinus. No glaucoma.

The floating anterior hyaloid membrane is drawn into folds at two places by zonule fibres (*F*). In the hyalocapsular sinus (at the ligamentum hyaloideocapsulare) and in the zonulocapsular sinus (at the dentate reflex-line) pigment has been deposited, forming two concentric rings in the periphery of the lens

Fig. 66. *Cystoid alterations in the region of the white midline* (F.H., 26 years of age, advanced myopia). Upper periphery at 12h.

The anterior hyaloid membrane is inserted at the white midline. There is a ridge of cystoid tissue, whose histological nature is unknown. There are two fine accessory lines. The tractus praeretinalis is split: one part following the typical direction parallel to the retina, the other one arching anteriorly, approaching the tractus medianus

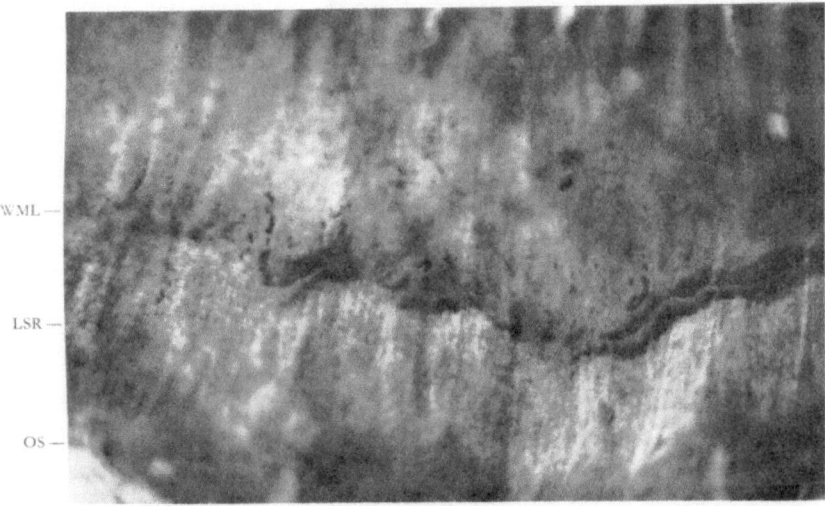

Fig. 67. *Deposition of blood at the white midline* (autopsy eye).
Blood is deposited at the white midline. (Notice: the position of the linea serrata is further posterior.) Anteriorly, the ciliary body is blurred by the opacities in the previtreal space. (By courtesy of Dr. B. Daicker)

139

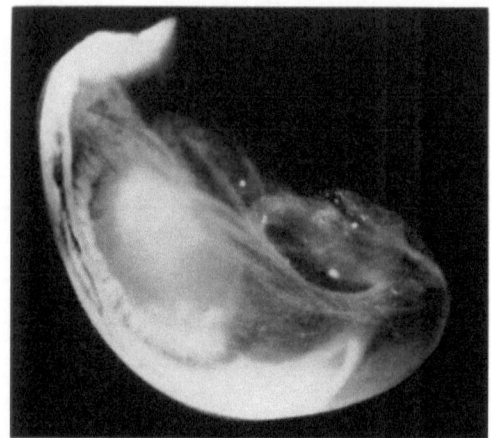

a

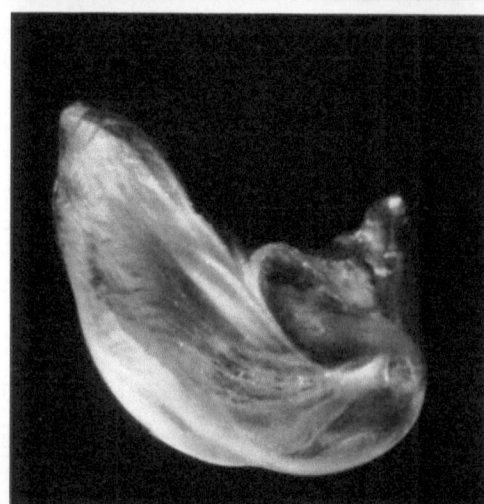

b

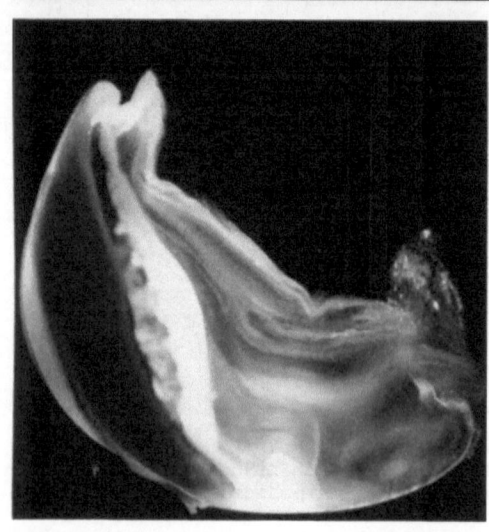

c

Fig. 68a–c. *Rhegmatogenous posterior vitreous detachment (detachment with collapse).*

Slit-lamp examination of an unfixed autopsy eye in which the retina has been removed. Appearance with various slit-beam widths.

a In diffuse illumination the prefoveal hole is readily recognizable.

b With a narrow slit beam the prefoveal hole is difficult to identify.

c In optical section the hole can scarcely be discerned

Fig. 69. *Rhegmatogenous posterior vitreous detachment (schematic drawing).*
The exchange of fluid between the vitreous body and the retrovitreal space takes place through the prefoveal hole. The main mass of the vitreous body rests on the lower half of the globe. The posterior hyaloid membrane falls steeply down from its upper insertion and is covered in the lower half of the globe by the prolapsed vitreous substance. The vitreal tracts run—as in every vitreous perforation—straight to the hole (prefoveal hole)

Fig. 70a–c. *Arrhegmatogenous posterior vitreous detachment (schematic drawing).*
The S-shaped course of the vitreal tracts is retained here.

a Partial posterior vitreous detachment.

b Subtotal arrhegmatogenous posterior vitreous detachment including the area of the prefoveal hole. The posterior boundary of the vitreous remains à niveau in the region of the hole. Such situations are exceptional at the prefoveal hole, but are predominantly met with at holes where the vitreous cortex is relatively broad, i.e. in the periphery (e.g. at chorioretinitic foci).

c Prolapse through the prefoveal hole. Here the prolapse is caused by a weakness in the vitreous wall, and not by an exchange of fluid into the retrovitreal space. The size of the prolapse does not correspond to the retrovitreal volume

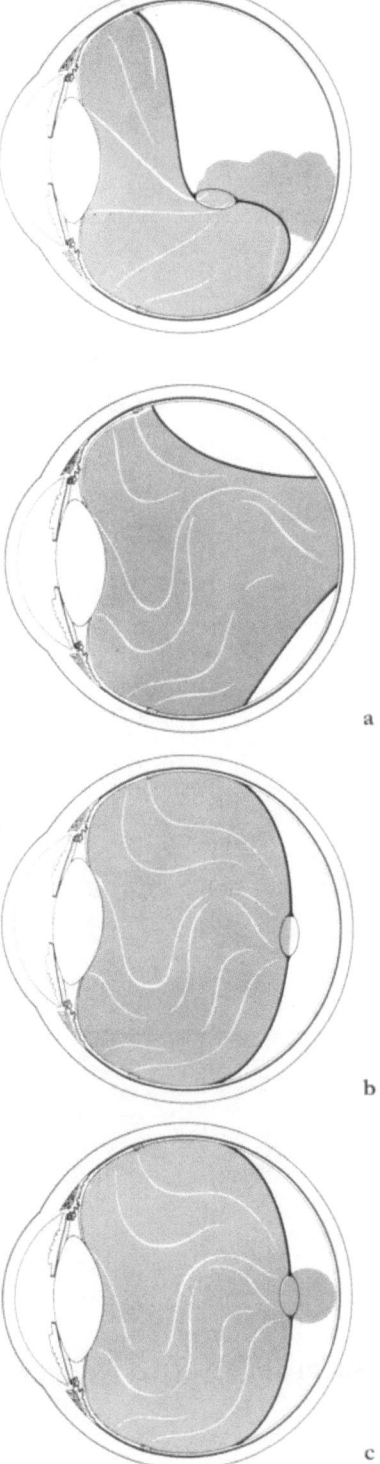

a

b

c

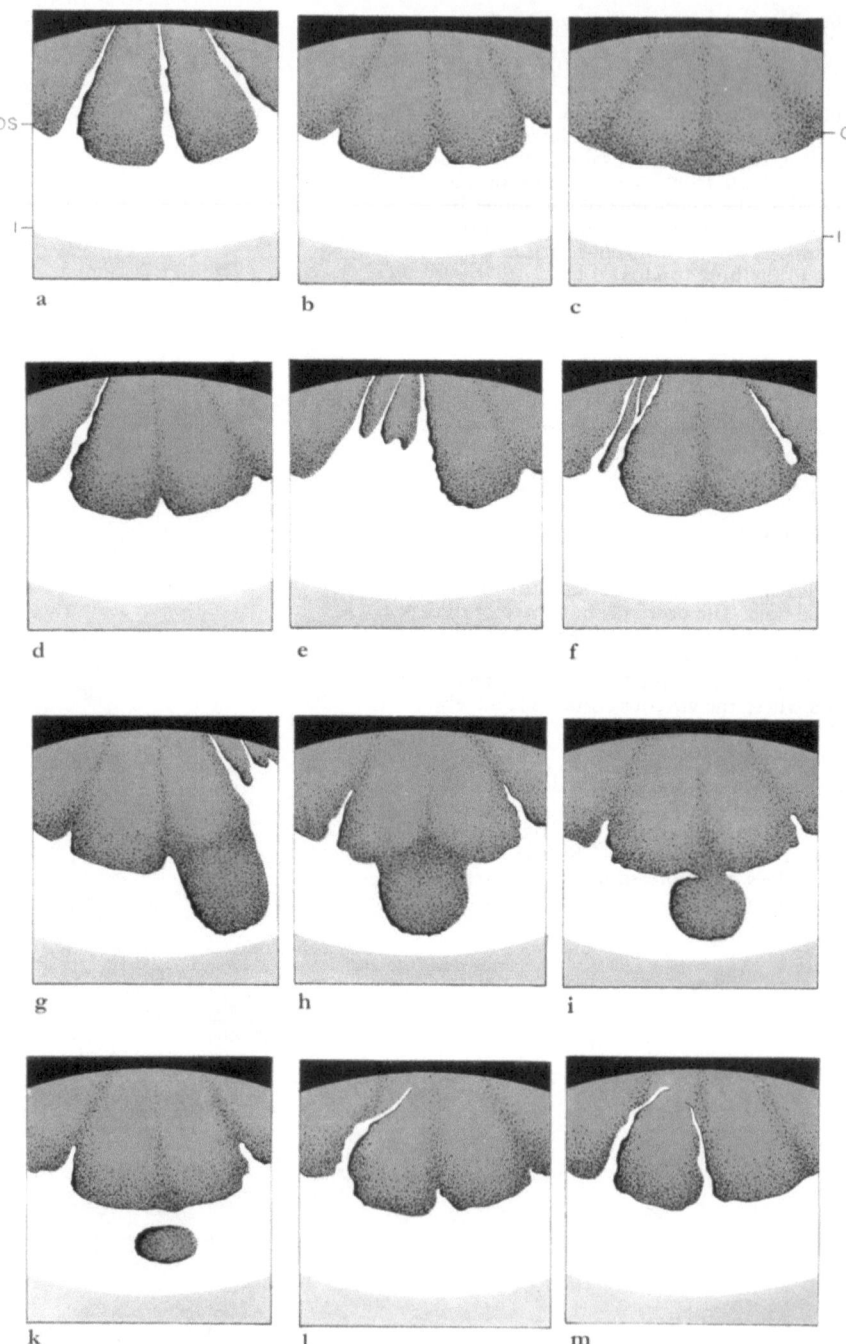

Fig. 71a–m. Legend see opposite page

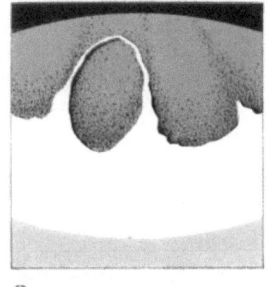 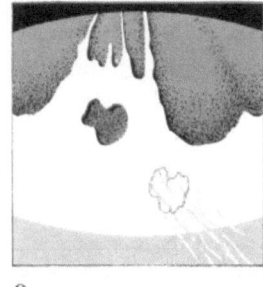

n   o

Fig. 71 a–o. *Variations of shape of the ora serrata.*

a Long teeth: upon the striae ciliares long processes extend anteriorly from the retinal border.

b Short ora teeth: at the striae ciliares the retinal border is stretched only slightly anteriorly·

c The retinal border has a smooth course and is not deformed at the striae ciliares.

d Among several short teeth, there is a single longer tooth.

e Confluent teeth: the retinal border is displaced anteriorly, not only at the striae ciliares but also in the intervals, and is irregularly serrated.

f Ramified tooth and isolated tooth.

g Abnormally deep ora bay: adjacent to confluent teeth, the retinal border is displaced posteriorly in the space between two striae ciliares.

h Abnormally deep bay: in contrast to Fig. 71 g, the very deep bay is not situated between two striae, but opposite a stria ciliaris, i.e. where a tooth would normally be expected.

i Incompletely enclosed bay.

k Enclosed ora bay. An "island" is formed in the retina, made of pars-plana tissue, posterior to the ora serrata.

l Curved ora teeth.

m Two curved, converging ora teeth.

n Formation of a "pars-plana island" by confluence of curved ora teeth. This type of "island" is situated anterior to the ora serrata, in the pars plana.

o Tear in an abnormally broad confluent ora tooth. This is a tongue-like protrusion above a normal pars plana; therefore, if a hole occurs in the "tongue", the normal ciliary epithelium is exposed at the bottom

J	Summit of indented area
L	Light of slit beam on retina and ciliary body
OS	Ora serrata
TP	Tractus praeretinalis
WML	White midline

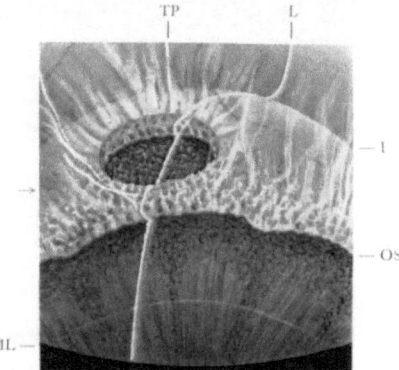

Fig. 72. *Enclosed ora bay* (M.G., 50 years of age).
Superficial examination might lead to the retinal defect being mistaken for a round retinal hole. It is distinguished from the latter, however, by the brown granular surface of the pars plana, seen at the bottom of the "hole". The edge of the "hole" exhibits, as does the ora serrata, coarse cystoid spaces. The tractus praeretinalis is a transparent, folded membrane inserted at the edges of the "hole", in the same way as at the ora serrata. Above the enclosed ora bay, there is thus a defect in the vitreous cortex

143

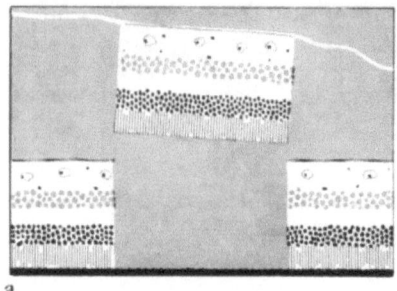
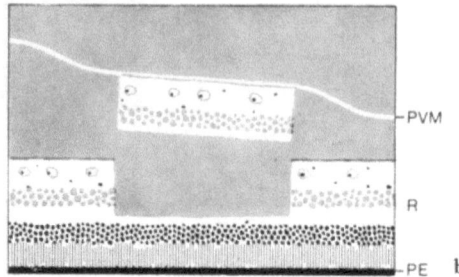

a

b — PVM

R

PE

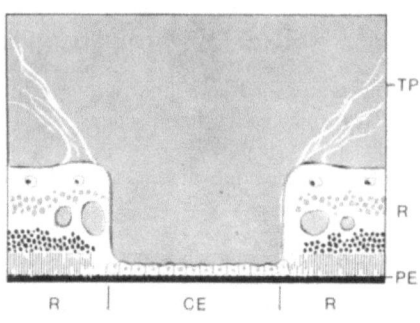

TP

R

PE

R | CE | R

c

Fig. 73a–c. *Schematic drawing of retinal defects.*

a Full-thickness retinal defect caused by traction of the posterior hyaloid membrane. At the bottom of the hole the pigment epithelium lies exposed.

b Partial-thickness defect as a result of traction of the posterior hyaloid membrane.

c Enclosed ora bay: in contrast to Fig. 73a and b, the bottom of the retinal defect is covered by normal ciliary epithelium. The edges have the same configuration as at the ora serrata, and the tractus praeretinalis is inserted there

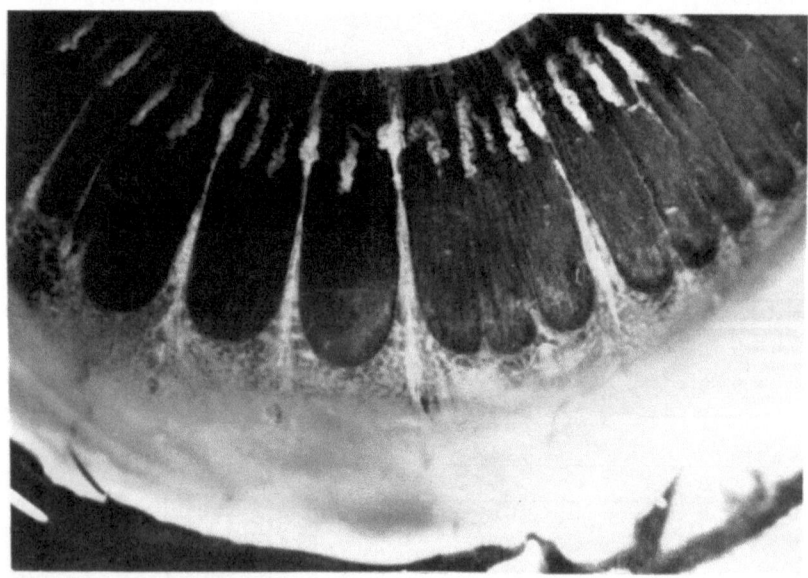

Fig. 74. *Meridional ridges and meridional complexes at the ora serrata* (autopsy eye).
Meridional ridges appear as protrusions of the retinal surface at ora teeth. Their axis therefore is the same as that of the ciliary valleys. Meridional complexes have basically the same structure but may be distinguished from single meridional ridges by an abnormally long ora tooth which is not extending into ciliary valleys but to an abnormally large ciliary process. Posterior to the meridional complex there is a patchy attenuation of the retina ("peripheral retinal excavation"). (By courtesy of Dr. B. Daicker)

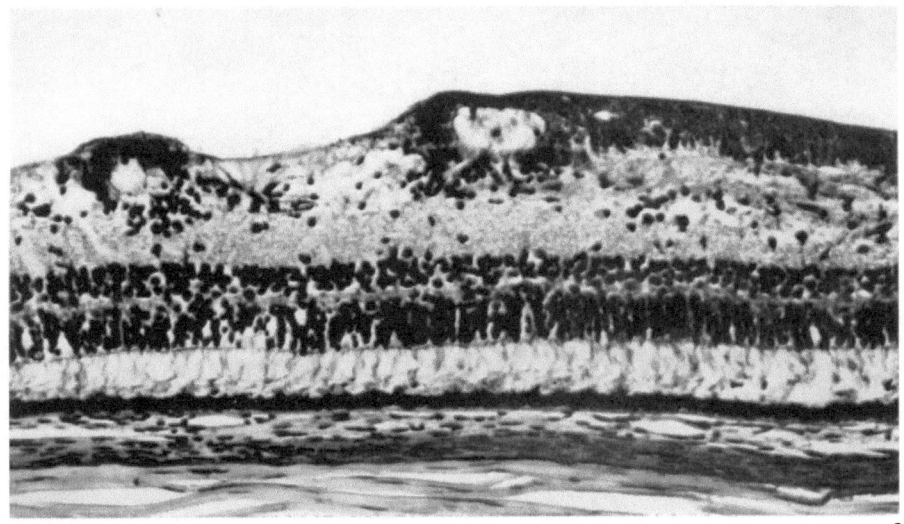

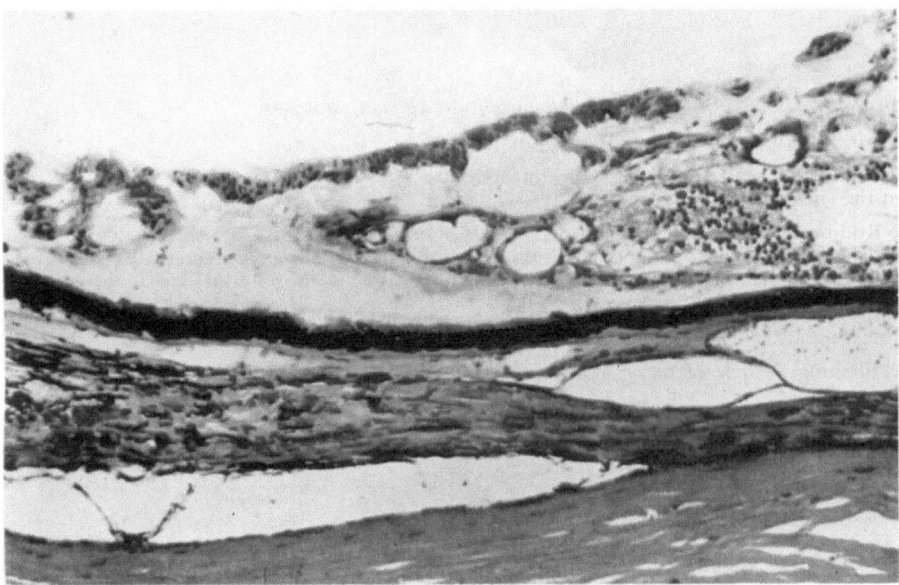

Fig. 75a and b. *Histological section through meridional ridges.* (By courtesy of Dr. B. Daicker.)

a In the child the meridional ridge is an epiretinal apposition of epithelial tissue similar to ciliary epithelium.

b In old age the epithelial cap is still present; however, the cells are more irregular in shape, though still in a single row. In the retina underneath there are numerous cyst-like spaces and a marked gliosis

CE	Ciliary epithelium
PE	Pigment epithelium
PVM	Posterior vitreous (hyaloid) membrane
R	Retina
TP	Tractus praeretinalis

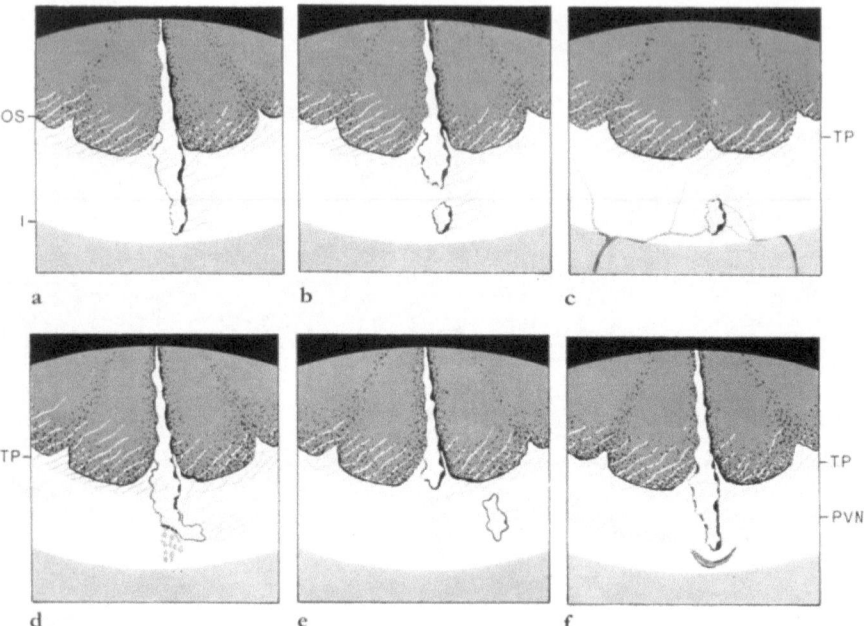

Fig. 76a–f. *Meridional ridges and their variations (schematic drawing).*

a Meridional ridge at an ora tooth.

b Meridional ridge interrupted by intact retina. The tractus praeretinalis is also inserted at the small isolated patch.

c Rudimentary meridional ridge: on the axis of an ora tooth there is a small patch of tissue of a structure similar to that of a meridional ridge, where the tractus praeretinalis is inserted. Atypical vessels penetrate the patch, probably forming a chorioretinal anastomosis.

d Partial-thickness defect at the posterior edge of a meridional ridge, the tractus praeretinalis inserting at the "flap".

e Floating particle of tissue at the posterior edge of a meridional ridge ("Pseudo-operculum").

f Horseshoe tear posterior to a meridional ridge. There is a full-thickness retinal horseshoe tear in an eye with a posterior vitreous detachment. At its operculum the posterior hyaloid membrane is inserted

---

Fig. 78a–c. *Variations of meridional ridges and ora teeth* (S.I., 22 years of age).

a O.s., upper periphery at 12h. In the temporal and superior periphery, the ora serrata has a smooth edge with slight coarse cystoid degeneration. On the pars plana there are oblong cystic agglomerations in a meridional direction, which are probably ectopic retinal tissue (isolated ora teeth)

b O.s., nasal periphery at 9h. In the centre, confluent ora teeth with a ridge-like protrusion of irregular shape. The retinal vessels do not penetrate it but pass over its surface; consequently, this might be a genuine retinal fold. The nature of the striate structure at the ora bay on the left is not known.

c O.d., nasal periphery at 3h. Moderate coarse cystoid degeneration along the retinal border. Several long ora teeth at regular intervals. Two meridional ridges at ora bays; one of them following a meridional, the other one an oblique direction.

146

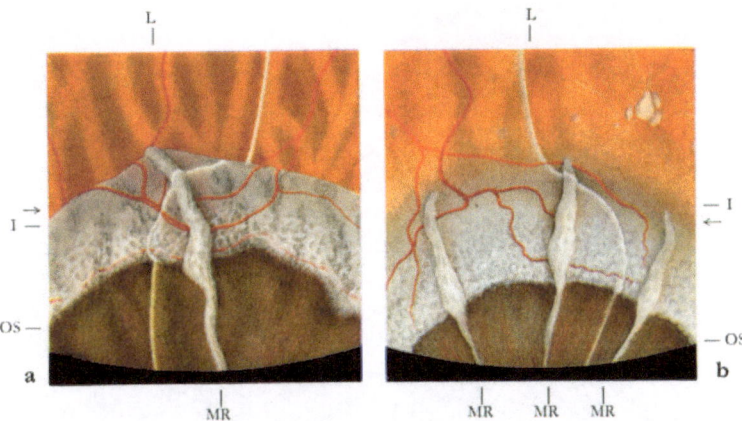

Fig. 77a and b. *Vascular anomalies, chorioretinal anastomosis* (M.O., 36 years of age).

a O.s., nasally at 9h. A single meridional ridge passes across the ora serrata. Under the ridge vessels of varying calibres disappear; the relation between their branches on either side of the ridge is indefinite. Presumably this is a case of retinochoroidal anastomosis.

b O.d., nasally at 3h. From the ora serrata spindle-shaped meridional ridges of a cystic structure run anteriorly and posteriorly at regular intervals. One of the ridges is penetrated by retinal vessels, all of which emerge obviously unchanged except for one that does not reappear. In the marginal retina there is a coarse cystoid degeneration. In the equatorial retina there are several drusen-like granules

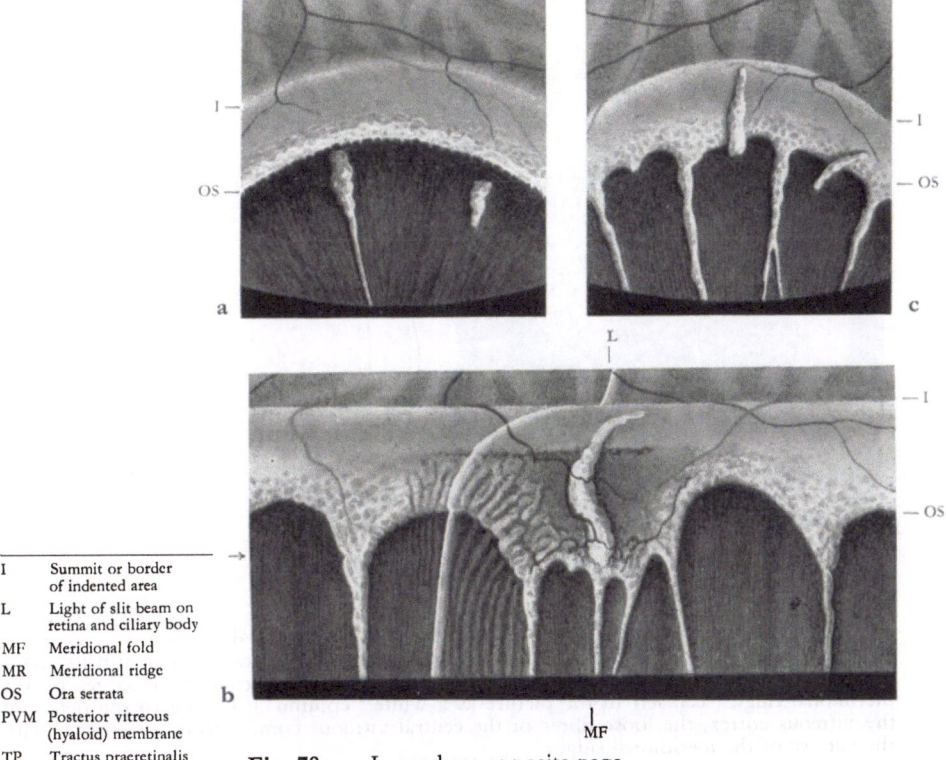

I	Summit or border of indented area
L	Light of slit beam on retina and ciliary body
MF	Meridional fold
MR	Meridional ridge
OS	Ora serrata
PVM	Posterior vitreous (hyaloid) membrane
TP	Tractus praeretinalis

Fig. 78a–c. Legend see opposite page

147

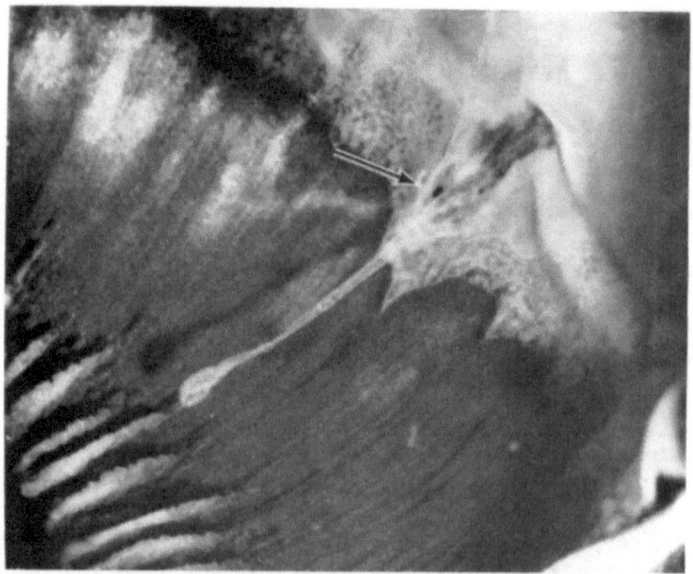

Fig. 79. *Zonular traction tuft* (autopsy eye). (By courtesy of Dr. R. Y. Foos.)
An extremely long "zonular traction tuft" protrudes from the peripheral retina into the vitreous space. At its posterior end the retina is attenuated and partially infiltrated with pigment. The arrow points to a full-thickness retinal tear. In the living eye the "zonular traction tufts" are difficult to identify, as they lie closely along the indentation protuberance. For this reason they may be mistaken for long ora teeth or meridional ridges

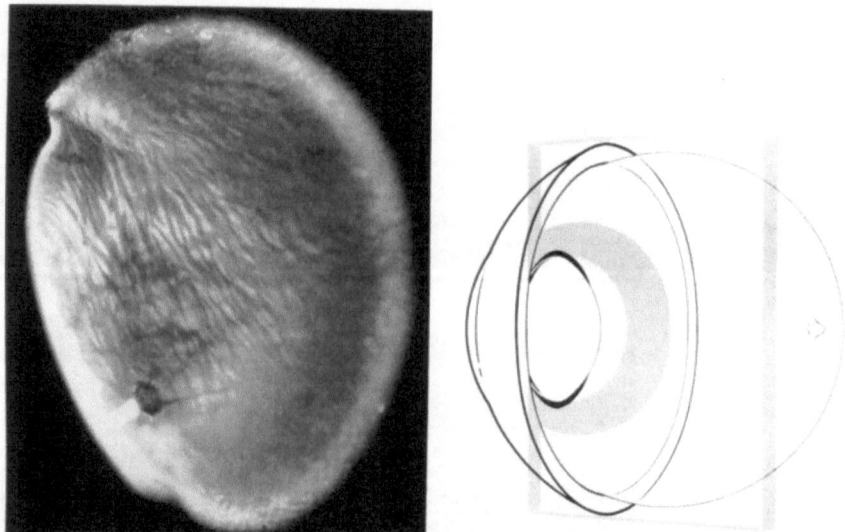

Fig. 80. *Hole in the vitreous cortex above an isolated meridional ridge* (see Fig. 76c). Autopsy eye, slit-lamp observation of an unfixed vitreous body. (Parasagittal section).
In the wide slit beam the vitreous cortex appears greyish, the tractus praeretinalis has a plicated, strongly reflecting surface. The preretinal tract is inserted at the edges of the meridional ridge (seen left in the picture as a white "column"). Owing to the defect in the vitreous cortex, the loose fibres of the central vitreous come into direct contact with the surface of the meridional ridges

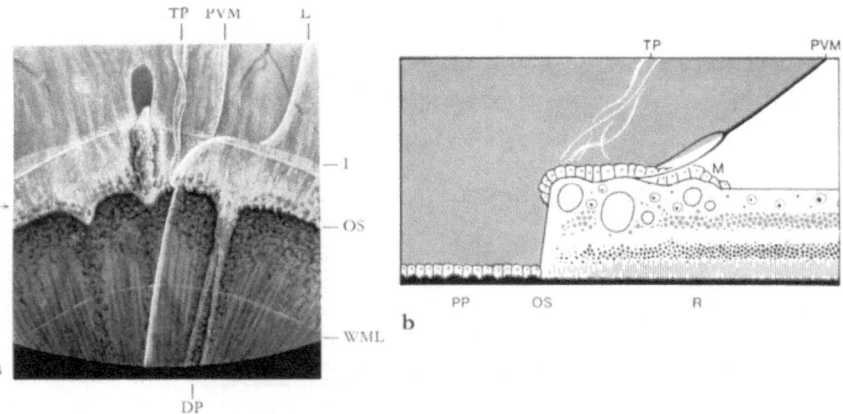

Fig. 81 a and b. *Detachment of the posterior hyaloid membrane at a meridional ridge* (H.B., 42 years of age).

Arrhegmatogenous posterior vitreous detachment in a case of periphlebitis.

a Upper periphery at 11 h. The posterior hyaloid membrane is drawn back tightly towards a periphlebitic scar in the posterior fundus (not visible in the picture). Its insertion line crosses the meridional ridge. The vitreous body is still attached in the anterior section of the meridional ridge. In the detached posterior hyaloid membrane there is a defect, the size and position of which correspond to the meridional ridge. In this defect no vitreous boundary is visible; the edges are densified. The defect in the hyaloid membrane must be distinguished from a defect in the cortex, which is present even when the vitreous is attached (Fig. 80).

b *Schematic drawing of the defect in the hyaloid membrane*

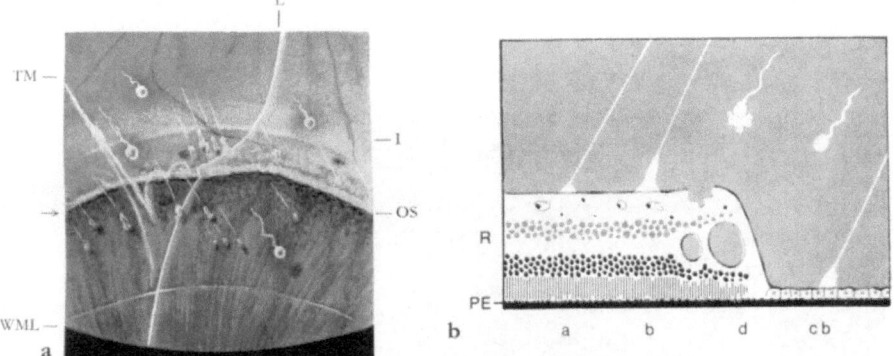

Fig. 82 a and b. *Micro-adhesions* (U. U., 33 years of age).

a The *attached adhesions* on the retina, right, are scarcely visible; only zonula-like vitreous fibres inserted there are recognizable. On the pars plana, however, owing to the better contrast, the micro-adhesions appear as greyish small protuberances, at which the typical vitreous fibres are inserted. When micro-adhesions are elongated, they form small "columns" on the retina and the pars plana. *Freely floating micro-adhesions* may be confused with small floating opercula; their edges are slightly thickened. The attached vitreous fibres are here twisted like corkscrews.

b *Schematic drawing of various forms of micro-adhesions on retina and pars plana.*
(*a*) Micro-adhesion adherent to the retinal surface. (*b*) Elongated micro-adhesion. (*c*) Freely floating micro-adhesion. (*d*) Extrusion of a micro-adhesion, with adherent retinal tissue, producing a partial-thickness defect in the retina

DP	Dentate process of the ora serrata	PP	Pars plana
I	Summit or border of indented area	PVM	Posterior vitreous (hyaloid) membrane
L	Light of slit beam on retina and ciliary body	R	Retina
M	Meridional ridge	TM	Tractus medianus
OS	Ora serrata	TP	Tractus praeretinalis
PE	Pigment epithelium	WML	White midline

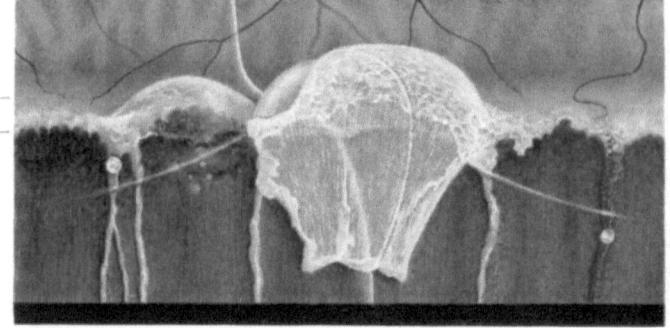

Fig. 83. *Drusen in ora teeth; vesicles of unknown origin at the ora serrata* (H.F., 37 years of age, normal eye).

Nasal upper periphery. Several long ora teeth and a branched ora tooth are infiltrated by pigment. In two of the teeth there is a "drusen" with a crystal-like gleam. The "drusen" are surrounded by a fine band of pigment. A further, fortuitous finding was a "cyst" with irregular edges. The surface of the "cyst" exhibits, like a cast, the pattern of the underlying tissues: coarse cystoid spaces in the posterior section, a clearly defined ora serrata boundary, marked striation over the pars plana. Close by, there is another, smaller cyst with less clearly defined wall structure. The midline of the pars plana is detached on both sides of the cyst but is invisible on its summit. The type of cyst remains undetermined. Since it has not changed in the course of time, and owing to the absence of other pathological findings in this eye, it is considered as a developmental variation

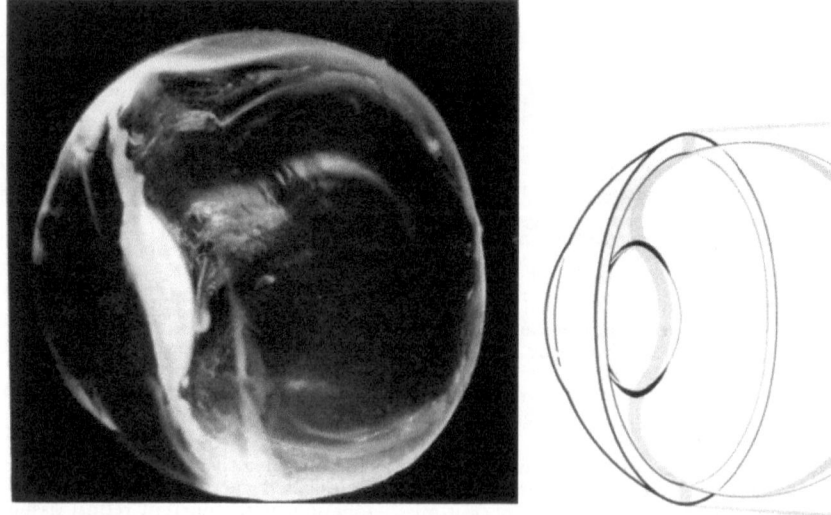

Fig. 84. *Ascension phenomenon of the tractus vitreales* (optical section of an unfixed autopsy eye). The tractus vitreales are forced upwards by soluble substances of higher specific gravity which accumulate in the lower half of the vitreous body. In experimental studies the centre of gravity of this eye proved to be shifted towards the bottom

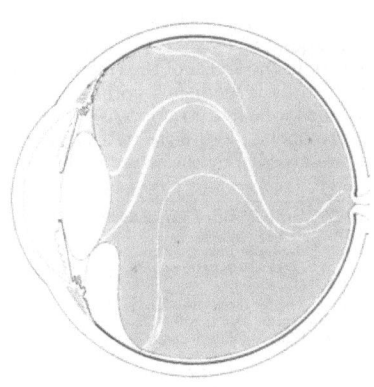

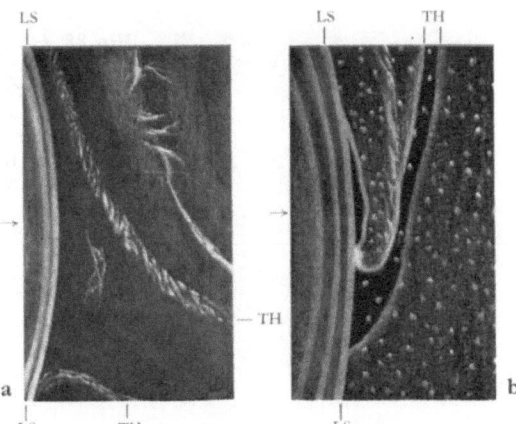

Fig. 85. *Ascension phenomenon of the tractus vitreales (schematic drawing).*
In chronic inflammatory processes the tractus vitreales are shifted upwards. The tractus hyaloideus and the tractus medianus rise steeply from their anterior insertion, passing through the upper half of the globe towards the posterior pole. The inferior previtreal space becomes enlarged by the ascension of the anterior hyaloid membrane

Fig. 86a and b. *Ascension phenomenon of the tractus hyaloideus* (slit-lamp observation without contact glass). (By courtesy of Professor Dr. H. Goldmann.)
a Normal course of the tractus hyaloideus; the superior plica drops after leaving the lens; the inferior plica first rises slightly and then also drops sharply towards the bottom.

b Inverse course of the tractus hyaloideus in diffuse uveitis. There is a distinct Tyndall phenomenon and marked cell content in the vitreous. Posterior to the lens the central canal, which appears to be optically empty, first runs upwards, instead of downwards. The inferior plica thus rises steeply; the superior plica first drops slightly, then turns abruptly upwards

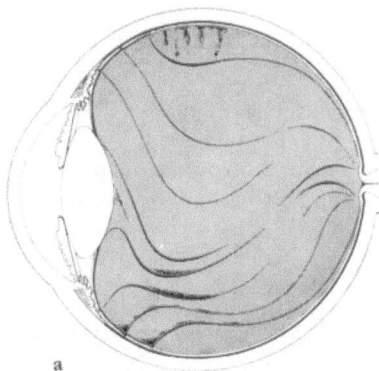

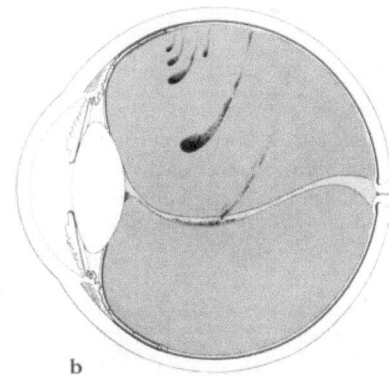

Fig. 87a and b. *Pattern of cell deposits in the vitreous body* (schematic drawing).

a Adult eye. Insoluble particles invading the vitreous body remain in the vicinity of their point of entry as long as they have not traversed the cortex (top of picture). After penetrating into the central vitreous they sink towards the bottom along the tractus vitreales, at whose lowest-lying parts they accumulate. Between the tractus praeretinalis and the tractus medianus they advance as far as the wall of the globe, thus forming an epiciliary hyphaemia or hypopyon. Those between the tractus medianus and the tractus hyaloideus remain within the vitreous, thus forming an intravitreal hyphaemia or hypopyon.

b In children's eyes the penetrating corpuscles follow the radial "fibres", accumulating in oblong sacs perpendicular to the retinal surface and in Cloquet's canal

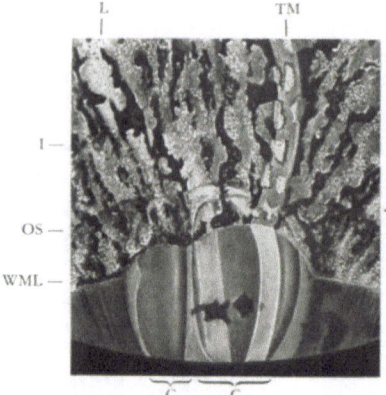

Fig. 88. *Haemorrhagic sediment in the lower fundus periphery* (L. Sch., 65 years of age).

Clouds of erythrocytes in the layers of the tractus vitreales. Those within the tractus medianus come into contact with the wall of the globe in the region of the white-midline. In the centre of the picture are two large pars plana cysts, which are crossed by the white midline

AVM	Anterior vitreous (hyaloid) membrane
C	Pars plana cysts
I	Border of indented area
L	Light of slit beam on retina and ciliary body
OS	Ora serrata
TM	Tractus medianus infiltrated with blood cells
TP	Tractus praeretinalis
WML	White midline

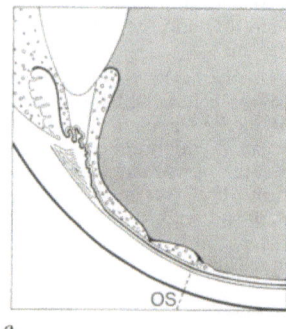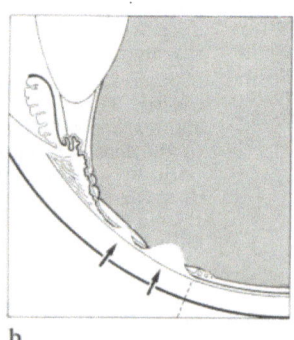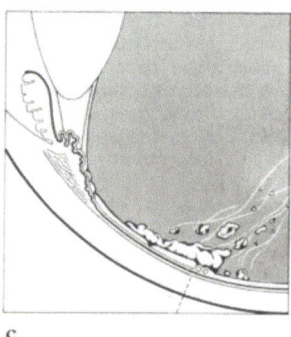

a   b   c

Fig. 89 a–c. *Origin of exudates in the outermost periphery* (schematic drawing).

a Precipitates in the previtreal space as a concomitant sign in uveitis anterior.

b Inflammatory foci of the uvea of the pars plana: true cyclitis posterior ("pars planitis").

c Exudates from the vitreous space accumulate in the lower vitreous base as a concomitant sign of posterior inflammation

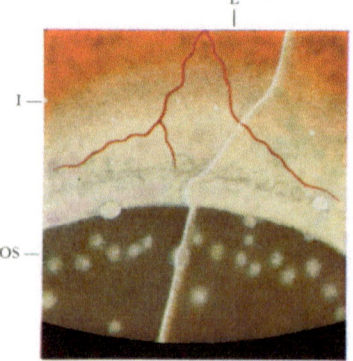

Fig. 90. *Precipitates on the pars plana in iridocyclitis* (N. G., 17 years of age).

Anterior uveitis of unknown aetiology with numerous mutton-fat precipitates on the posterior corneal surface. Posterior uvea unaffected.

In the whole circumference of the pars plana there are numerous mutton-fat precipitates of the same size and shape as the corneal precipitates. In the region of the midline they form a slightly denser girdle, anteriorly and posteriorly they are more scattered. The pars plana itself has the same normal structure as the unaffected right eye. In the anterior vitreous body no zones of discontinuity can be seen. At the retinal border there is a drusen-like body

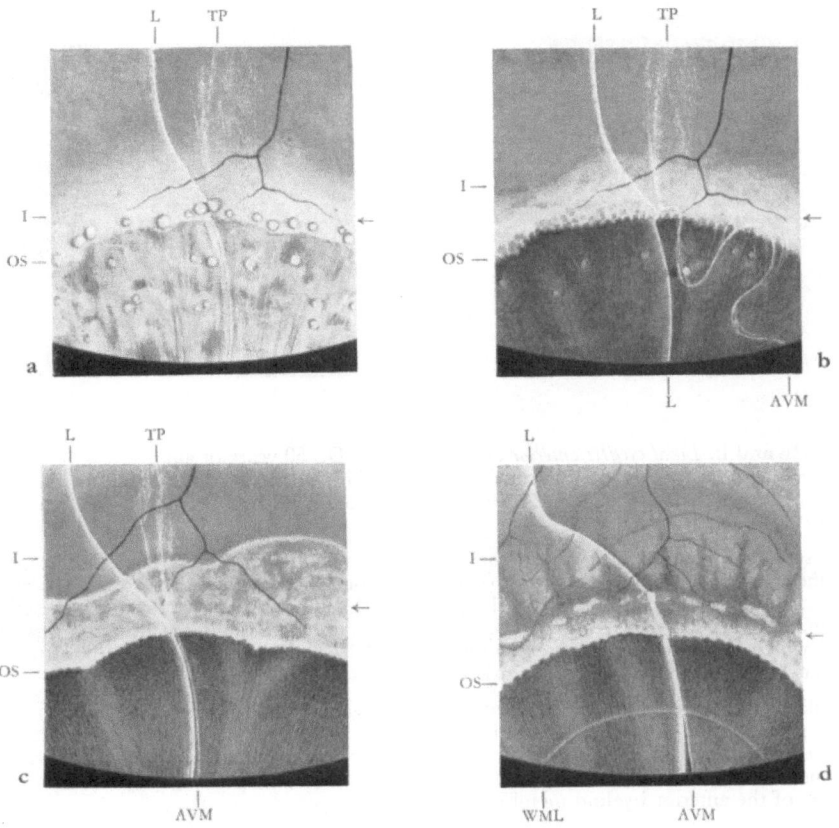

Fig. 91a–d. *Inflammatory changes of the pars plana in a case of iridocyclitis* (J.B., 34 years of age).
Unilateral iridocyclitis due to leptospirosis, which healed within 2 weeks.
a to c Right eye in various stages of inflammation. d Left (normal) eye.

a Acute phase: the pars plana has a greyish tint, its structure is blurred. In the optical section it appears to be thickened. Cells and precipitates are scattered all over the pars plana. The cells are too fine to be drawn in the picture. Above the ora serrata the precipitates accumulate in a narrow band which, on account of the perspective, appears in the picture to lie slightly posterior to the retinal border. In the anterior vitreous body no zones of discontinuity, hence no anterior hyaloid membrane, are visible.

b Healing phase: after the other clinical inflammatory symptoms subsided (retinal oedema and exudates in the anterior chamber), the oedema of the pars plana has also disappeared. The normal striate surface structure of the pars plana is visible again, but residues of precipitates are still there. The hyaloid membrane is floating, but only in the lower periphery, forming a wavy line there in optical section ("ascension phenomenon", see Fig. 85).

c Six months after the inflammation has healed, the last precipitates have also disappeared. Posterior to the ora serrata a more strongly reflecting zone remains ("pseudo-white with pressure"). The hyaloid membrane now lies quite close to the ciliary body. However, no white midline is to be seen.

d Unaffected left eye: Here the white midline is present. Moderate cystoid degeneration of the peripheral retina. Posteriorly, slight irregularity in pigment epithelium

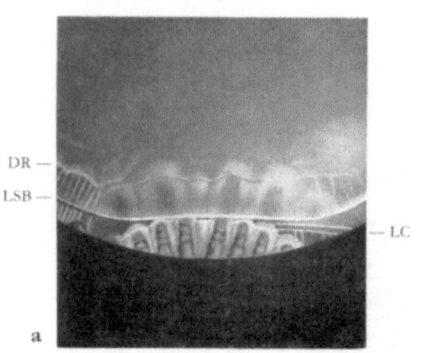

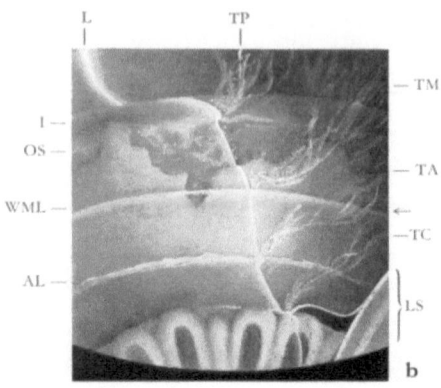

Fig. 92a and b. *Focal cyclitis anterior and posterior* (D.D., 50 years of age).
Bilateral chronic cyclitis of unknown aetiology. Mutton-fat precipitates in the anterior chamber, cystic macular oedema. In both eyes there are no other focal lesions than those on the ciliary body.

a Observation without indentation through the iridolenticular space. The ciliary body is tumified, the zonula has relaxed, and there is a deformation of the lens border. The ciliary processes are covered by a whitish, sharply defined cap of exudate. Anteriorly, the ciliary stroma lies exposed. Above the processes there are fibres of the ligamentum coronarium, from which single zonule fibres extend into the ciliary valleys (right). The same structures appear, more magnified, also in translental view.

b Indentation of the pars plana, translental observation. Sharply defined exudates cover large parts of the pars plana. Posteriorly, they are irregularly defined. The exudates are situated exclusively in the previtreal space. The anterior hyaloid membrane is intact, the tractus vitreales are normal; only at the site of their insertion is there a slight cellular infiltration of the anterior hyaloid membrane

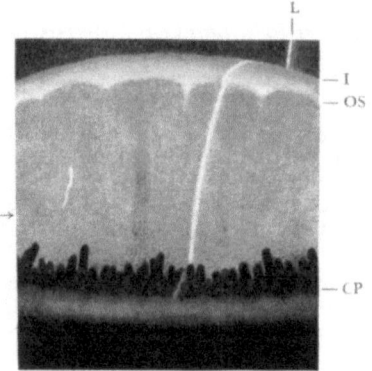

Fig. 93. *Diffuse scarring of the pars plana after severe panuveitis* (S.P., 27 years of age).
Bilateral extremely severe chronic recurrent panuveitis of unknown aetiology. Bilateral aphakia. Phthisis developed in the right eye; in the left eye, the heavily infiltrated vitreous body would clear occasionally, the fundus thus becoming visible. The retina then appeared diffusely thickened, but circumscribed foci were not found. The whole pars plana is a yellow scar without any surface structure. The processes, on the other hand, are apparently normal. In the vitreous body there is a striking Tyndall phenomenon, and no zones of discontinuity can be seen

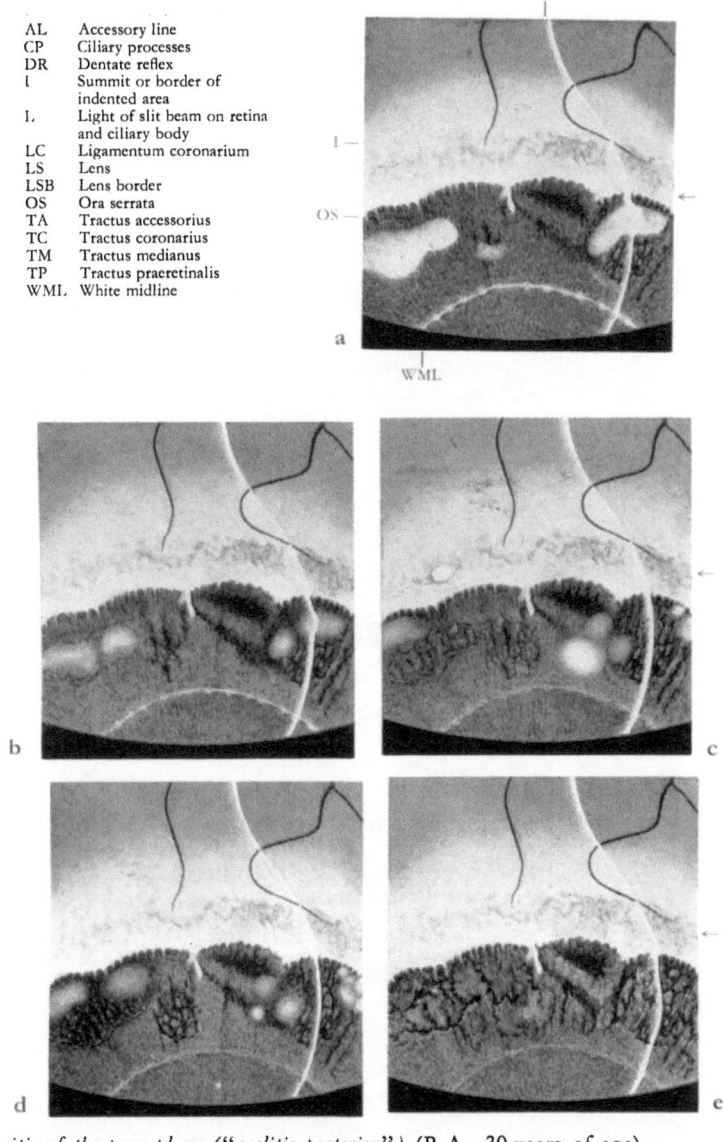

AL	Accessory line
CP	Ciliary processes
DR	Dentate reflex
l	Summit or border of indented area
L	Light of slit beam on retina and ciliary body
LC	Ligamentum coronarium
LS	Lens
LSB	Lens border
OS	Ora serrata
TA	Tractus accessorius
TC	Tractus coronarius
TM	Tractus medianus
TP	Tractus praeretinalis
WML	White midline

Fig. 94a–e. *Focal uveitis of the pars plana ("cyclitis posterior")* (R.A., 30 years of age).
Bilateral recurrent fibrinous iritis lasting for many years. Each time the anterior chamber had cleared, inflammatory exudates with surrounding pigmentation could be observed upon the pars plana. The posterior sections of the eye were also affected by an oedema of the macula and of the papilla.

a Fresh inflammatory foci on the pars plana among old pigmented scars. Accumulation of cells in the region of the white midline.

b The exudates are dissolved and form small isolated patches.

c Exacerbation with formation of new foci.

d Resorption of old and new foci.

e Healing with the formation of pigmented scars. The infiltration at the white midline has disappeared. Later on, pars plana cysts and a schisis retinae developed in the previously affected area

155

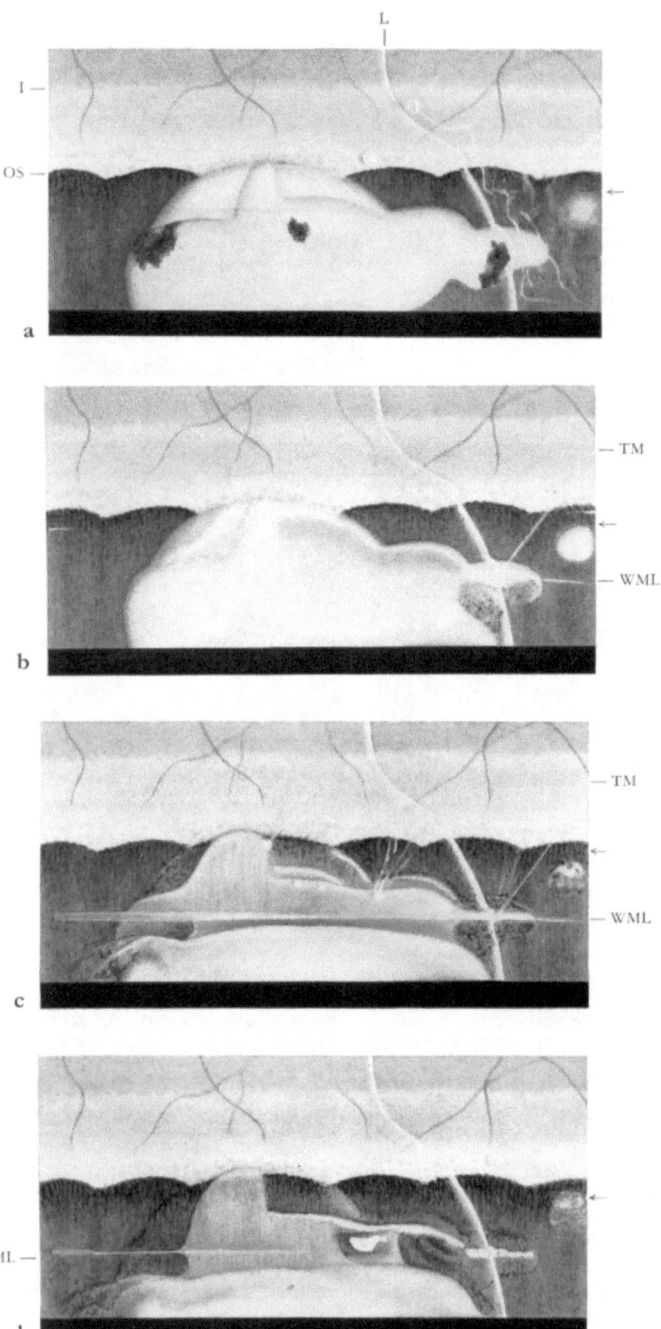

Fig. 95a–d. Legend see opposite page

Fig. 96a and b. *Cellular infiltration of the vitreous in uveitis posterior* (S.I., 50 years of age).
Acute chorioretinitis at the posterior pole. Aetiology unknown.

a Slight infiltration of the tractus praeretinalis and of the tractus medianus by cells and precipitates (lower periphery at 6h). At the edge of the retina, there is a vascularized scar probably due to an earlier attack.

b Fundus photograph of the chorioretinitic focus

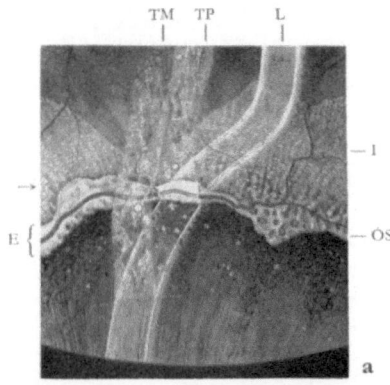

a

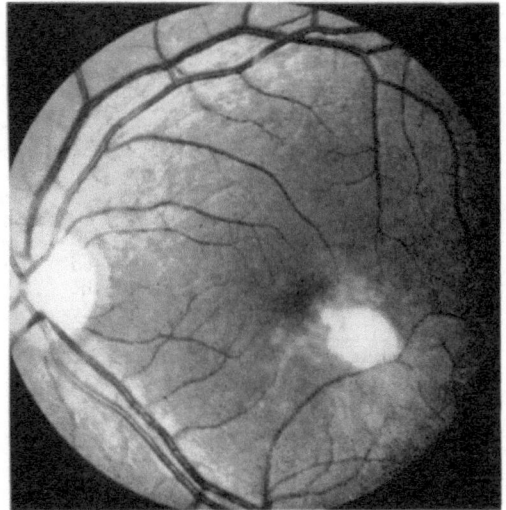

b

E	Exudate
1	Border of indented area
L	Light of slit beam on retina and ciliary body
OS	Ora serrata
TM	Tractus medianus
TP	Tractus praeretinalis
WML	White midline

◀

Fig. 95a–d. *Focal inflammation of the pars plana (cyclitis posterior)* (R.C., 23 years of age).
Unilateral subacute fibrinous iritis with haemorrhagic hypopyon. The posterior section of the globe was not affected. After clearing of the anterior chamber an examination of the peripheral fundus was possible. Anterior to the ora serrata at 1 and 6h, dense exudates were found whose topographical relation to the boundaries of the vitreous base could not be discerned initially. In the course of one year the exudates were resorbed. After the reappearance of the white midline the position of the exudates within the previtreal space could be distinctly made out. Later on, pigmented scars became visible on the pars plana. Our picture shows various stages of the exudative foci at 6h.

a Acute phase: the vitreous base above the pars plana is infiltrated with inflammatory exudates. On the surface of the exudates there are small haemorrhages (black in the picture). In the vitreous body no distinct structures are identifiable.

b The haemorrhages have disappeared. Scars begin to form at the edge of the large exudative focus. This is covered by the white midline and by the tractus medianus, which are visible again. The exudation at the small adjacent focus has increased.

c Further regression of the focus. All of the white midline is now again visible, as well as the membranelles of the tractus medianus. The adjacent exudative focus has scarred.

d The focus is surrounded by a pigmented scar. In its centre there are still exudates

157

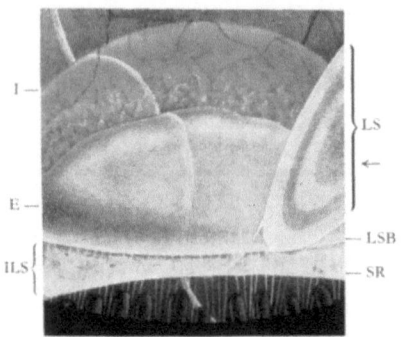

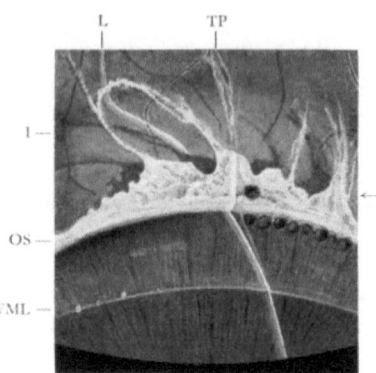

Fig. 97. *Exudative sediments in uveitis posterior* (K.M., 24 years of age).
Unilateral chronic uveitis of unknown aetiology. The anterior chamber remained unaffected. The vitreous body, however, was clouded by opacities consisting of exudates, cells, and pigment. Four months later, the vitreous body had slightly cleared, but in the lower periphery a large exudative sediment remained. In translental view its position erroneously might have been located upon the pars plana. But seen through the iridolenticular space, the opacity was clearly delimited by the anterior hyaloid membrane, the ciliary body being entirely free from any inflammatory changes

Fig. 98. *Scarring of the vitreous base in the lower periphery* (F. B., 23 years of age, no ocular complaints).
In the course of a routine examination sheathing of the peripheral vessels was observed as well as some single cells and a moderate vitreous destruction. In the inferior periphery, there is a sharply defined fibrous condensation of the tractus praeretinalis. Anteriorly, upon the pars plana coarse clumps of pigment

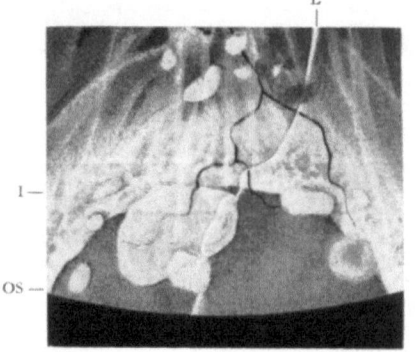

E	Exudate
I	Summit or border of indented area
ILS	Iridolenticular space
L	Light of slit beam on retina and ciliary body
LS	Lens
LSB	Lens border
OS	Ora serrata
SR	Silhouette reflex
PVM	Posterior vitreous (hyaloid) membrane
TM	Tractus medianus
TP	Tractus praeretinalis
WML	White midline

Fig. 99. *Fundus periphery in severe panuveitis* (E. E., 21 years of age).
Unilateral severe inflammation, affecting all sections of the eye: nodules on the iris and in the chamber angle, massive exudation in the vitreous body, disseminated chorioretinitic foci. In the tractus praeretinalis and on the pars plana there are large quantities of exudative deposits, some of which have become vascularized by retinal vessels. At the right edge of the picture there is a greyish inflammatory focus with poorly defined boundaries, which probably originates in the pars plana itself. Following intravenous injection of fluorescein there was a rapid and very intense staining of the focus, whereas the other exudates fluoresced neither in the early nor in the late phases

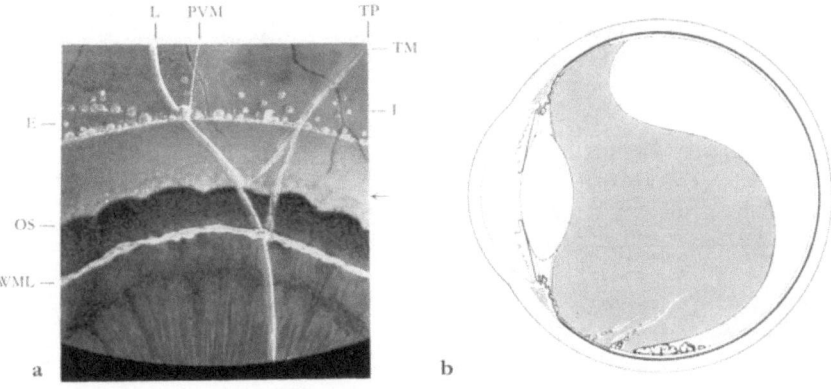

Fig. 100a and b. *Exudative sediments after a posterior vitreous detachment (hypopyon praeretinale)* (L. Sch., 46 years of age).
Recurrence of a unilateral chorioretinitis juxtapapillaris.

a Hypopyon-like sediment at the lower boundary of the retrovitreal space. Within the vitreous, there is a slight infiltration also into the tractus vitreales. Exudative sediments at the ora serrata and at the white midline.

b Schematic drawing of the hypopyon praeretinale and of the infiltration of the tractus vitreales

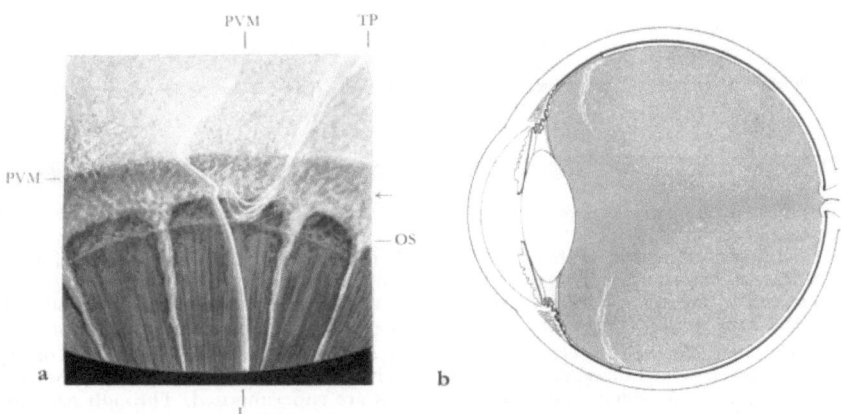

Fig. 101a and b. *Heavy infiltration of the retrovitreal space* (E. H., 54 years of age).
Bilateral panuveitis with slight symptoms of inflammation in the anterior sections, but with complete clouding of the posterior fundus.

a The retrovitreal space is entirely filled with opaque exudates. The retina is visible only in the outermost periphery, in the region of the posterior vitreous base.

b Schematic drawing of the infiltration of the retrovitreal space

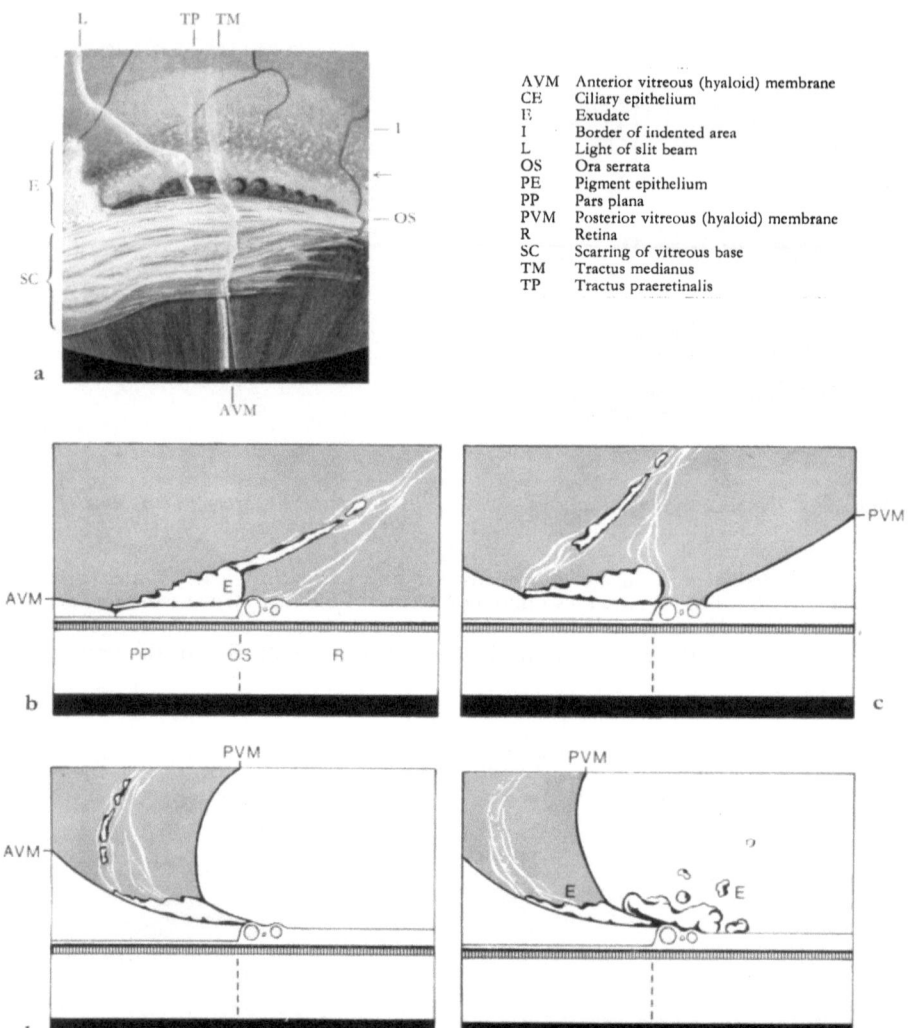

AVM	Anterior vitreous (hyaloid) membrane
CE	Ciliary epithelium
E	Exudate
I	Border of indented area
L	Light of slit beam
OS	Ora serrata
PE	Pigment epithelium
PP	Pars plana
PVM	Posterior vitreous (hyaloid) membrane
R	Retina
SC	Scarring of vitreous base
TM	Tractus medianus
TP	Tractus praeretinalis

Fig. 102a–e. *Inflammatory sediments in the lower periphery ; organization of the vitreous base* (S.G., 8 years of age).

At the first examination of this child a scarcely distinguishable chorioiditic focus was found posterior to the equator. This focus healed completely after a short time, leaving practically no traces. In the lower periphery, however, exudates had accumulated and an inflammatory process kept smouldering there for several years. The picture shows the periphery at 6h.

a Early phase. At the ora serrata the retina has increased in thickness, and cysts of different sizes are interspersed there. Anteriorly, at the vitreous base, there are fibrous condensations, at some places of which fresh cloudy exudates are superimposed. Through gaps in these opacities the unaffected pars plana can be recognized. With observation through the irido-lenticular space, a similar picture as that in Fig. 97 is seen. The posterior hyaloid membrane is not yet detached.

b Status of Fig. a in schematic drawing.

c Posterior vitreous detachment. A posterior vitreous detachment having developed subsequently, the intravitreal exudates are displaced anteriorly.

d Organization and shrinking of the vitreous base. The posterior hyaloid membrane has been drawn so far anteriorly that it appears to be inserted anterior to the ora serrata.

e With the next recurrence, the posterior hyaloid membrane being displaced anteriorly, the preretinal hypopyon now overlies even the ora serrata

160

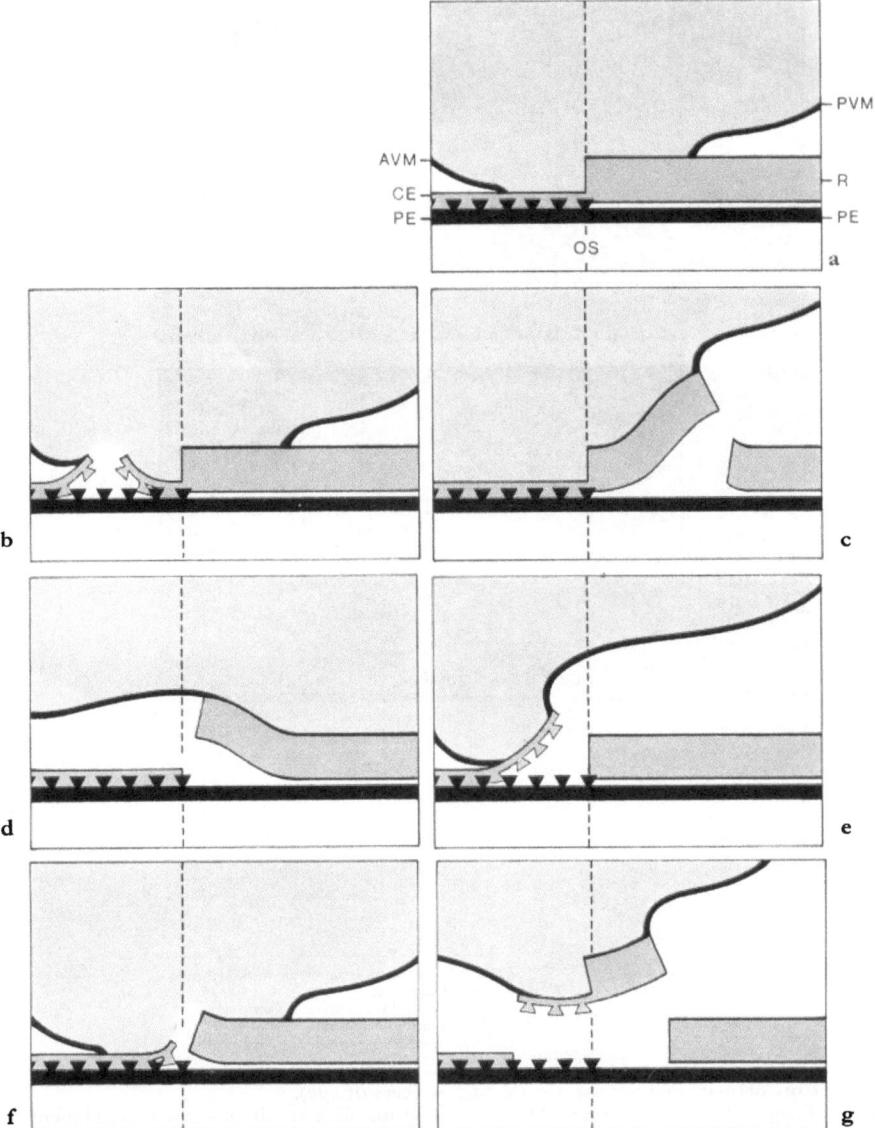

Fig. 103a–g. *Amotio retinae. Various types of tears.*

a Vitreous base and retroretinal interstice in a normal eye.

b Tear in the ciliary epithelium at the pars plana (in the region of the retroretinal adhesion).

c Tear in the retina at the posterior boundary of the vitreous base (in the region of the retroretinal interstice).

d Prebasal ora tear: the anterior hyaloid membrane is inserted at the posterior edge of the tear. The site of rupture is above the retroretinal interstice.

e Retrobasal ora tear: the posterior hyaloid membrane is inserted at the anterior edge of the tear. The traction works in the direction of the zone of retroretinal adhesion.

f Intrabasal ora tear. The hyaloid membranes are not in direct contact with the edges of the tear.

g Avulsion of the vitreous base. The tears are situated at the anterior and the posterior edges of the vitreous base. A strip of tissue containing ciliary epithelium and retina is torn out. Thus a defect is formed, where no hyaloid membranes are attached at the anterior and posterior edges. Traction may be expected, if at all, at the lateral edges of the defect, where the extruded strip is re-inserted in the retina

161

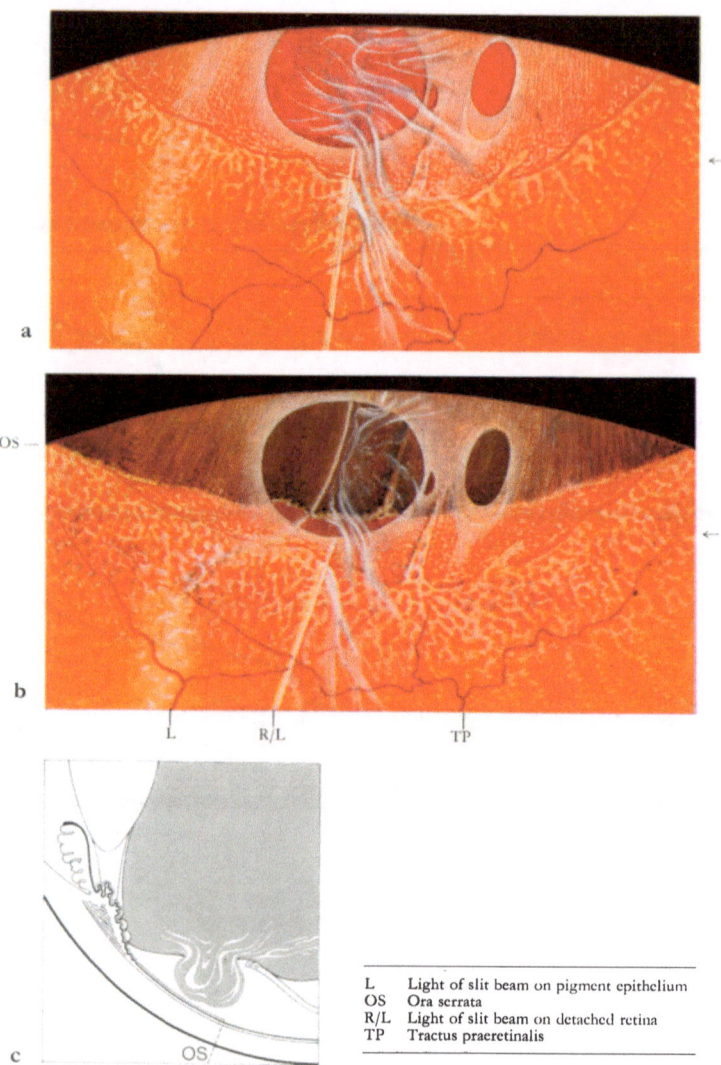

a

OS —

b

L   R/L   TP

L	Light of slit beam on pigment epithelium
OS	Ora serrata
R/L	Light of slit beam on detached retina
TP	Tractus praeretinalis

c   OS

Fig. 104a–c. *Prebasal ora tear* (V.M., 34 years of age).
Temporal upper quadrant. Decrease of vision as a result of retinal detachment. No indication of previous trauma.

a With the ophthalmoscope and with the three-mirror contact glass, a retinal detachment with atrophy of the retina was diagnosed. In the detached lamina there is still the pattern of the ora serrata region with cystoid spaces, dentate processes, and a granular and striate structure of the pars plana. Anterior to the ora serrata there are two round holes. These findings might be interpreted as a retinal detachment extending beyond the ora serrata into the ciliary body.

b Indentation shows, however, that the ciliary epithelium is still attached to the ciliary body. This can be ascertained in optical section from a step at the ora serrata between the uncovered pigment epithelium and the ciliary epithelium. On the still attached ciliary epithelium there is the typical granular and striate pattern of the pars plana and even an intact ora tooth is still there. This is a typical prebasal ora tear. The anterior hyaloid membrane is condensed, and the surface structures of the pars plana are cast onto it. It is perforated in two places. As regards treatment, closing the two "round holes" would not have sufficed. The entire ora tear, comprising almost half the circumference, had to be treated.

c Schematic drawing

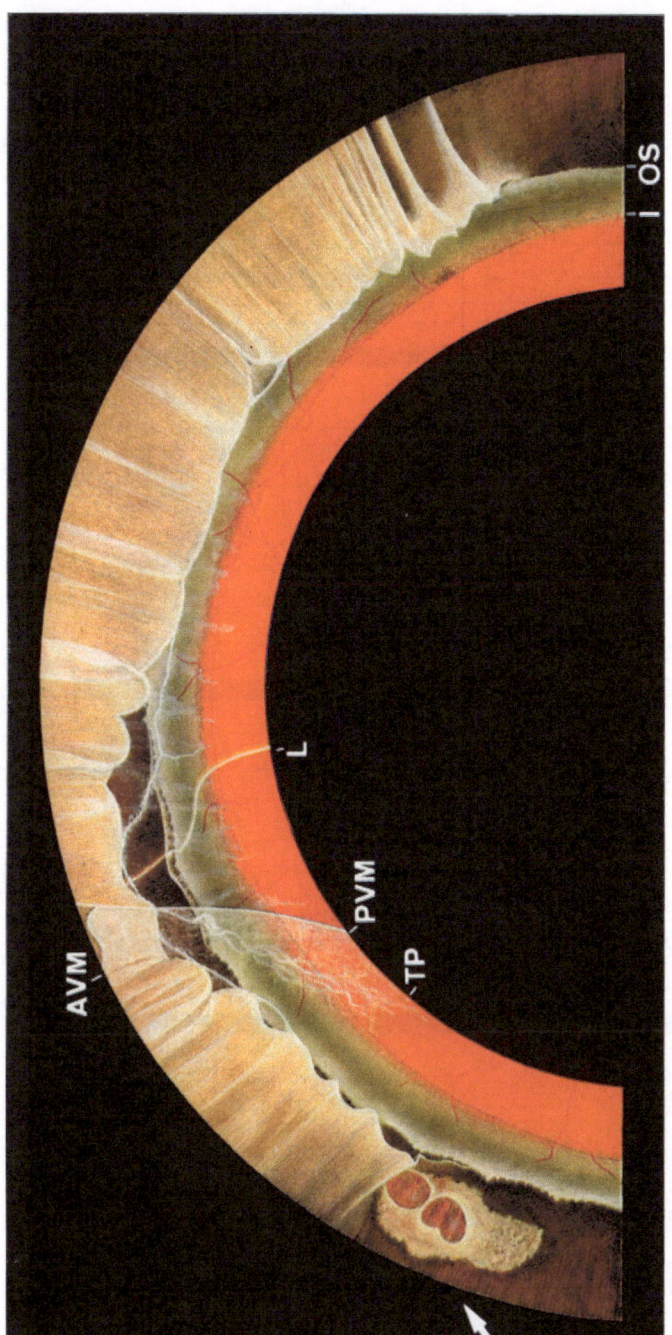

AVM	Anterior vitreous (hyaloid) membrane
I	Border of indented area
L	Light of slit beam on retina and ciliary body
OS	Ora serrata
PVM	Posterior vitreous (hyaloid) membrane
TP	Tractus praeretinalis

Fig. 105a and b. *Retrobasal ora tear* (B.L., 25 years of age).

Large pars plana cysts developed secondary to an intense inflammatory vitreous exudation. By coalescence of the cysts the ciliary epithelium detached in the whole upper circumference. Following a posterior vitreous detachment, a giant ora tear developed from 10–12h, and the cysts collapsed. The ciliary epithelium—formerly the inner wall of the cysts—became detached. The posterior edges of the tear were traction-free.

a Upper fundus periphery. The detached ciliary epithelium appears as a yellowish, semitransparent membrane with the typical striate pattern. It covers a large part of the ora tear, which is visible only in the centre of the picture. Here the slit beam is reproduced. At the anterior detached edge of the tear the posterior hyaloid membrane and the tractus praeretinalis insert. The attached pars plana appears dark brown. At the left edge of the picture are two round defects in the ciliary epithelium, surrounded by a flat detachment with incipient scarring of the edges.

b Schematic drawing. The vitreous base adheres to the detached ciliary epithelium, the anterior hyaloid membrane is floating

163

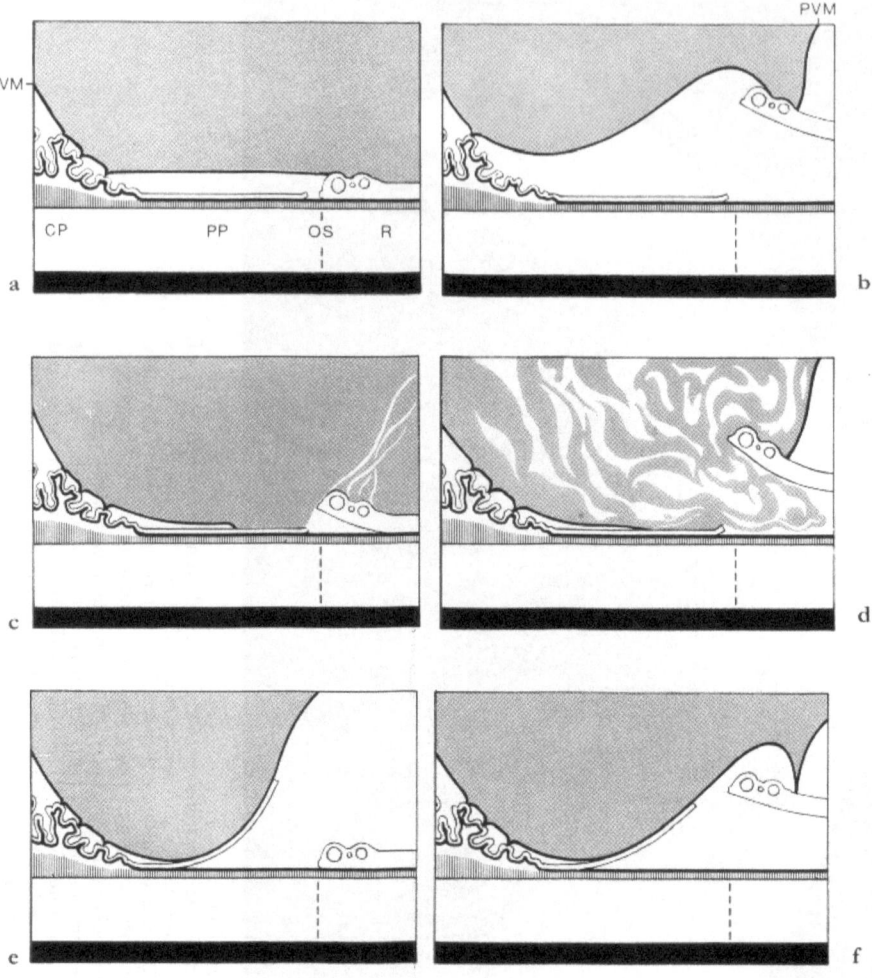

Fig. 106a–f. *Effect of traction and adhesion in ora tears.*

a and b Prebasal tear.

a The anterior hyaloid membrane is still fixed at the ciliary body, inducing only a slight traction.

b The anterior hyaloid membrane is floating. The vitreous is destroyed, the posterior hyaloid membrane is detached. There is now a stronger traction at the edges, and the retina becomes detached.

c and d Intrabasal ora tear.

c Vitreous structure intact. Minimal effect of traction.
d Vitreous destroyed. The traction of the posterior hyaloid membrane is transferred to the edge of the tear. Large quantities of destroyed vitreous penetrate into the retroretinal space.

e and f Retrobasal ora tear.

e In the absence of retinal adhesions, no amotio retinae develops. Traction, however, must be reckoned with at the lateral edges of the tear.
f A small residual adhesion on the retina is sufficient to cause detachment

164

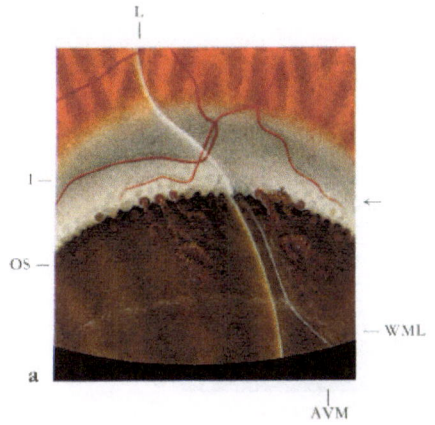

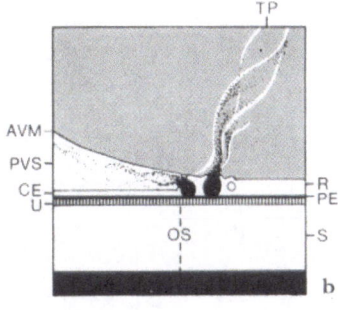

Fig. 107a and b. *Rupture of cysts at the retinal border* (W.B., 40 years of age).
Contusio bulbi with hyphaemia, tears in the ciliary body band, and Berlin's oedema at the posterior pole. Two months post trauma, brown pigmented granules were still found posterior to the lens, at the insertion of the anterior hyaloid membrane, between the zonular fibres, as well as in the vitreous body.

a In the temporal upper periphery some cysts at the retinal border are ruptured, with pigment leaking out in clouds. Here, the anterior hyaloid membrane, along with the white midline, is detached from the ciliary epithelium. The previtreal space is enlarged posteriorly as far as the ora serrata.

b Migration of pigment from ruptured cysts of the retinal border (schematic drawing). Depending on the position of the rupture, the pigment may leak either into the previtreal space or into the vitreous body

AVM	Anterior vitreous (hyaloid) membrane
CE	Ciliary epithelium
CP	Ciliary processes
I	Border of indented area
L	Light of slit beam on retina and ciliary body
OS	Ora serrata
PE	Pigment epithelium
PP	Pars plana
PVM	Posterior vitreous membrane
PVS	Previtreal space
R	Retina
S	Sclera
TP	Tractus praeretinalis
U	Uvea
WML	White midline

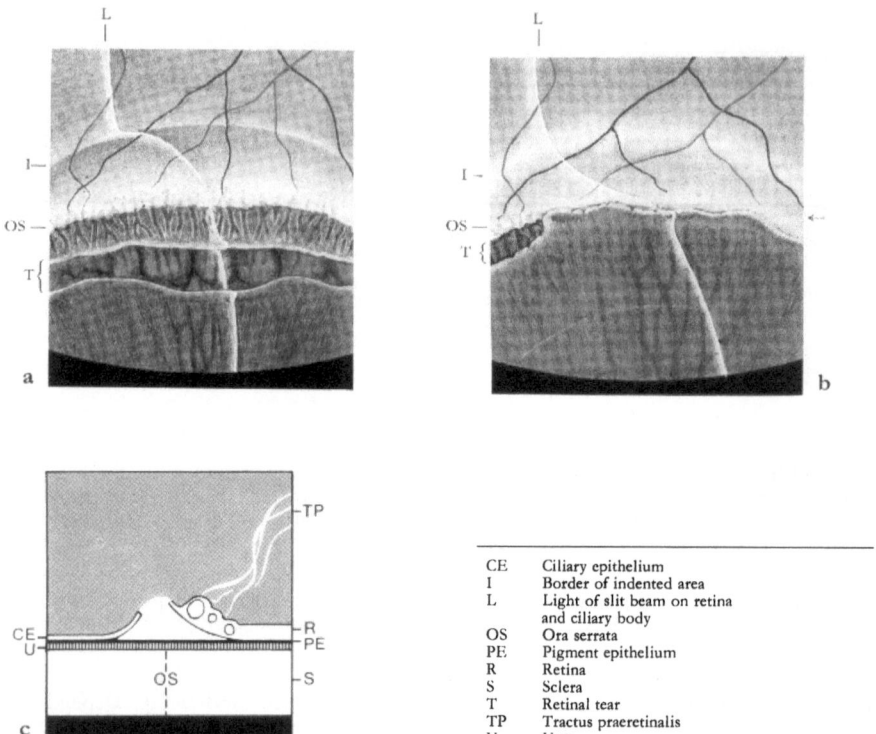

CE	Ciliary epithelium
I	Border of indented area
L	Light of slit beam on retina and ciliary body
OS	Ora serrata
PE	Pigment epithelium
R	Retina
S	Sclera
T	Retinal tear
TP	Tractus praeretinalis
U	Uvea

Fig. 108a–c. *Traumatic tear of the ciliary epithelium* (B.M., 17 years of age).
6 years before the examination, the patient suffered from an ocular contusion with hyphaemia, tears in the ciliary body band, subluxation of the lens, peripapillary choroidal rupture, secondary glaucoma.

a A gaping tear is clearly visible on the anterior surface of the indentation protuberance. At the bottom of the tear, the pigment epithelium lies exposed.

b With the indenter shifted the tear may disappear from view. Only diligent examination in optical section may reveal its presence.

c Schematic drawing of the ciliary epithelium tear

166

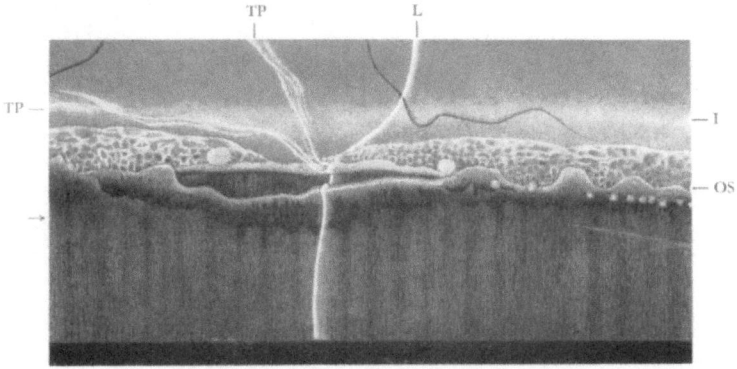

Fig. 109. *Tear of the ciliary epithelium* (W. Sch., 9 years of age).
Contusio bulbi, with hyphaemia, massive vitreous haemorrhage, and lesions at the posterior pole. Brown pigmented granules are dispersed in the vitreous body. The ciliary epithelium is torn from 8–11 h immediately anterior to the ora serrata. The bottom of the tear is visible only in the centre of the picture; on either side it is hidden by the detached anterior edge of the tear. The tractus praeretinalis is inserted at the posterior edge of the tear

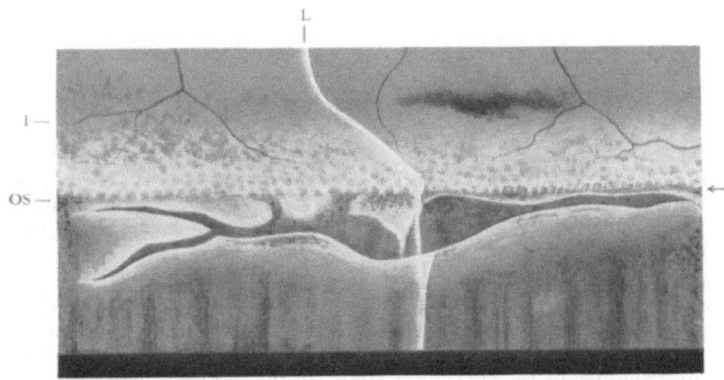

Fig. 110. *Ramified tear of the ciliary epithelium* (F. Sch., 39 years of age).
Contusio bulbi with slight hyphaemia, Berlin's oedema. Pigmented cells in the vitreous. On the pars plana at 12 h there is a large ramified tear of the ciliary epithelium. In the early stages, the edges of the tear were slightly prominent, later they became re-attached. Pre-retinal haemorrhage in the pre-equatorial retina

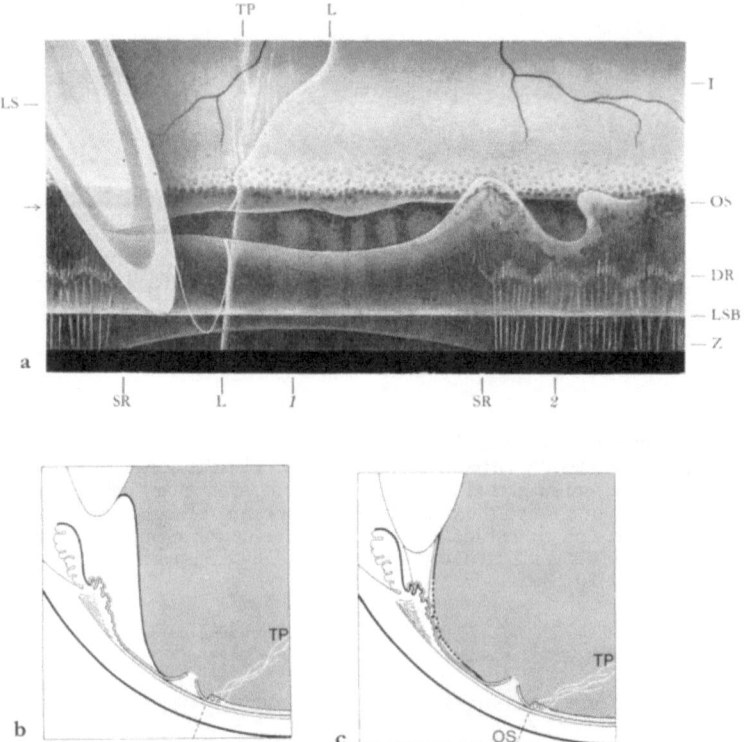

Fig. 111a–c. *Tear in the ciliary epithelium and the zonule* (E. E., 18 years of age)
Status after two contusions inducing a disturbance of pupillary motility and a recession of the angle. Slight deformation of the lens, hypotonia. Brown pigmented granules in the vitreous.

a From 8–11h on the pars plana there is a rupture of the ciliary epithelium, with raising of the anterior edge of the tear. In the same meridian, zonule fibres are interrupted, those running to the lens as well as those which attach the hyaloid membrane to the ciliary body. The anterior hyaloid membrane has therefore retracted here towards the centre of the eye. (Recognizable by the curvilinear course of the silhouette reflex.)

b and c Schematic drawings of a meridional section at the points *1* and *2* of Fig. a

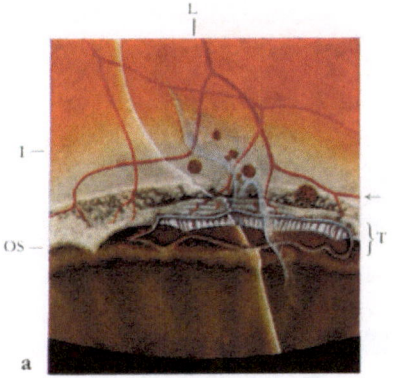

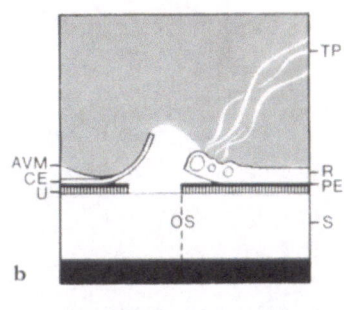

Fig. 112a and b. *Intrabasal tear with choroidal rupture* (A.M., 9 years of age).
Contusio bulbi with detachment of the ciliary body band from the scleral spur. Transitory macular oedema; brown granules in the vitreous.

a At 12h, at the ora serrata, the ciliary epithelium is torn. The edges of the tear have already slightly re-attached. At the bottom of the tear, there are two zones: anterior, the evenly brown pigment epithelium; posterior, a choroidal defect, with the white sclera covered by some large choroidal vessels. Posterior to the ora serrata, slight retinal scarring. In the vitreous there are pigmented, precipitate-like deposits.

b Schematic drawing of a rupture of the ciliary epithelium and the choroid

AVM	Anterior vitreous (hyaloid) membrane		PE	Pigment epithelium
CE	Ciliary epithelium		R	Retina
DR	Dentate reflex		S	Sclera
I	Border of indented area		SR	Silhouette reflex on AVM
L	Light of slit beam on retina and ciliary body		T	Retinal tear
LS	Lens		TP	Tractus praeretinalis
LSB	Lens border		U	Uvea
OS	Ora serrata		Z	Zonule

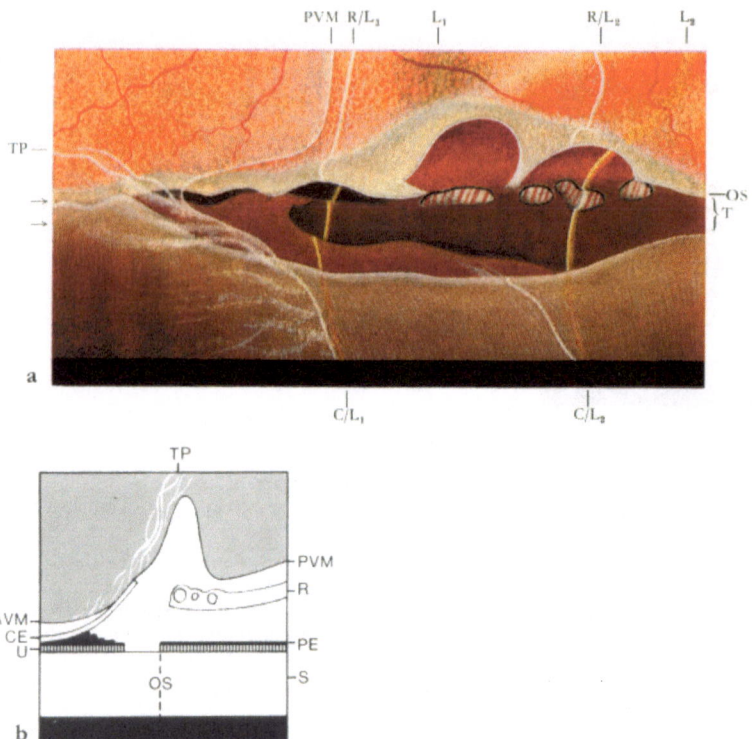

Fig. 113a and b. *Retrobasal ora tear with choroidal rupture* (J.J., 34 years of age).
By the time symptoms appeared, the detached retina had already undergone marked atrophy. The amotio had obviously spread gradually. Although no trauma could be elicited in the history, a previous contusion must be postulated, since choroidal ruptures are present.

a The retina and the ciliary epithelium are detached. There is an oblong tear at the ora serrata, with some connecting strands from the retina towards the pigment epithelium. At the bottom of the tear the ora serrata boundary may be recognized by the transition from red to brown colouring. At this site there are several elongated choroidal defects in which the sclera lies exposed, with large choroidal vessels overlying it. The posterior hyaloid membrane is inserted at the anterior edge of the tear first running in a curve towards the centre of the globe and then re-approaching the retina.

b Schematic drawing of the sagittal section through the tear

170

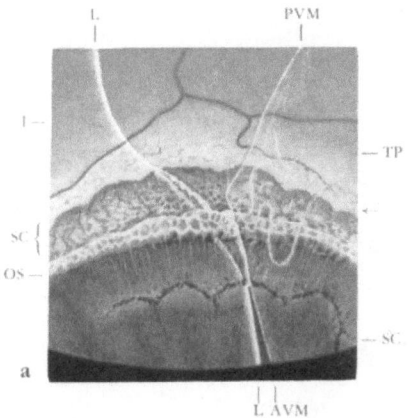

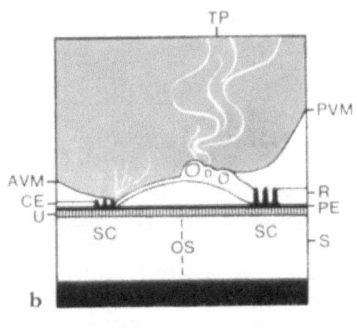

Fig. 114a and b. *Incomplete avulsion of the vitreous base* (B.H., 36 years of age).
Ocular contusion with parapapillary choroidal ruptures. Two months post trauma, the periphery of the retina was examined, and a small avulsion of the vitreous base from 9–11h was discovered. The adjoining areas could not be examined because of vitreal haemorrhages.

a Five months later, the avulsed vitreous base had re-attached and tears were no longer apparent. The edges of the anterior tear form an irregularly pigmented band. Posterior to this, a strip of pars plana epithelium and retinal tissue is slightly raised. The vitreous base adheres to this strip. Posterior to the raised strip the posterior tear is closed by pigmented scarring. Examinations during the next 5 years showed no traces of retinal detachment.

b Schematic drawing of sagittal section through the raised strip

AVM	Anterior vitreous (hyaloid) membrane	PVM	Posterior vitreous (hyaloid) membrane
CE	Ciliary epithelium	R	Retina
C/L$_1$ and C/L$_2$	Light of slit beams on detached ciliary epithelium	R/L$_1$ and R/L$_2$	Light of slit beams on detached retina
I	Border of indented area	S	Sclera
L	Light of slit beam on retina and ciliary body	SC	Scar
L$_1$ and L$_2$	Light of slit beams on pigment epithelium	T	Tear
OS	Ora serrata	TP	Tractus praeretinalis
PE	Pigment epithelium	U	Uvea

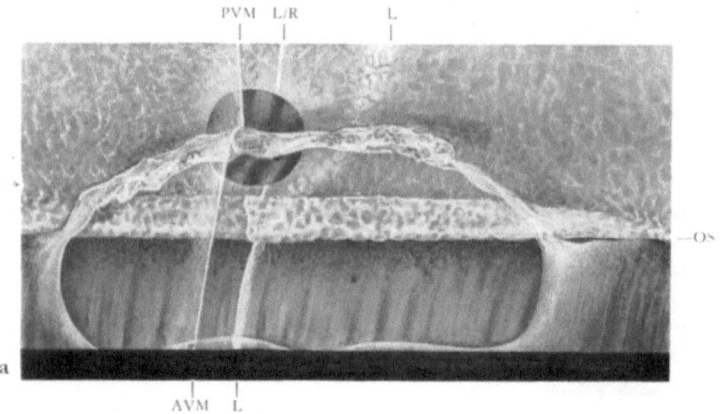

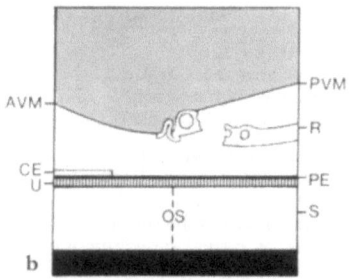

Fig. 115a and b. *Complete avulsion of the vitreous base after contusio bulbi* (P.H., 18 years of age).

a Three weeks post trauma, following resorption of the vitreous haemorrhage, an amotio retinae was diagnosed. There is a peripheral circular hole, at whose edges, however, no hyaloid membrane is inserted. The main cause of the amotio is a large defect at the ora serrata extending from 5–7h. From the nasal edge of this defect a strip of retinal and ciliary tissue, densely covered with pigment granules, projects into the vitreous space. Temporally, this strip has torn loose from the ciliary epithelium and is connected with it only by a densified fibrous strand. At this strip the anterior and posterior hyaloid membranes insert.

b Schematic drawing of sagittal section through the avulsed strip

AVM Anterior vitreous (hyaloid) membrane
CE   Ciliary epithelium
L   Light of slit beam on pigment epithelium and ciliary body
L/R   Light of slit beam on detached retina
LS   Lens
OS   Ora serrata
PE   Pigment epithelium
PVM   Posterior vitreous (hyaloid) membrane
R   Retina
S   Sclera
TP   Tractus praeretinalis

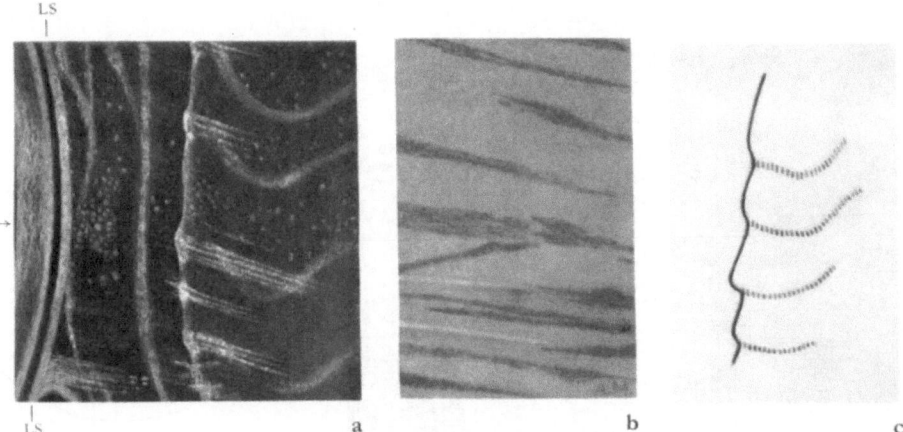

LS

LS   a   b   c

Fig. 116a–c. *Change of the vitreous structure after perforation.* (By courtesy of Professor Dr. H. Goldmann.) Examination without contact glass.

a Translental view. The membranelles of the tractus hyaloideus situated immediately posterior to the lens follow their normal course. In between there are irregularly dispersed erythrocytes. Further posteriorly new vitreous membranelles have been formed, starting perpendicularly from a normal tractus vitrealis. In the folds of the newly formed membranelle system, the sedimented blood forms "hyphaemia".

b Translental observation in reflected light. Blood deposits in the newly formed vitreal tracts. In the sectors behind the lens they are almost parallel, laterally they converge to the site of the perforation ("arrows" pointing to the site of the perforation).

c Schematic drawing

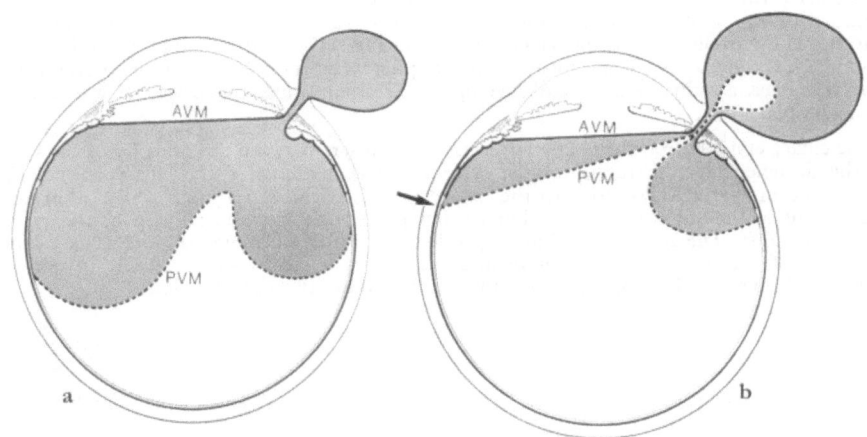

Fig. 117a and b. *Incarceration of hyaloid membranes in a perforation near the limbus* (schematic drawing after Goldmann [58]).

a Only the anterior hyaloid membrane is incarcerated in the wound.

b Incarceration of the anterior and posterior hyaloid membranes following abundant los of vitreous. In case of vitreous shrinkage, the retina becomes detached by traction of the posterior hyaloid membrane, on the side opposite the perforation (arrow)

173

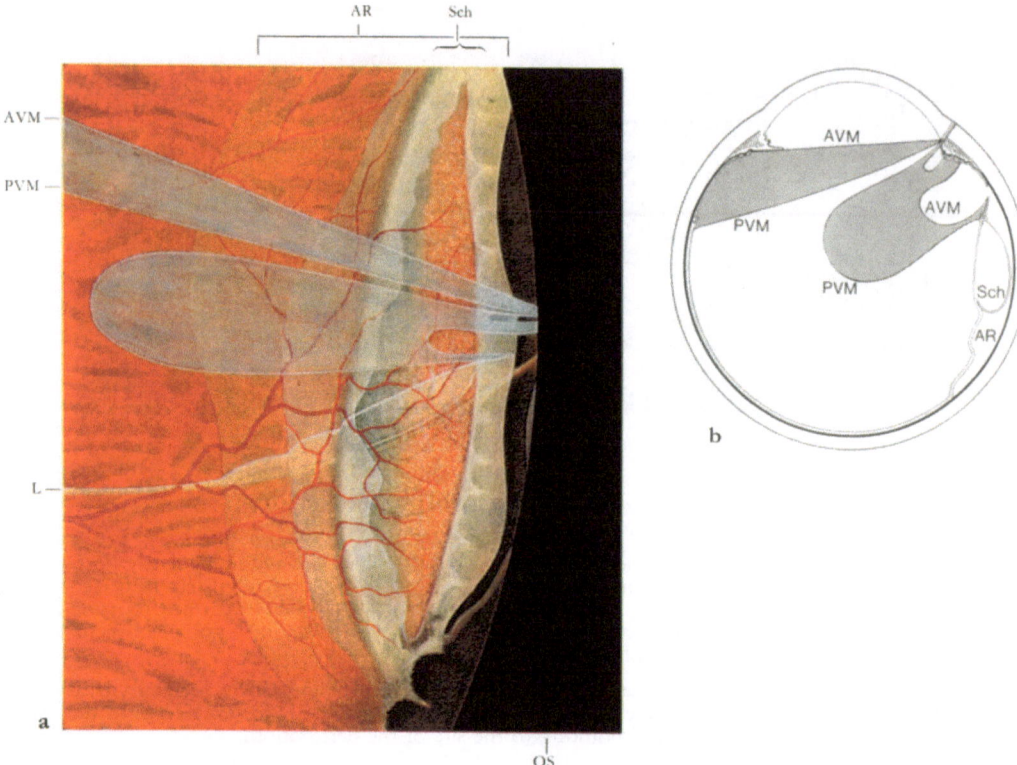

Fig. 118a and b. *Vitreous traction at the edges of a pars plana tear after perforation. Development of an amotio retinae* (F. Sch., 20 years of age). Horizontal slit beam.
Rupture of the globe at the temporal limbus from 12–5h with traumatic aphakia and aniridia. The vitreous body is characteristically (see Fig. 117) incarcerated in the perforation wound. Gradually, a schisis developed in the peripheral retina on the side of the perforation. One year later, a retinal detachment developed, spreading under the schisis. It was caused by a pars plana tear.

a The ciliary epithelium is torn. The vitreous base is inserted at the posterior lip of the tear. In the detached layer there appear the typical surface patterns of the ciliary epithelium and of the ora serrata. Posterior to the ora serrata is a schisis. Its inner wall is thin and transparent in the anterior sections, but further posteriorly, beyond a sharp boundary, it appears opaque. The retinal detachment produces two folds posterior to the schisis. The extension of the retinal detachment behind the schisis is clearly demonstrable in optical section. b Schematic drawing of a horizontal cross-section through the globe

AR	Amotio retinae
AVM	Anterior vitreous (hyaloid) membrane
CE	Ciliary epithelium
L	Light of slit beam on retina and ciliary body
OS	Ora serrata
PVM	Posterior vitreous (hyaloid) membrane
Sch	Schisis retinae
VM	Tractional vitreous membranules

174

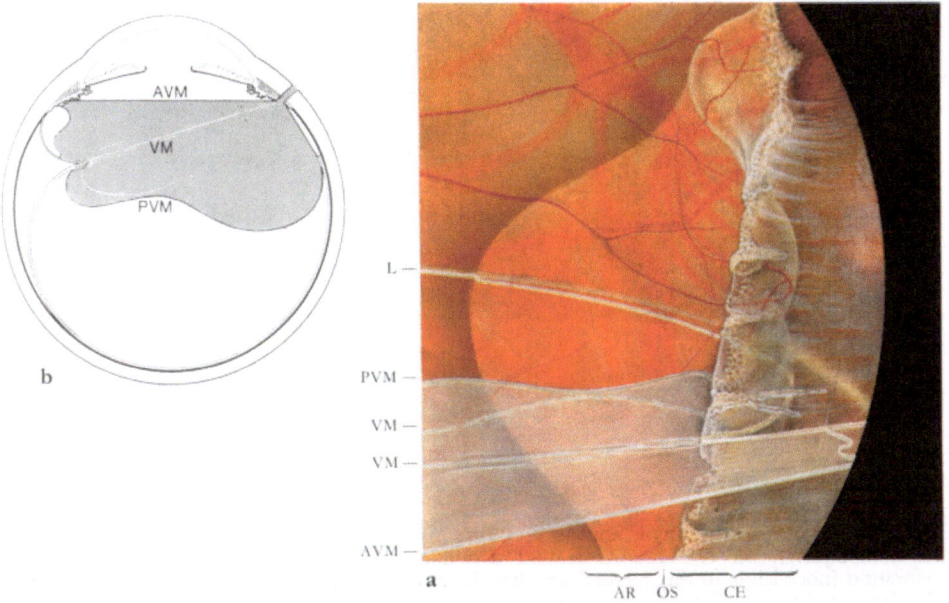

Fig. 119a and b. *Amotio retinae due to traction by newly formed vitreous strands* (I.B., 64 years of age). Horizontal slit beam.

Four years previously, perforation of the globe by wood splinters piercing the eye nasally in the region of the pars plicata of the ciliary body. Several operations for secondary glaucoma, later cataract extraction. Six months post trauma, after the vitreous haemorrhages had resorbed, a detachment of the ciliary epithelium was seen on the side opposite the perforation. Diagnosis of a retrobasal ora tear was then made (see Fig. 115). After removal of the lens the traction of the vitreous increased. Thus the stretched ciliary epithelium became atrophic and transparent; the retina behind it was discovered to be detached. Contrary to the former diagnosis there was no tear, but the retina and the ciliary epithelium had been drawn up into a fold.

a Temporal periphery at 3h. The crest of the fold lies at the ora serrata. The anterior surface is formed of ciliary epithelium, the posterior surface of retina. The vitreous traction responsible for the fold is not, as usually, produced by the posterior hyaloid membrane, but by a newly formed intravitreal membrane (tractional vitreous membrane).

At a superficial examination, this picture might be mistaken for a retrobasal ora tear with detachment of the ciliary epithelium. The crest of the fold might be misinterpreted as the anterior edge of an ora tear. Yet a correct diagnosis can be made even without the ciliary epithelium becoming transparent: the crest of the fold runs in a straight line and is not serrated as in an ora tear. The ora teeth overlap the crest anteriorly, the ora bays, on the other hand, posteriorly. The main clue for differential diagnosis, however, is provided by the insertion line of the posterior hyaloid membrane. In a retrobasal ora tear this line is at the ora serrata. In the present case, however, the site of insertion lies further posteriorly.

b Schematic drawing

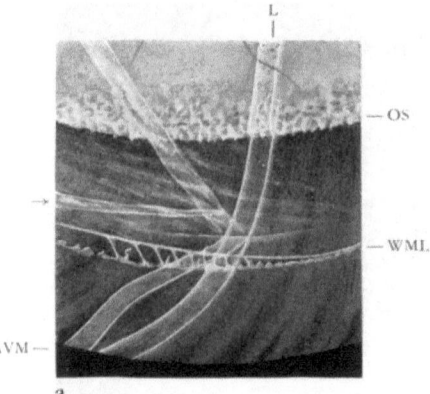

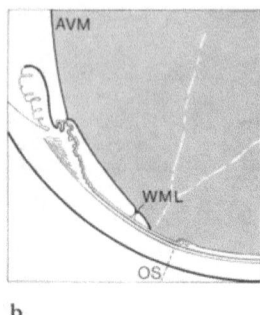

Fig. 120a and b. *Partial detachment of the vitreous body from its anterior base* (R.S., 63 years of age).
Perforating injury with traumatic aniridia and vitreous prolapse 46 years previously. Since then no complications. The anterior hyaloid membrane is dragged towards the site of the perforation (not visible in this picture) and has therefore become detached from the ciliary epithelium in the area of the anterior base.
a The lateral edge of the anterior vitreous detachment is shown. The white midline is detached from the ciliary epithelium, but there remain connecting strands at regular intervals. The tractus medianus is not visible. New vitreous membranelles have been formed·
b Schematic drawing of sagittal section

AVM	Anterior vitreous (hyaloid) membrane
OS	Ora serrata
WML	White midline

Fig. 121. *Complete detachment of the vitreous body from its base. Retinal detachment caused by a tear in the pars plana* (M.M., 31 years of age).
Perforatio bulbi by an intra-ocular foreign body. After resorption of the haemorrhage, vitreous strands are seen converging to the site of the perforation. Three years later a flat retinal detachment, unnoticed by the patient himself, is detected in the inferior periphery. It was caused by a long tear in the ciliary epithelium, whose posterior edge was inserted at the hyaloid membrane of the detached vitreous body.
Left, the vitreous body is entirely detached from its base (*I*). The surface patterns of the pars plana and the ora serrata underneath are cast upon the membranous vitreous surface. From this membrane dense fibres extend towards the ciliary body; some of them are torn and twisted like corkscrews.
The hyaloid membrane approaches the ciliary body in the right side of the picture (*III*). At the white midline there are bright spots probably formed by connecting strands like those in Fig. 120.
In the centre of the picture (*II*) there is a tear in the ciliary epithelium at the white midline. The posterior edge adheres to the detached hyaloid membrane. The retinal detachment extends posteriorly beyond the ora serrata.
I, II, III Schematic drawings of sagittal sections whose sites are indicated by the corresponding numbers in the figure

176

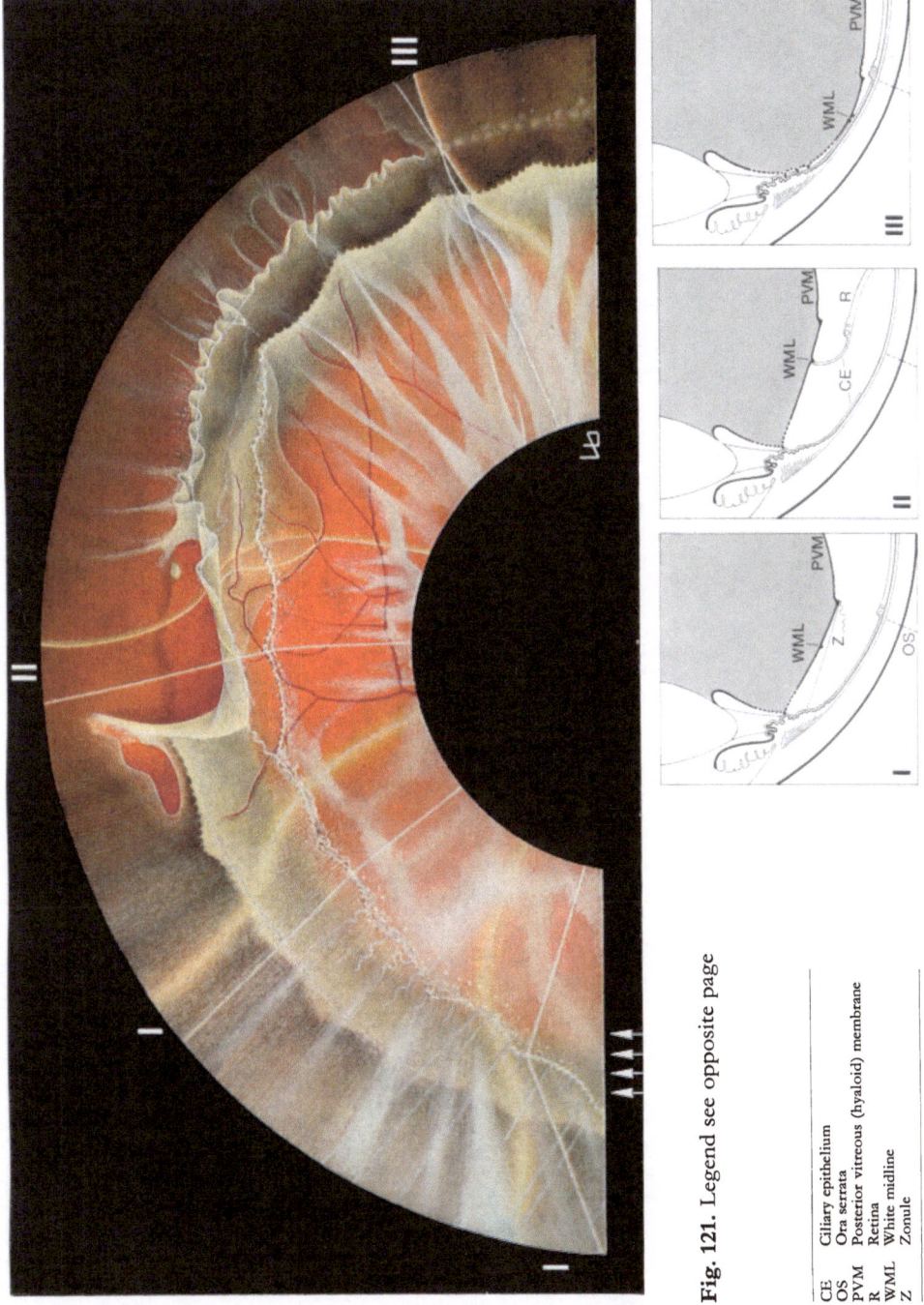

Fig. 121. Legend see opposite page

CE	Ciliary epithelium
OS	Ora serrata
PVM	Posterior vitreous (hyaloid) membrane
R	Retina
WML	White midline
Z	Zonule

References

1. Adam, S. T.: Pars plana cysts. Arch. Ophthal. (Chic.) **58**, 328–330 (1957).
2. Allen, R. A., Miller, D. H., Straatsma, B. R.: Cysts of the posterior ciliary body (pars plana). Arch. Ophthal. (Chic.) **66**, 302–313 (1961).
3. Alper, M. G.: Contusion angle deformity and glaucoma. Gonioscopic observations and clinical course. Arch. Ophthal. (Chic.) **69**, 455–467 (1963).
4. Amsler, M., Klöti, R.: Welches sind die gefährlichen Fundusherde, die mit der Lichtkoagulation anzugehen sind? Ophthalmologica (Basel) **141**, 329–333 (1961).
5. Ashton, N.: Ocular changes in multiple myelomatosis. Arch. Ophthal. (Chic.) **73**, 487–494 (1965).
6. Balazs, E. A.: Die Mikrostruktur und Chemie des Glaskörpers. Ber. dtsch. ophthal. Ges. **68**, 536–572 (1967).
7. Balazs, E. A.: The molecular biology of the vitreous. In: New and controversal aspects of retinal detachment. New York-Evanston-London: Hoeber Med. Division. Harper & Roy 1968.
8. Balazs, E. A., Toth, L. Z., Eckl, E. A., Mitchell, A. P.: Studies on the structure of the vitreous body XII; cytological and histochemical studies on the cortical tissue layer. Exp. Eye Res. **3**, 57–71 (1964).
9. Beauvieux: La zonule. Arch. Ophthal. (Paris) **29**, 410–427, 484–502 (1922).
10. Belmonte, N.: Nuevo Dispositivo de Indentacion variable durante el examen biomicroscopico de la periphería del fondo. Arch. Soc. esp. Oftal. **31**, 533–544 (1971).
11. Berliner, M. L.: Biomicroscopy of the eye. New York: P. B. Hoeber 1949.
12. Brini, A., Bronner, A., Gerhard, J. P., Nordmann, J.: Biologie et chirurgie du corps vitré. Paris: Masson 1968.
13. Brini, A., Porte, A., Stoeckel, M. E.: Morphologie et structure du vitré adulte. In: Rapport Soc. franç. d'Ophtal. Paris: Masson 1968.
14. Brockhurst, R. J., Schepens, Ch. L., Okamura Schiro, D.: Uveitis. I. Gonioscopy. Amer. J. Ophthal. **42**, 545–554 (1956).
15. Brockhurst, R. J., Schepens, Ch. L., Okamura Schiro, D.: II. Peripheral uveitis: clinical description, complications and differential diagnosis. Amer. J. Ophthal. **49**, 1257–1266 (1960).
16. Brockhurst, R. J., Schepens, Ch. L., Okamura Schiro, D.: III. Peripheral uveitis: pathogenesis, etiology and treatment. Amer. J. Ophthal. **51**, 19–26 (1961).
17. Brockhurst, R. J., Schepens, Ch. L., Okamura Schiro, D.: IV. Peripheral uveitis: the complication of retinal detachment. Arch. Ophthal. (Chic.) **80**, 747–753 (1968).
18. Burian, H., Allen, L.: Mechanical changes during accommodation observed by gonioscopy. Arch. Ophthal. (Chic.) **54**, 66–72 (1955).
19. Busacca, A.: Un nouveau phénomène observé dans le corps vitré antérieur au cours des uvéites. Ophthalmologica (Basel) **126**, 355–360 (1953).
20. Busacca, A.: Biomicroscopie et histopathologie de l'oeil, vol. I, II, III. Zürich: Schweiz. Druck- & Verlagshaus AG 1957.
21. Busacca, A., Goldmann, H., Schiff-Wertheimer, S.: Biomicroscopie du corps vitré et du fond de l'oeil. Paris: Masson 1957.
22. Byer, N. E.: Clinical study of lattice degeneration of the retina. Trans. Amer. Acad. Ophthal. **69**, 1064–1077 (1965).
23. Byer, N. E.: Clinical study of retinal breaks. Trans. Amer. Acad. Ophthal. Otolaryng. **71**, 461–473 (1967).
24. Byer, N. E.: Clinical study of senile retinoschisis. Arch. Ophthal. (Chic.) **79**, 36–44 (1968).
25. Cibis, P. A.: Vitroretinal pathology and surgery in retinal detachment. St. Louis: C. V. Mosby 1965.
26. Cockerham, W. D., MacKenzie Freeman, H.: Molehills, mountains and prophylaxis of retinal detachment. Arch. Ophthal. (Chic.) **79**, 655–656 (1968).
27. Colyear, B. H., Pischel, D. K.: Clinical tears in the retina without detachment. Amer. J. Ophthal. **41**, 773–792 (1956).

28. Cox, M. S., Schepens, C. L., Freeman, H. M.: Retinal detachment due to ocular contusion. Arch. Ophthal. (Chic.) **76**, 678–685 (1966).
29. Daicker, B.: Iuxtavenöse Netzhautgruben. Albrecht v. Graefes Arch. klin. exp. Ophthal. **171**, 292–299 (1967).
30. Daicker, B.: Zur Pathomorphologie und Pathogenese der pars-plana Zysten. Ophthalmologica (Basel) **156**, 289–296 (1968).
31. Daicker, B.: Retinochorioidale Venenanastomosen an der Ora serrata. Albrecht v. Graefes Arch. klin. exp. Ophthal. **175**, 28–33 (1968).
32. Daicker, B.: Anatomie und Pathologie der menschlichen retinociliaren Fundusperipherie. Basel-New York: S. Karger 1972.
33. Daicker, B.: Zur Kenntnis von Substrat und Bedeutung der sogenannten Schneckenspuren der Retina. Ophthalmologica (Basel) **165**, 360–365 (1972).
34. Daicker, B., Eisner, G.: Die Drusen der Ora serrata, ihre Klinik und pathologische Anatomie. Albrecht v. Graefes Arch. klin. exp. Ophthal. **174**, 336–343 (1968).
35. Delori, F., Pomerantzeff, O., Cox, M. S.: Deformation of the globe under high-speed impact: Its relation to contusion injuries. Invest. Ophthal. **8**, 290–301 (1969).
36. Dobbie, J. G., Phillips, C. I.: Detachment of ora serrata and pars ciliaris retinae in "idiopathic" retinal detachment. Arch. Ophthal. (Chic.) **68**, 610–614 (1962).
37. Duke-Elder, W. S.: System of ophthalmology, vol. II. St. Louis: C. V. Mosby 1961.
38. Dumas, J. J.: Retinal detachment following contusion of the eye. Int. Ophthal. Clinc. **7**, 19–38 (1967).
39. Dumas, J., Schepens, C. L.: Chorioretinal lesions predisposing to retinal breaks. Amer. J. Ophthal. **61**, 620–630 (1966).
40. Eisner, G.: Biomikroskopische Untersuchungen nach Fluoreszeininjektion. Ophthalmologica (Basel) **150**, 371–385 (1965).
41. Eisner, G.: Traumatische Veränderungen der pars plana corporis ciliaris. Ophthalmologica (Basel) **154**, 311–317 (1967).
42. Eisner, G.: Attachment for Goldmann three mirror contact glass. Amer. J. Ophthal. **64**, 467–468 (1967).
43. Eisner, G.: Zur Spaltlampenmikroskopie der Ora serrata und pars plana corporis ciliaris. I. Albrecht v. Graefes Arch. klin. exp. Ophthal. **176**, 223–231 (1969).
44. Eisner, G.: II. Albrecht v. Graefes Arch. klin. exp. Ophthal. **176**, 283–304 (1969).
45. Eisner, G.: III. Albrecht v. Graefes Arch. klin. exp. Ophthal. **177**, 232–247 (1969).
46. Eisner, G.: IV. Albrecht v. Graefes Arch. klin. exp. Ophthal. **177**, 248–260 (1969).
47. Eisner, G.: V. Albrecht v. Graefes Arch. klin. exp. Ophthal. **177**, 283–304 (1969).
48. Eisner, G.: VI. Albrecht v. Graefes Arch. klin. exp. Ophthal. **178**, 187–210 (1969).
49. Eisner, G.: VII. Albrecht v. Graefes Arch. klin. exp. Ophthal. **178**, 211–229 (1969).
50. Eisner, G.: VIII. Albrecht v. Graefes Arch. klin. exp. Ophthal. **178**, 230–245 (1969).
51. Eisner, G.: Zusatztricher zum 3-Spiegelkontaktglas mit verschieblichem Indentator. Albrecht v. Graefes Arch. klin. exp. Ophthal. **178**, 183–186 (1969).
52. Eisner, G.: Autoptische Spaltlampenuntersuchung des Glaskörpers I–III. Albrecht v. Graefes Arch. klin. exp. Ophthal. **182**, 1–40 (1971).
53. Eisner, G.: Biomicroscopy of the peripheral fundus. Surv. Ophthal. **17**, 1–28 (1972).
54. Eisner, G.: Autoptische Spaltlampenuntersuchung des Glaskörpers, IV–V. Albrecht v. Graefes Arch. klin. exp. Ophthal. **187**, 1–20 (1973).
55. Fankhauser, F.: Zur Klinik der pars-plana-Abhebung. Ophthalmologica (Basel) **145**, 411–418 (1963).
56. Fankhauser, F., Lotmar, W.: Methods of photocoagulation through the Goldmann contact lens. Mod. Probl. Ophthal. (Basel) **7**, 256–272 (1968).
57. Fankhauser, F., Lotmar, W.: A contact glass with an adjustable indentator. Description of a prototype. Docum. ophthal. (Den Haag) **26**, 295–299 (1969).
58. Fankhauser, F., Lotmar, W.: Skleraindentation und Photokoagulation. Acta ophthal. (Kbh.) **48**, 253–260 (1970).
59. Fanta, A.: Diskussionsbemerkung zu einem Vortrag von Eisner. Ophthalmologica (Basel) **154**, 316 (1967).
60. Favre, M.: Démonstration d'un verre de contact pour la pars plana. Club Gonin 1966.
61. Favre, M., Goldmann, H.: Zur Genese der hinteren Glaskörperabhebung. Ophthalmologica (Basel) **132**, 87–97 (1956).
62. Fine, B. S.: Retinal structure: Light- and Electromicroscopic observations, Chap. II.2. New York-Evanston-London: Hoeber Medical division. Harper & Row 1968.
63. Fine, B. S., Tousimis, A. J.: The structure of the vitreous body and the suspensory ligaments of the lens. Arch. Ophthal. (Chic.) **65**, 95–110 (1961).
64. Fine, B. S., Zimmerman, C. E.: Müller's cells and the "middle limiting membrane" of the human retina. Invest. Ophthal. **1**, 304–326 (1962).

65. Fine, B. S., Zimmerman, C. E.: Light and electromicroscopic observations on the ciliary epithelium in man and rhesus monkey. Invest. Ophthal. **2**, 105–137 (1963).
66. Fischer, F. P.: Netzhautcysten und cystoide Degeneration der Netzhaut. Docum. ophthal. (Den Haag) 5/6, 12–72 (1951).
67. Foos, R. Y.: Zonular traction tufts of the peripheral retina in cadaver eyes. Arch. Ophthal. (Chic.) **82**, 620–632 (1969).
68. Foos, R. Y.: Senile Retinoschisis: relationship to cystoid degeneration. Trans. Amer. Acad. Ophthal. Otolaryng. **74**, 33–51 (1970).
69. Foos, R. Y., Allen, R. A.: Retinal tears and lesser lesions of the peripheral retina in autopsy eye. Amer. J. Ophthal. **64**, part II, 643–655 (1967).
70. Foos, R. Y., Allen, R. A.: Opaque cysts of the ciliary body (pars ciliaris retinae). Arch. Ophthal. (Chic.) **77**, 559–568 (1968).
71. Foos, R. Y., Spencer, L. M., Straatsma, B. R.: Trophic degenerations of the peripheral retina. In: Symposium on retina and retinal surgery, p. 90–120. St. Louis: C. V. Mosby 1969.
72. Foos, R. Y., Feman, St. S.: Reticular cystoid degeneration of the peripheral retina. Amer. J. Ophthal. **69**, 392–403 (1970).
73. François, J.: La Gonioscopie. Louvain: R. Fonteyn 1948.
74. Frisen, L.: An adjustable biomicroscopy contact glass with erect imagery. Arch. Ophthal. (Chic.) **87**, 202–205 (1972).
75. Fuchs, E.: Über den anatomischen Befund einiger angeborener Anomalien der Netzhaut und des Sehnerven. Albrecht v. Graefes Arch. Ophthal. **93**, 1–48 (1917).
76. Gärtner, J.: Histologische Beobachtungen über physiologische vitreovaskuläre Adherenzen. Klin. Mbl. Augenheilk. **141**, 530–545 (1962).
77. Gärtner, J.: Elektronenmikroskopische Untersuchungen über die Feinstruktur der normalen und pathologisch veränderten vitreoretinalen Grenzschicht. Albrecht v. Graefes Arch. Ophthal. **165**, 71–102 (1962).
78. Gärtner, J.: Histologische Beobachtungen über das Verhalten der vitreoretinalen Grenzschicht bei Glaskörperabhebung. Klin. Mbl. Augenheilk. **142**, 769–792 (1963).
79. Gärtner, J.: Über persistierende periphere vitreochorioidale Gefäßanastomosen. Albrecht v. Graefes Arch. Ophthal. **166**, 475–493 (1964).
80. Gärtner, J.: Die Feinstruktur der Glaskörperrinde des menschlichen Auges an der Ora serrata im Alter. Albrecht v. Graefes Arch. klin. exp. Ophthal. **168**, 529–562 (1965).
81. Gärtner, J.: The fine structure of the vitreous base of the human eye and pathogenesis of pars planitis. Amer. J. Ophthal. **71**, 1317–1327 (1971).
82. Gärtner, J.: Pars plana cysts. Amer. J. Ophthal. **73**, 971–984 (1972).
83. Gloor, B. P.: Clinical application of contact lens. In: Current concepts in ophthalmology, ed. B. Becker, p. 31–48. St. Louis: C. V. Mosby 1969.
84. Gloor, B. P., Niesel, P., Gloor, M.-L.: Selektive Verschlüsse der Retinagefäße bei der Katze. I. Technik und ophthalmoskopische Befunde. Albrecht v. Graefes Arch. klin. exp. Ophthal. **181**, 344–362 (1971).
85. Goldmann, H.: Zwei Vorlesungen über Biomikroskopie des Auges. Bern: Haag-Streit 1954.
86. Goldmann, H.: Zur Biomikroskopie des Glaskörpers. Ophthalmologica (Basel) **127**, 334–339 (1954).
87. Goldmann, H.: Biomicroscopie du corps vitré et du fond de l'oeil. In: Busacca, Goldmann et Schiff-Wertheimer. Paris: Masson 1957.
88. Goldmann, H.: Diskussionsbemerkungen zu einem Vortrag von Amsler und Klöti. Ophthalmologica (Basel) **141**, 331–332 (1961).
89. Goldmann, H.: Seneszenz des Glaskörpers. Ophthalmologica (Basel) **143**, 253–279 (1962).
90. Goldmann, H.: Glaskörperabhebung. Ophthalmologica (Basel) **154**, 324–327 (1967).
91. Goldmann, H.: Biomikroskopie des normalen menschlichen Glaskörpers während des Lebens. Ber. dtsch. ophthal. Ges. **68**, 15–29 (1967).
92. Goldmann, H.: Biomicroscopy of the eye. Amer. J. Ophthal. **66**, 789–804 (1968).
93. Goldmann, H., Schmidt, Th.: Ein Kontaktglas zur Biomikroskopie der Ora serrata und pars plana. Ophthalmologica (Basel) **149**, 481–483 (1965).
94. Goldmann, H., Favre, M.: Demonstration eines neuen Spiegelkontaktglases. Mod. Probl. Ophthal. (Basel) **3**, 210 (1965).
95. Goldmann, H., Lotmar, W., Schröder, W.: Eine Vorrichtung zur Erleichterung der Untersuchung seitlicher Partien der Fundusperipherie. Albrecht v. Graefes Arch. klin. exp. Ophthal. **183**, 40–46 (1971).
96. Göttinger, W.: Beidseitig symmetrische idiopathische Netzhautcysten. Albrecht v. Graefes Arch. klin. exp. Ophthal. **183**, 81–96 (1971).

97. Gottlieb, F., Harris, D., Stratford, Th. P.: The peripheral eyeground in chronic respiratory disease. Arch. Ophthal. (Chic.) **82**, 611–619 (1969).
98. Grignolo, A., Schepens, C. L., Heath, P.: Cysts of the pars plana ciliaris. Arch. Ophthal. (Chic.) **58**, 530–543 (1957).
99. Hagler, W. S., North, A. W.: Retinal dialyses and retinal detachment. Arch. Ophthal. (Chic.) **79**, 376–388 (1968).
100. Havener, W. H.: Atlas of diagnostic techniques and treatment of retinal detachment. St. Louis: C. V. Mosby 1967.
101. Havener, W. H.: Atlas of diagnostic techniques and treatment of intraocular foreign bodies. St. Louis: C. V. Mosby 1969.
102. Hayreh, S. S.: Posterior drainage of the intraocular fluid from the vitreous. Exp. Eye Res. **5**, 123–144 (1966).
103. Hogan, M. J.: The vitreous, its structure and relation to the ciliary body and retina. Invest. Ophthal. **2**, 418–445 (1963).
104. Hogan, M. J., Kimura, S. J., Thygeson, Ph.: Signs and symptoms of uveitis. I. Anterior uveitis. Amer. J. Ophthal. **47**, part II, 155–170 (1959).
105. Hogan, M. J., Kimura, S. J.: Cyclitis and peripheral chorioretinitis. Arch. Ophthal. (Chic.) **66**, 667–677 (1961).
106. Hogan, M. J., Kimura, S. J., O'Connor, R. G.: Peripheral retinitis and chronic cyclitis in children. Trans. ophthal. Soc. U.K. **85**, 39–52 (1965).
107. Hogan, M. J., Alvarado, J. A., Weddell, J. E.: Histology of the human eye. Philadelphia-London-Toronto: W. B. Saunders 1971.
108. Hovland, K. R., Elzeheiny, I. H., Schepens, C. L.: Clinical evaluation of the small-pupil binocular indirect ophthalmoscope. Arch. Ophthal. (Chic.) **82**, 466–477 (1969).
109. Howard, G. M., Ellsworth, R. M.: Findings in the peripheral fundi of patients with retinoblastoma. Amer. J. Ophthal. **62**, 243–251 (1966).
110. Hruby, R.: Spaltlampenmikroskopie. Wien: Urban & Schwarzenberg 1950.
111. Jaffé, N. S.: Macula retinopathy after separation of vitroretinal adherence. Arch. Ophthal. (Chic.) **78**, 585–591 (1967).
112. Jaffé, N. S.: Complications of acute posterior vitreous detachment. Arch. Ophthal. (Chic.) **79**, 568–571 (1968).
113. Jaffé, N. S.: The vitreous in clinical ophthalmology. St. Louis: C. V. Mosby 1969.
114. Johnson, B. L., Storey, J. D.: Proteinaceous cysts of the ciliary epithelium I. Arch. Ophthal. (Chic.) **84**, 166–170 (1970).
115. Johnson, B. L.: Proteinaceous cysts of the ciliary epithelium II. Arch. Ophthal. (Chic.) **84**, 171–175 (1970).
116. Jokl, A.: Vergleichende Untersuchungen über den Bau und die Entwicklung des Glaskörpers und seiner Inhaltsgebilde bei Wirbeltieren und beim Menschen. Uppsala-Stockholm: Almquist & Wiksells 1927.
117. Jütte, A., Lemke, L., Opitz, J.: Chronische Zyklitis im Kindesalter. Ophthalmologica (Basel) **157**, 169–177 (1969).
118. Iwanoff, A.: Beiträge zur normalen und pathologischen Anatomie des Auges. Arch. Ophthal. (Berl.) **11**, (1) 136–170 (1865).
119. Iwanoff, A.: Beiträge zur normalen und pathologischen Anatomie des Auges. Das Ödem der Netzhaut. Arch. Ophthal. (Berl.) **15** (2), 88–105 (1859).
120. Keith, C. C.: Retinal cysts and retinoschisis. Brit. J. Ophthal. **50**, 617–628 (1966).
121. Kimura, S. J., Thygeson, Ph., Hogan, M. J.: Signs and symptoms of uveitis. II. Classification of the posterior manifestations of uveitis. Amer. J. Ophthal. **47**, Part II, 171–176 (1959).
122. Kimura, S. J., Hogan, M. J.: Chronic cyclitis. Arch. Ophthal. (Chic.) **71**, 193–201 (1964).
123. Kolmer, W.: Die Netzhaut. Handbuch der mikroskopischen Anatomie des Menschen, Bd. 3, Teil 2, S. 364–365. Berlin: Springer 1936.
124. Kyrieleis, E.: Über die cyclitis anularis pseudotumorosa exsudativa. Klin. Mbl. Augenheilk. **150**, 216–221 (1967).
125. Lauber, H.: Anatomie des Ciliarkörpers der Aderhaut und des Glaskörpers. Handbuch der gesamten Augenheilkunde, Bd. 1, Teil 2. Berlin: Springer 1931. S. 6 u. S. 57.
126. Lee, P., Pomerantzeff, O., Schepens, C. L.: New contact lens for peripheral fundus examination and photocoagulation. Arch. Ophthal. (Chic.) **84**, 650–654 (1970).
127. Leffertstra, L. J.: Disinsertions at the Ora serrata. Ophthalmologica (Basel) **119**, 1–16 (1950).
128. Liesenhoff, H.: Über erweiterte Möglichkeiten der Funduskopie mit dem Dreispiegelkontaktglas nach Goldmann. Klin. Mbl. Augenheilk. **151**, 382–385 (1967).

129. Linder, B.: Personal communication.
130. Long, J. C., Danielson, R. W.: Traumatic detachment of retina and of pars ciliaris retinae. Amer. J. Ophthal. **36**, 515–516 (1953).
131. Lonn, L. J., Smith, T. R.: Ora serrata pearls. Arch. Ophthal. (Chic.) **77**, 809–813 (1967).
132. Lotmar, W.: A theoretical eye model with aspheres. J. opt. Soc. Amer. **61**, 1522–1529 (1971).
133. McCulloch, W.: The zonula Zinn. Trans. Amer. ophthal. Soc. **52**, 525–585 (1954).
134. Machemer, R.: A new concept for vitreous surgery (2 and 3). Amer. J. Ophthal. **74**, 1022–1056 (1972).
135. Maggiore, L.: L'ora serrata nell'occhio umano. Ann. Ottal. **52**, 625–723 (1924).
136. Mann, I.: The development of the human eye. London: Butler & Tanner 1964.
137. Martenet, A. C.: A propos d'un terme nouveau dans le cadre des uvéites: La «pars planitis». Ophthalmologica (Basel) **147**, 282–290 (1964).
138. Maumenee, A. E.: Clinical entities in "uveitis". Amer. J. Ophthal. **69**, 1–27 (1970).
139. Okun, E.: Gross and microscopic pathology in autopsy eyes. Part I: Introduction and long posterior ciliary nerves. Amer. J. Ophthal. **50**, 424–429 (1960).
140. Okun, E.: Part II: Peripheral chorioretinal atrophy. Amer. J. Ophthal. **50**, 574–583 (1960).
141. Okun, E.: Part III: Retinal breaks without detachment. Amer. J. Ophthal. **51**, 369–391 (1961).
142. Okun, E.: Part IV: Pars plana cysts. Amer. J. Ophthal. **51**, 1221–1228 (1961).
143. Okun, E., Cibis, P.: Retinoschisis. Classification, Diagnosis and Management. In: McPherson, A., New and controversal aspects of retinal detachments, p. 424–434. New York-Evanston-London: Harper & Row 1968.
144. O'Malley, P. F., Allen, R. A., Straatsma, B. R., O'Malley, C. C.: Pavingstone degeneration of the retina. Arch. Ophthal. (Chic.) **73**, 169–182 (1965).
145. O'Malley, P. F., Allen, F. A.: Peripheral cystoid degeneration of the retina. Arch. Ophthal. (Chic.) **77**, 769–776 (1967).
146. Pape, R.: Postkontusionelle Ziliarkörperabhebung. Klin. Mbl. Augenheilk. **147**, 730–741 (1965).
147. Pau, H.: Zur Histologie der „cystoiden Degenerationen" in der Netzhautperipherie. Albrecht v. Graefes Arch. Ophthal. **158**, 558–567 (1957).
148. Pau, H.: Die Bedeutung der embryonalen Blutgefäße für die Struktur sowie für degenerative und entzündliche Veränderungen des Glaskörpers. Klin. Mbl. Augenheilk. **147**, 335–348 (1965).
149. Pau, H.: Die Beziehungen der embryonalen Blutgefäße zur Pathologie und Anatomie des Glaskörpers. Ber. dtsch. ophthal. Ges. **68**, 380 (1966).
150. Pei Fen Yen, Smelser, G. K.: Some fine structural features of the ora serrata region in primate eyes. Invest. Ophthal. **7**, 672–688 (1968).
151. Redslob, E.: Le corps vitré. Paris: Masson 1932.
152. Reichling, W., Klemens, F.: Über eine gefäßführende Bindegewebsschicht zwischen dem Pigmentepithel der Retina und der Lamina vitrea. 1. Mitt. Albrecht v. Graefes Arch. Ophthal. **137**, 515–526 (1937).
153. Reichling, W., Klemens, F.: II. Mitt. Albrecht v. Graefes Arch. Ophthal. **141**, 500–512 (1940).
154. Rieger, H.: Zur Histologie der Glaskörperabhebung. I. Mitt.: Über das Wesen und die Entstehung der „geformten Glaskörpertrübungen". Albrecht v. Graefes Arch. Ophthal. **146**, 305–335 (1944).
155. Rieger, H.: II. Mitt.: Über die Beziehungen des abgehobenen Glaskörpers zur Netzhaut. Albrecht v. Graefes Arch. Ophthal. **146**, 447–462 (1944).
156. Rohen, J. W.: Das Auge und seine Hilfsorgane. Handbuch der mikroskopischen Anatomie des Menschen, Bd. 3, Teil 4. Berlin-Göttingen-Heidelberg-New York: Springer 1964.
157. Rohen, J. W., Rentsch, F. J.: Der konstruktive Bau des Zonulaapparates beim Menschen und dessen funktionelle Bedeutung. Albrecht v. Graefes Arch. klin. exp. Ophthal. **178**, 1–19 (1969).
158. Rohen, J. W., Zimmermann, A.: Altersveränderungen des Ciliarepithels beim Menschen. Albrecht v. Graefes Arch. klin. exp. Ophthal. **179**, 302–317 (1970).
159. Rosen, E.: I. Biomicroscopic examination of the zonules without a contact lens. Amer. J. Ophthal. **53**, 345–351 (1962).
160. Rosen, E.: II. In Krukenberg spindles and annular pigment rings of the lens. Amer. J. Ophthal. **53**, 845–853 (1962).
161. Rosen, E.: Ascension Phenomenon. Amer. J. Ophthal. **53**, 55–65 (1962).

162. Rosen, E.: Further studies on the ascension phenomenon. Amer. J. Ophthal. **55**, 597–605 (1963).
163. Rosen, E.: The Shatz phenomenon. Amer. J. Ophthal. **57**, 305–310 (1964).
164. Rosen, E.: Anterior hyaloid membrane. Amer. J. Ophthal. **59**, 1069–1079 (1965).
165. Rosen, E.: Detachment of the anterior hyaloid membrane. Amer. J. Ophthal. **62**, 1185–1194 (1966).
166. Rosen, E.: Vibration of the anterior hyaloid membrane. Amer. J. Ophthal. **68**, 133–143 (1969).
167. Rosen, E.: Zonulo-hyaloideo ligament. Ann. Ophthal. **2**, 857–862 (1970).
168. Rosen, E., Lyne, A.: Uveal effusions. Amer. J. Ophthal. **65**, 509–518 (1968).
169. Rutnin, U., Schepens, C. L.: Fundus appearance in normal eye. II. The standard peripheral fundus and development variations. Amer. J. Ophthal. **64**, 840–852 (1967).
170. Rutnin, U., Schepens, C. L.: III. Peripheral degenerations. Amer. J. Ophthal. **64**, 1041–1062 (1967).
171. Rutnin, U., Schepens, C. L.: IV. Retinal breaks and other findings. Amer. J. Ophthal. **64**, 1063–1078 (1967).
172. Salzmann, M.: Anatomie und Histologie des menschlichen Augapfels. Leipzig-Wien: Franz Deuticke 1912.
173. Sampaolesi, R.: Le glaucome pigmentaire; son rapport avec le glaucome. Bull. Soc. franç. Ophtal. **81**, 434–455 (1968).
174. Sanders, T. E., Podos, S.: Pars plana cysts in multiple myeloma. Trans. Amer. Acad. Ophthal. Otolaryng. **70**, 951–958 (1966).
175. Schepens, C. L.: L'inflammation de la région de l'ora serrata et ses séquelles. Bull. Soc. franç. Ophtal. **63**, 113–125 (1950).
176. Schepens, C. L.: Retinal detachment and aphakia. Arch. Ophthal. (Chic.) **45**, 1–17 (1951).
177. Schepens, C. L.: Subclinical retinal detachments. Arch. Ophthal. (Chic.) **47**, 593–606 (1952).
178. Schepens, C. L.: Diagnostic and prognostic factors as found in preoperative examination. Trans. Amer. Acad. Ophthal. **56**, 398–418 (1952).
179. Schepens, C. L.: Clinical aspects of pathologic changes in the vitreous body. Amer. J. Ophthal. **38**, II, 8–21 (1954).
180. Schepens, C. L.: Examination of the ora serrata-region: Its clinical significance. Conc. Ophthal. Brittania 1950, p. 1384–1393.
181. Schepens, C. L.: Present Day Treatment of Retinoschisis: An evaluation. In: McPherson, A., New and controversal aspects of retinal detachments. New York-Evanston-London: Harper & Row 1968.
182. Schepens, C. L., Bahn, G. C.: Examination of the ora serrata. Its importance in retinal detachment. Arch. Ophthal. (Chic.) **44**, 677–690 (1950).
183. Schepens, C. L., Dobbie, J. G., McMeel, J. W.: Retinal detachments with giant breaks. Preliminary report. Trans. Amer. Acad. Ophthal. Otolaryng. **66**, 471–479 (1962).
184. Schepens, C. L., Regan, Ch. J. D.: Controversal aspects of the management of retinal detachment. Boston: Little, Brown & Company 1965.
185. Schepens, C. L., Brockhuist, R. J.: Uveal effusion I. Clinical picture. Arch. Ophthal. (Chic.) **70**, 189–201 (1963).
186. Schirmer, K. E.: Transillumination and visualisation of the anterior fundus. Arch. Ophthal. (Chic.) **71**, 475–580 (1964).
187. Shea, M., Schepens, C. L., Pirquet, S. R.: Retinoschisis. Arch. Ophthal. (Chic.) **63**, 25–33 (1960).
188. Slansky, H. H., Bronstein, M., Gärtner, S.: Ciliary body cysts in multiple myeloma. Their relation to urthane, hyperproteinaemia and duration of the disease. Arch. Ophthal. (Chic.) **76**, 686–689 (1966).
189. Slezak, H.: Biomikroskopische Untersuchungen bei peripherer Uveitis. Klin. Mbl. Augenheilk. **140**, 88–95 (1962).
190. Slezak, H.: Spaltlampenuntersuchung des ligamentum hyaloideocapsulare. Albrecht v. Graefes Arch. Ophthal. **166**, 112–118 (1963).
191. Slezak, H.: Die vordere retrozonuläre und ciliare Glaskörperabhebung. Albrecht v. Graefes Arch. Ophthal. **167**, 89–98 (1964).
192. Slezak, H.: Ein Kontaktglas zur binokularen Untersuchung der nasalen und temporalen Fundusperipherie an der Spaltlampe (Äquatorimpressionsglas). Albrecht v. Graefes Arch. klin. exp. Ophthal. **171**, 169–172 (1966).
193. Slezak, H.: Zur Klinik, Pathogenese und Differentialdiagnose der peripheren Uveitis. Albrecht v. Graefes Arch. klin. exp. Ophthal. **174**, 9–33 (1968).

194. Slezak, H.: Der Äquatorimpressionstrichter und seine Anwendung bei der Biomikroskopie der Fundusperipherie. Klin. Mbl. Augenheilk. **152**, 533–537 (1968).
195. Slezak, H.: Der Ciliarkörperimpressionstrichter zur Biomikroskopie der corona ciliaris linsenhaltiger Augen. Albrecht v. Graefes Arch. klin. exp. Ophthal. **176**, 349–351 (1968).
196. Slezak, H.: Über Fluorescein in der Hinterkammer des menschlichen Auges. Albrecht v. Graefes Arch. klin. exp. Ophthal. **178**, 260–267 (1969).
197. Slezak, H.: Die Fluoresceinfärbung der Cysten der orbiculus ciliaris. Klin. Mbl. Augenheilk. **156**, 372–376 (1970).
198. Slezak, H.: Gefäßentzündung der Netzhautrandzone. Albrecht v. Graefes Arch. klin. exp. Ophthal. **180**, 267–272 (1970).
199. Slezak, H.: Periphere gürtelförmige Netzhautatrophie bei Ablatio retinae. Albrecht v. Graefes Arch. klin. exp. Ophthal. **180**, 31–37 (1970).
200. Slezak, H.: Impressionsbiomikroskopie der Hinterkammer (Gonioskopia posterior). I. Mitt. Albrecht v. Graefes Arch. klin. exp. Ophthal. **183**, 53–61 (1971).
201. Spee, F. Graf: Über den Bau der Zonulafasern und ihre Anordnung im menschlichen Auge. Anat. Anz. Zbl. ges. wiss. Anat. **21**. Erg.-H., 236–241 (1902).
202. Spencer, L. M., Straatsma, B. R., Foos, R. Y.: Tractional degenerations of the peripheral retina. In: Symposium on retina and retinal surgery, p. 103–127. St. Louis: C. V. Mosby 1969.
203. Spencer, L. M., Foos, R. Y., Straatsma, B. R.: Meridional folds and meridional complexes of the peripheral retina. Trans. Amer. Acad. Ophthal. Otolaryng. **73**, 204–217 (1969).
204. Spencer, L. M., Foos, R. Y., Straatsma, B. R.: Meridional folds, meridional complexes and associated abnormalities of the peripheral retina. Amer. J. Ophthal. **70**, 697–714 (1970).
205. Spencer, L. M., Foos, R. Y., Straatsma, B. R.: Enclosed bays of the ora serrata. Arch. Ophthal. (Chic.) **83**, 421–426 (1970).
206. Spencer, L. M., Foos, R. Y.: Paravascular vitreoretinal attachment. Arch. Ophthal. (Chic.) **84**, 557–564 (1970).
207. Stein, R.: Beiträge zur Topographie und Anatomie der Ora serrata und des orbiculus ciliaris. Arch. Augenheilk. (München) **106**, 145–184 (1932).
208. Straatsma, B. R., Allen, R. A.: Lattice degeneration of the retina. Trans. Amer. Acad. Ophthal. Otolaryng. **66**, 600–613 (1962).
209. Straatsma, B. R., Landers, M. B., Kreiger, A. E.: The ora serrata in the adult human eye. Arch. Ophthal. (Chic.) **80**, 3–20 (1968).
210. Straatsma, B. R., Allen, B. A., O'Malley, P., O'Malley, C. C.: Pathologic and clinical manifestations of paving-stone degeneration of the retina. In: McPherson, New and controversal aspects of retinal detachment, Chap. V, p. 76. New York-Evanston-London: Hoeber 1968.
211. Sullivan, G. L., Pirquet, S. R.: Retinoschisis. Perimetry as a clue to diagnosis. Trans. Amer. ophthal. Soc. **59**, 80–95 (1961).
212. Szent Györgyi, A.: Untersuchungen über den Bau des Glaskörpers des Menschen. Arch. mikr. Anat. **89**, 324–386 (1917).
213. Tasman, W.: Retinal detachment with breaks in the pars plana. Brit. J. Ophthal. **52**, 181–183 (1968).
214. Tasman, W.: Posterior vitreous detachment and peripheral retinal breaks. Trans. Amer. Acad. Ophthal. Otolaryng. **72**, 217–224 (1968).
215. Teng, C. C., Katzin, H. M.: An anatomic study of the peripheral retina. Part I: Non pigmented epithelial cell proliferation and hole formation. Amer. J. Ophthal. **34**, 1237–1248 (1951).
216. Teng, C. C., Katzin, H. M.: Part II: Peripheral cystoid degeneration of the retina, formation of cysts and holes. Amer. J. Ophthal. **36**, 29–39 (1953).
217. Teng, C. C., Katzin, H. M.: Part III: Congenital retinal rosettes. Amer. J. Ophthal. **36**, 169–185 (1953).
218. Thiel, H. L.: Zur topographischen und histologischen Situation der Ora serrata. Albrecht v. Graefes Arch. Ophthal. **156**, 590–629 (1955).
219. Tolentino, F. I., Kietzler, X., Pomerantzeff, O.: Adjustable mirror contact lens for fundus and vitreous examinations. Ann. Ophthal. **4**, 95–98 (1972).
220. Trantas, A.: Moyens d'explorer par l'ophtalmoscope — et par translucidité — la partie antérieure du fond oculaire, le cercle ciliare y compris. Arch. Ophtal. (Paris) **20**, 314–326 (1900).
221. Trantas, A.: Excroissances de l'ora serrata et leur aspect ophtalmologscopique. Clin. Ophtal. **12**, 115–119 (1906).

222. Trantas, A.: Ophtalmoscopie de la région ciliaire et rétrociliare. Bull. Soc. franç. Ophtal. **24**, 546–592 (1907).
223. Velicky, J.: Iridocyclitische Retinopathie. Stuttgart: F. Enke 1968.
224. Vogt, A.: Spaltlampenmikroskopie des lebenden Auges, Bd. 1–2, Berlin: Springer 1931. Bd. 5, Zürich: Schweizer Druck- & Verlagshaus 1941.
225. Vrabec, F.: Neurohistology of cystoid degeneration of the peripheral human retina. Amer. J. Ophthal. **64**, 90–99 (1967).
226. Wagner, H.: Bestimmung der linearen Masse auf der Bulbusoberfläche vom Limbus bis zur Ora serrata, zum hinteren Pol und zur Papille. Albrecht v. Graefes Arch. Ophthal. **127**, 103–136 (1931).
227. Watzke, R. C.: The ophthalmoscopic sign "white with pressure", a clinicopathologic correlation. Arch. Ophthal. (Chic.) **66**, 812–823 (1961).
228. Weber, E.: Spaltlampenmikroskopische Untersuchungen über die vordere Glaskörperbegrenzung und deren Beziehung zur Linse. I. Mitt. Klin. Mbl. Augenheilk. **108**, 710–761 (1942).
229. Weber, E.: Der vordere Glaskörperabschluß. Die spontane Linsenblattablösung im Senium, eine neue Spaltlampendiagnose. Ophthalmologica (Basel) **107**, 108–115 (1944).
230. Weidenthal, D. T.: Experimental ocular contusion. Arch. Ophthal. (Chic.) **71**, 77–81 (1964).
231. Weidenthal, D. T., Schepens, C. L.: Peripheral fundus changes associated with ocular contusion. Amer. J. Ophthal. **62**, 465–477 (1966).
232. Welch, R. B., Maumenee, E. A., Wahlen, H. E.: Peripheral posterior segment inflammation, vitreous opacities and edema of the posterior pole. "Pars planitis". Arch. Ophthal. (Chic.) **64**, 540–549 (1960).
233. Witmer, R., Körner, G.: Uveitis im Kindesalter. Ophthalmologica (Basel) **152**, 277–282 (1966).
234. Wolff, St. M., Zimmerman, L.: Chronic secondary glaucoma associated with retrodisplacement of iris root and deepening of the anterior chamber angle secondary to contusion. Amer. J. Ophthal. **54**, 547–563 (1962).
235. Wollensak, J.: Zonula zinni. Fortschr. Augenheilk. **16**, 240–335 (1965).
236. Wolter, R. J., Wilson, W. W.: Degeneration of the peripheral retina. Amer. J. Ophthal. **47**, 153–165 (1959).
237. Yanoff, M., Tsou, K. C.: Demonstration of ocular reduced diphosphopyridine nucleotide (DPNH) and triphosphopyridine nucleotide (TPNH) diaphorases using tetrazelium salts. Amer. J. Ophthal. **60**, 310–317 (1965).
238. Zimmerman, L. E., Straatsma, B. R.: Anatomic relationships of the retina to the vitreous body and to the pigment epithelium. In: Schepens, C. L., Importance of the vitreous body in retina surgery with special emphasis in reoperations. St. Louis: C. V. Mosby 1960.
239. Zimmerman, L. E., Spencer, L. M.: The pathologic anatomy of retinoschisis. Arch. Ophthal. (Chic.) **63**, 34–43 (1960).
240. Zimmerman, L. E., Fine, B. S.: Production of hyaluronic acid by cysts and tumors of the ciliary body. Arch. Ophthal. (Chic.) **72**, 365–379 (1964).
241. Zimmerman, L. E., Nauman, G.: The pathology of retinoschisis. In: McPherson, New and controversal aspects of retinal detachment. New York-Evanston-London: Harper & Row 1968.
242. Zollinger, H. U.: Die Beziehungen zwischen Gefäßsystem und peripherer cystoider Degeneration der Netzhaut. Albrecht v. Graefes Arch. Ophthal. **143**, 403–423 (1944).

Subject Index*

---

* Figures in *italics* refer to the illustrations.